AFTER THE ICU

NOTICE

Medicine is an ever-changing science. As new research and clinical experience broaden our knowledge, changes in treatment and drug therapy are required. The authors and the publisher of this work have checked with sources believed to be reliable in their efforts to provide information that is complete and generally in accord with the standards accepted at the time of publication. However, in view of the possibility of human error or changes in medical sciences, neither the authors nor the publisher nor any other party who has been involved in the preparation or publication of this work warrants that the information contained herein is in every respect accurate or complete, and they disclaim all responsibility for any errors or omissions or for the results obtained from use of the information contained in this work. Readers are encouraged to confirm the information contained herein with other sources. For example and in particular, readers are advised to check the product information sheet included in the package of each drug they plan to administer to be certain that the information contained in this work is accurate and that changes have not been made in the recommended dose or in the contraindications for administration. This recommendation is of particular importance in connection with new or infrequently used drugs.

AFTER THE ICU
Multidisciplinary Perspectives on Supporting Critical Illness Survivors

EDITORS

Meghan B. Lane-Fall, MD, MSHP
Associate Professor
Department of Anesthesiology and Critical Care
Department of Biostatistics, Epidemiology, and Informatics
Perelman School of Medicine, University of Pennsylvania
Philadelphia, Pennsylvania

David S. Shapiro, MD, MHCM
Chief Quality Officer
Vice Chairman, Surgery Service Line
Chief, Surgical Critical Care
Saint Francis Hospital and Medical Center
Hartford, Connecticut
Associate Professor of Surgery
University of Connecticut School of Medicine
Farmington, Connecticut
Frank H. Netter MD School of Medicine
Quinnipiac University
Hamden, Connecticut

Lewis J. Kaplan, MD, FACS, FCCP, FCCM
Professor of Surgery
Perelman School of Medicine, University of Pennsylvania
Department of Surgery
Division of Trauma, Critical Care and Emergency Surgery
Philadelphia, Pennsylvania
Section Chief, Surgical Critical Care
Medical Director, Surgical ICU
Corporal Michael J Crescenz VA Medical Center
Philadelphia, Pennsylvania

New York Chicago San Francisco Athens London Madrid
Mexico City New Delhi Milan Singapore Sydney Toronto

After the ICU: Multidisciplinary Perspectives on Supporting Critical Illness Survivors

1 2 3 4 5 6 7 8 9 LKV 28 27 26 25 24 23

ISBN 978-1-260-46925-7
MHID 1-260-46925-5

This book was set in Minion Pro by MPS Limited.
The editors were Timothy Y. Hiscock and Peter J. Boyle.
The production supervisor was Richard Ruzycka.
Project management was provided by Himanshu Abrol, MPS Limited.
The cover designer was W2 Design.

Library of Congress Control Number: 2023944850

Dedication

The editors dedicate this book to the following people:

- Our patients, both those who did and did not survive their critical illness. Your stories inspire us to be better clinicians. We are honored to have been part of your journey.
- Family caregivers and friends, without whom surviving and thriving after critical illness would not be possible.
- Our colleagues, who bring their intellect, empathy, passion, and grace to the care of the most vulnerable patients.
- The people who generate and curate the knowledge needed to care for critically ill and injured patients, including researchers and the members of professional medical societies that create practice guidance and guidelines.
- Our families, who support us as professionals and teach us through our shared experiences. Thank you for helping us undertake the vitally important work of supporting critical illness survivors.

Contents

Contributors

Sean Malone Alexander
Chapter 1

Jeff F. Barletta, BS, PharmD
Professor & Vice Chair of Pharmacy
  Practice
Midwestern University, College of
  Pharmacy
Glendale, Arizona
Chapter 6

Gary Alan Bass, MD, MS, MBA,
MRCSI, PhD, FEBS (Em Sure)
Perelman School of Medicine
University of Pennsylvania
Department of Surgery
Division of Trauma
Surgical Critical Care and
  Emergency Surgery
Philadelphia, Pennsylvania
Chapter 22

Andrew Bergman, MSN, RN, CCRN
Cooper University Healthcare
Camden, New Jersey
Chapter 4

Toba Bolaji, DO
Resident
ChristianaCare
Wilmington, Delaware
Chapter 24

Mary Elizabeth Bouchard, MS,
CCC-SLP, CBIS
Saint Francis Hospital
Hartford, Connecticut
Chapter 7

J. Christian Brown, MD
Department of Surgery
Cleveland Clinic Foundation
Cleveland, Ohio
Chapter 5

Katherine R. Casey, AGACNP-BC
Emory Critical Care Center
Emory University
Atlanta, Georgia
Chapter 16

Craig M. Coopersmith, MD
Director, Emory Critical Care Center
Emory University
Atlanta, Georgia
Chapter 16

Caoimhe Carmel Duffy, MD, MSc,
FCAI
Perelman School of Medicine
University of Pennsylvania
Department of Anesthesiology and
  Critical Care
Philadelphia, Pennsylvania
  Chapter 22

Amy L. Dzierba, PharmD
Clinical Pharmacy Manager
New York-Presbyterian Hospital
Columbia University Irving Medical
    Center
New York, New York
Chapter 6

Philip Efron, MD
University of Florida
Department of Surgery
Division of Acute Care Surgery
Gainesville, Florida
Chapter 5

Paula Ferrada, MD
INOVA Trauma Center
Falls Church, Virginia
Chapter 24

Julie Fuller, MS, RD, CNSC
Saint Francis Hospital
Chapter 11

Garret Garborcauskas, BA
Frank H. Netter School of Medicine
Quinnipiac University
North Haven, Connecticut
Chapter 23

Rebecca Anna Gersten, MD
Division of Pulmonary and Critical
    Care Medicine
Department of Medicine
Johns Hopkins University School of
    Medicine
Baltimore, Maryland
Chapter 8

Allison Gonzalez, LCSW
Johns Hopkins University Medical
    Center
Baltimore, Maryland
Chapter 12

Jafar Haghshenas, MD
Advocate Christ Medical Center
Oak Lawn, Illinois
Chapter 21

Neil Halpern, MD, MCCM
Director, Critical Care Center
Department of Anesthesiology and
    Critical Care
Memorial Sloan Kettering Cancer
    Center
New York, New York
Chapter 25

Jason Hansen, RRT
UF Health
Gainesville, Florida
Chapter 5

Bradley J. Heyward, MD
Division of Pulmonary and Critical
    Care Medicine
Department of Medicine
Weill Cornell Medicine
New York City, New York
Chapter 8

Sara Holland, DNP, RN
University of Pennsylvania Health
    System
Philadelphia, Pennsylvania
Chapter 17

Patrick Holman, MD
Division of Internal
  Medicine-Pediatrics
UCLA Medical Center
Los Angeles, California
Chapter 15

Anand S. Iyer, MD, MSPH
Division of Pulmonary, Allergy, and
  Critical Care Medicine
Center for Palliative and Supportive
  Care
Division of Gerontology, Geriatrics,
  and Palliative Care
Department of Medicine
School of Nursing
University of Alabama at Birmingham
Birmingham, Alabama
Chapter 8

**Juliane Jablonski, DNP, RN,
CCRN-K, CCNS**
University of Pennsylvania Health
  System
Philadelphia, Pennsylvania
Chapter 17

**Lewis J. Kaplan, MD, FACS, FCCP,
FCCM**
Professor of Surgery
Perelman School of Medicine
University of Pennsylvania
Department of Surgery
Division of Trauma, Critical Care
  and Emergency Surgery
Philadelphia, Pennsylvania
Section Chief, Surgical Critical Care
Medical Director, Surgical ICU
Corporal Michael J Crescenz VA
  Medical Center
Philadelphia, Pennsylvania
Chapters 2 and 22

Colleen Kelly Alexander
Chapter 1

Zhan Liang, PhD, MSN, RN
Assistant Professor
University of Miami
School of Nursing and Health Studies
Miami, Florida
Chapter 13

Camille Lineberry, MSN, ACNP-BC
Department of Anesthesiology and
  Critical Care Medicine
Memorial Sloan-Kettering Cancer
  Center
New York, New York
Chapter 25

**Linda Mackay-Morgan, MA,
CCC-SLP, BCS-S, CBIST**
HealthPRO Heritage at Masonicare
  Home Health and Hospice
Hartford, Connecticut
Chapter 7

Jason H. Maley, MD
Director, Critical Illness and
  COVID-19 Survivorship Program
Division of Pulmonary, Critical
  Care, and Sleep Medicine
Beth Israel Deaconess Medical Center
Harvard Medical School
Boston, Massachusetts
Chapter 15

John McGill, MSN, RN, CCRN
Penn Presbyterian Medical Center
University of Pennsylvania Health
  System
Philadelphia, Pennsylvania
Chapter 14

Heather Meissen, DNP, ACNP-BC, FAANP
Emory Critical Care Center
Emory University
Atlanta, Georgia
Chapter 16

Mark E. Mikkelsen, MD, MSCE
Associate Chief Medical Officer,
    Critical Care
Associate Professor of Medicine
University of Colorado Anschutz
    School of Medicine
Aurora, Colorado
Chapter 14

Alexis Moren, MD, MPH
Salem Health Hospitals & Clinics
Salem, Oregon
Chapter 23

Vinay Nadkarni, MD, MS
Department of Pediatric Critical
    Care Medicine
Children's Hospital of Philadelphia
Philadelphia, Pennsylvania
Chapter 18

Brandon Oto, PA-C, NREMT
Bridgeport Hospital
Bridgeport, Connecticut
UConn Health
Farmington, Connecticut
Chapter 3

Tina Palmieri, MD
Professor, Division of Burn Surgery
UC Davis
Sacramento, California
Chapter 20

Neethi P. Pinto, MD, MS
Department of Anesthesiology and
    Critical Care

Children's Hospital of Philadelphia
Philadelphia, Pennsylvania
Chapter 18

Asanthi Ratnasekera, DO
Christiana Hospital
Surgery Surgical Services
Newark, Delaware
Chapter 24

Nina Raoof, MD
Department of Anesthesiology and
    Critical Care Medicine
Memorial Sloan-Kettering Cancer
    Center
New York, New York
Chapter 25

Jamie L. Rubino, DPT, PT
Cooper University Healthcare
Camden, New Jersey
Chapter 4

Kim Sabino, MS, RD, CNSC
Department of Food and Nutrition
Trinity Health of New England
Saint Francis Hospital and Medical
    Center
Hartford, Connecticut
Chapter 11

Joseph V. Sakran, MD, MPH, MPA
Johns Hopkins Hospital
Baltimore, Maryland
Chapter 21

Peter Sandor, MBA, PA-C, DFAAPA
St. Francis Hospital
Hartford, Connecticut
Quinnipiac University
North Haven, Connecticut
Chapter 3

Gloria M. Satriale, Ed.D, JD, LBS-PA, ACRE, QM, MCPP
Preparing Autistic Adolescents for Life School
Downingtown, Pennsylvania
Chapter 22

Christa A. Schorr, DNP, MSN, RN, NEA-BC
Cooper University Healthcare
Cooper Medical School at Rowan University
Camden, New Jersey
Chapter 4

Kristin E. Schwab, MD
Co-director, Post-ICU Recovery Clinic
Division of Pulmonary, Critical Care, and Sleep Medicine
UCLA Medical Center
Los Angeles, California
Chapter 15

Kimberly Sena Moore, PhD, MT-BC
Florida Gulf Coast University
Bower School of Music & the Arts
Fort Myers, Florida
Chapter 13

David S. Shapiro, MD, MHCM
Chief Quality Officer
Vice Chairman, Surgery Service Line
Chief, Surgical Critical Care
Saint Francis Hospital and Medical Center
Hartford, Connecticut
Associate Professor of Surgery
University of Connecticut School of Medicine
Frank H. Netter MD School of Medicine

Quinnipiac University
Hamden, Connecticut
Chapter 23

Annalise N. Slicer, RPT
School of Health Sciences
Quinnipiac University
Hamden, Connecticut
Chapter 7

Keturah M. Sloan, FNP
Shriners Hospital for Children Northern California
Sacramento, California
Chapter 20

Randi N. Smith, MD, MPH
Grady Memorial Hospital
Department of Surgery
Emory University School of Medicine
Atlanta, Georgia
Chapter 2

Reka Somodi, DNP, CRNP
Corporal Michael J. Crescenz VA Medical Center
Surgical Services
Section of Surgical Critical Care
Philadelphia, Pennsylvania
Chapter 2

Deborah Stein, MSN, ACNP-BC, CCRN
Department of Anesthesiology and Critical Care Medicine
Memorial Sloan-Kettering Cancer Center
New York, New York
Chapter 25

Jessica E. Taylor, MD, MBA
University of Florida
Department of Surgery
Division of Acute Care Surgery
Gainesville, Florida
Chapter 5

Caitlin C. ten Lohuis, ACNP-BC
Emory Critical Care Center
Emory University
Atlanta, Georgia
Chapter 16

Ashley M. Thompson, MD
Memorial Health
Savannah, Georgia
Chapter 5

Christine C. Toevs, MD
Clinical Associate Professor of
  Surgery
Indiana University School of
  Medicine
Terre Haute, Indiana
Chapter 9

Crisanto Torres, MD
Johns Hopkins Hospital
Baltimore, Maryland
Chapter 21

Arthur Jason Vaught, MD
Robert E. Meyerhoff Professor
Assistant Professor of Gynecology
  and Obstetrics
Assistant Professor of Surgery
Johns Hopkins Medicine
Department of Gynecology and
  Obstetrics – Maternal Fetal
  Medicine

Director, Labor and Delivery
Director, Advanced Obstetric
  Surgery Center
Baltimore, Maryland
Chapter 19

Courtney Wagner, MD
Tinsley Harrison Internal Medicine
  Residency Program
Department of Medicine
University of Alabama at
  Birmingham
Birmingham, Alabama
Chapter 8

Aron Wahrman, MD, MBA, MHCDS
Section Chief, Plastic Surgery
Clinical Associate Professor of
  Plastic Surgery
Perelman School of Medicine,
  University of Pennsylvania
Corporal Michael J. Crescenz VA
  Medical Center
Philadelphia, Pennsylvania
Chapter 10

Hilary Yip, MM, MT-BC
Assistant Professor and Program
  Director, Music Therapy
Music Therapist-Board Certified
California State University,
  Northridge
Los Angeles, California
Chapter 13

Megan K. Zielke, PharmD, BCCCP
University of Pittsburgh Medical
  Center
Pittsburgh, Pennsylvania
Chapter 14

Foreword

■ INTO AND THROUGH THE POST-INTENSIVE CARE SYNDROME: A PATIENT'S JOURNEY

Lying in bed on the sixth floor of Yale-New Haven Hospital, I watched as snow fell outside the window. It was the first weekend in March 2009, and the weather was typical of early springtime in New England: gray overcast skies peppered with spiky ice particles. I know I had regained consciousness a few days earlier, but my first post-trauma memory is that view of the snow falling.

It was almost three months since I had arrived in the ER, and just a few days since I had been moved out of ICU. IVs and other tubes and wires were attached to my body, and monitors beeped behind my head. Propped up with pillows, there was a rigid collar around my neck and my left leg was gone. I knew then that my life—as I had known it—was over. Nothing would be the same as it had been before.

I was the first amputee I'd ever met. Not only had my body been broken, my life plan had been shattered, and I had no idea what the future held. Faced with unknowns, a muddled brain and battered body, it was tough to imagine my future. I asked myself, "Is my life over?"

Eight months earlier I had traveled to Bandiagara, Mali, a rural village in one of the least developed countries in Africa, to begin a 15-month volunteer post as a business advisor to an eco-tourism development project. One morning in early December the project coordinator and I traveled to another small village to follow up on an irrigation project. While we were there, a water tower collapsed, crushing both of us. Local workers lifted slabs of stone and concrete to find me alive but unconscious. Tragically, my colleague did not survive. I regained consciousness as the men loaded me into a pickup truck for the 40-minute drive over rough terrain back to the village hospital.

Local Peace Corps Volunteers and friends mobilized to help me, despite their grief over our friend's death. They contacted the US Embassy and arranged for me to be medevacked to the nearest trauma center, the American Hospital in Paris. I have no recollections of the time I was hospitalized in Paris, nor the medevac transfer to the United States, but when I woke up in a bed at Yale-New Haven Hospital (YNHH), I was not surprised to see that my leg was gone—I had seen my broken body after the accident.

My medical history still shocks me: nearly every vertebra fractured, including C1; several broken ribs; punctured spleen and gall bladder; head injury; broken bones, including an open fracture of my left femur and multiple fractures of the left tibia and fibula. On arrival at YNHH, the trauma surgeon knew immediately that my left leg could not be saved and performed an emergency amputation.

Complications arose as an infection of unknown origin spread through my body. I was in ICU as my dedicated medical team combatted the infection, performing surgeries nearly every day in December, January, and February—including holidays Christmas Eve, Christmas Day, and New Year's Day. While they searched for effective treatment, my body was nearly overcome by the infection. Abdominal compartment syndrome threatened multiple organ failure. Once the foreign origin of the infection was finally identified, life-saving treatment was administered.

By the time I regained consciousness in mid-March, my broken bones had healed (except for the C1 fracture—I had to wear the rigid collar for a while longer), the infection had been defeated, and my body began to recover. Because of the multiple debridement procedures, skin had to be grafted onto my left residual limb. There was also a temporary patch of grafted skin on my belly, a consequence of surgery to relieve pressure in the abdomen. Both the grafts and the graft donor sites were still bandaged when I was released to a rehabilitation hospital and remained bandaged for months afterward.

My Life, As I Had Known It, Was Over

After three months in ICU, I had wasted away. I'm a small person to begin with, just over five feet tall. I was strong and healthy when I was injured, but by the time I was released from the hospital I had shrunk to 85 pounds and my calf was the size of my wrist. For several days my hands were too weak to open a bottle of water, and were not coordinated enough to write my name. With the aid of a walker I could stand for a short time and take a few hops. Besides my physical weakness and the unfamiliar hospital environment, I just didn't feel quite like myself. It was difficult to pinpoint and difficult to explain to others, but something wasn't quite right in my head: it felt like there were spots of my brain that had gone dark and I couldn't find the light switch. My memory was unreliable. Word finding, focus, and concentration were all damaged. Reading was tiring. I felt vaguely muddled overall, and sometimes it was not easy to differentiate between real and false memories.

I couldn't deny my feelings of hopelessness. I was emotionally delicate and physically fragile. Before the accident, I had been on the threshold of a meaningful career track. Now those dreams were dashed and my life plan was erased.

There are so many questions, and as patients with a new disability we don't know where to find answers. After long-term ICU stays, whether from trauma or disease, anxiety about an uncertain future is to be expected. Not knowing when I'd be able to walk again, live independently, care for my dog, drive a car, get a job—all of these unknowns caused a constant hum of anxiety with the potential to spiral into depression.

Post-ICU Syndrome

My symptoms were typical of long-term ICU patients, a constellation of symptoms known as Post-ICU Syndrome, or PICS. Similar to PTSD, PICS patients typically suffer from brain fog, memory loss, physical weakness, depression, nightmares, or night terrors. They can be in danger of being unable to move beyond their fear and experience anxiety as endless uncertainties tumble like a hamster wheel in their head.

Compounded by the physical, mental, and emotional impacts of a long-term ICU stay, anxiety and depression are common symptoms of PICS. Advice that I received—and that I now share with new amputees and trauma patients—is to focus on the present, especially during your initial recovery. Start by tackling today's challenges. Take one step at a time. Regain your health and mobility first. When you're relearning the basic activities of daily living, it's too early to worry about your long-term future. To keep myself occupied and avoid dwelling on the big questions about my future, I tried to focus on my recovery and rehabilitation program.

Key factors that can aid in PICS recovery include social connection, supportive communities, and individual purpose. I may never fully recover from the traumatic experience that left my body disfigured and my mind scrambled, but by accepting help from others, staying connected with friends, and finding new activities and interests, I began to live and eventually to thrive[1] despite my disability and the side-effects of PTSD and PICS. Unwittingly, the actions I took mirrored the recommendations of Watkins-Hayes' model, moving from "dying from" to "living with" to "thriving despite": those steps include education about and self-advocacy for my needs, establishment of formal and informal support networks, and a newfound sense of purpose.

First Steps

Why didn't I fall into a black pool of hopelessness? With the love of my family and friends, medical support by physicians and therapists, mental health counseling, amputee support groups, and disabled sports clinics, I was able to gradually make progress toward accepting my body and regaining my life. I recognize my good fortune and am grateful: everything has changed, yet I am determined to continue to move *forward*, to love life and have new adventures.

To learn to live with my disability, move forward, and thrive, several factors were key for me:

- **As a foundation, access to proper medical care, including appropriate assistive devices and therapies, physical therapy, and a healthy diet and exercise.** I was fortunate to have good medical insurance coverage through my employer, then extended with COBRA, and in 2014 passage of the Affordable Care Act assured my continued access to healthcare. An additional formal support system was sessions with a therapist who specialized in working with people with disabilities.
- **A solid support system from my family, friends, counseling, peer visits and support groups.** While I was hospitalized, family members visited every day. They brought my laptop and I was able to catch up with friends on social media and email. These informal support networks grew as I became more independent and began to build new friendships and connections within my local community.
- **Discovering a purpose I felt passionate about.** I describe my entry into advocacy for people with limb loss as "accidental" because my interest grew after being stopped several times on the street and in parking lots, to be asked questions about my prosthesis. In response, I spoke frankly about my experiences as an amputee and trauma survivor. Often people were curious because they had a friend or family member who was struggling with limb loss. It was rewarding to be able to offer advice or guidance, or simply to point them to other resources. Eventually this led to deeper involvement with peer visits and legislative advocacy.

I also learned some key lessons:

Learn to Ask for Help

While hospitalized, my brother managed my care. After I was released, I lived with his family for six months while I received at-home nursing and physical therapy visits. My first—and most challenging—lesson was learning to ask for help. I've always been independent. At first, I tried to do everything myself but quickly learned that I couldn't. I didn't like feeling needy or bothering others with my problems; I felt diminished whenever I had to ask for help. But ultimately, I learned that those feelings and fears were mine alone, generated by my ego that insisted on trying to be self-sufficient. My family and friends *wanted* to help, and after a while I realized that their offers to help were truly expressions of caring. Now I tell others in the same situation, "The people who want to help you are the people who care most about you. By allowing them to help you, you are giving them a gift by allowing them to express their love for you."

Talk to Peers

Peer communities and support groups exist for many groups: cancer survivors, stroke survivors, Alcoholics Anonymous, and also for trauma survivors and people with limb loss. As a new amputee, I knew nothing about my new state, nothing about what would happen next, how to manage it, or whether my life would ever return to normal. While in-patient at Gaylord Hospital (a rehabilitation facility), a physical therapist recommended I attend an amputee support group meeting that was scheduled for the following Thursday. I didn't know what to expect, wondering how meeting others with limb loss (and possibly nothing else in common) could help me. At the meeting I learned that everyone else had had those same questions, was learning how to move forward, and had, to varying degrees, regained their lives. They knew what I was going through physically and emotionally because they had been in my shoes. In the support group we spoke freely about realistic expectations for prosthetics, working with a prosthetist, managing physical challenges, and treating discomfort and pain. They assured me that my fears about living with a disability were normal. We compared our "gear," our replacement joints and sockets, and discussed the latest prosthetic technology.

The first person I met at the support group meeting was Todd, whose physical presence complemented his big personality. He had a custom foot and ankle that allowed him to return to his lifelong sport, golfing. I also met Mildred, age 93, who had lost her leg 26 years earlier yet still went square-dancing with her husband every weekend. These people and others I have met at support groups across Connecticut are my heroes. They continue to face challenges and every day decide to continue their lives doing what they love.

I had searched online and read about people living with limb loss; I had researched prosthetic limbs and sought counsel for mental health. But reading and watching videos was not as powerful as meeting and talking with other amputees. By having this traumatic experience in common, we were able to open up to each other. Like any painful life experience, it's a relief to talk to someone who really knows what you've been through, a relief to know you're not alone.

Meeting people who had returned to their favorite activities and actively regained their lives helped to alleviate my anxieties. This is one reason why support group meetings are highly effective, whether for amputee, trauma, cancer, or long-term ICU survivors. Meeting others who have had similar experiences, seeing that people have moved forward to live productive and satisfying lives, is reassuring. Seeing that others have overcome similar challenges, we know that we can too. This forward-looking perspective is an essential step in moving beyond "my life is over," or "I may as well be dead," or "I can't survive this trauma," to thinking, "I'm going to be able to live with this challenge."

Try New Activities

Recreational activities I participated in pre-injury were downhill skiing, mountain biking (in CO and UT), and rock-climbing. I ran for exercise and practiced yoga every morning. While still in-patient at Yale-New Haven Hospital, the surgeon Dr. Kaplan, in response to my panicky question "What will I do now?" replied "You will be able to do anything you want." Startled, and doubtful, I challenged him. "Really? How long before I can bike and ski again?" I asked. "Two years," he replied confidently. Trusting his assurance helped me to look for a path forward, for specific steps I could take to return to my favorite outdoor activities. It took longer than he predicted, closer to five years, for me to return to outdoor sports, but his confidence gave me the encouragement to believe I could do it. I worked with a personal trainer to get strong again and swam regularly to build fitness. I attended adaptive recreation events to explore outdoor activities in a supportive environment: rock-climbing, kayaking, golfing, bicycling. Now that I live on the shoreline, kayaking has become a favorite. By 2010 I was skiing in Vermont and by 2018 I was surfing in Costa Rica. In 2019 I obtained Scuba certification and in 2022 I went diving in the Caribbean.

In addition to outdoor recreation, I returned to earlier creative interests like painting and knitting. I gave myself permission to try new things, such as silversmithing and mosaics. Even though I may not be able to ski or bicycle as well as I used to, I can learn to enjoy them at my current ability level and explore new activities.

One Step at a Time

Following my injury, I didn't see much of a future, but over the next several months I learned to adapt. Post-hospitalization, my focus turned to regaining life skills that would allow me to live independently. I learned to walk with a prosthesis— at first with crutches, then with a cane, and then one day I left my cane in the car and I didn't pick it up again. I relearned how to accomplish daily chores such as cooking, shopping, vacuuming—normal home tasks, whether standing or in a wheelchair. I found a job, moved into my own apartment, and my dog came to live with me again. Caring for him was a big step in learning the power of focus outside of myself as part of the healing process. Every day he needed a walk, giving me a reason to get out of bed and out of the house. Day by day, my life settled into a new normal as I learned to live with my disability.

Many friends, when they learned of my injury, called my family or sent notes of encouragement and—oddly, it seemed to me—congratulations on my bravery. They told me how strong I was to have survived, how I was a hero for my courage to face my disability. I didn't feel like a hero and I didn't feel strong. I felt weak and vulnerable and, honestly, afraid of the world. I knew that I was lucky, not strong or brave or courageous. I was lucky to survive, as my friend had not. I was lucky to have a future, whatever it may turn out to be.

Recovery and rehabilitation are a process—progression from injury or illness back to life, from fear and despair back to hope. It starts with one step—followed by another step, and another—to move forward.

My "New Normal" Life

By 2014, six years after my injury, I had settled into a new life, my "new normal." I moved to a cottage in a small coastal town in Connecticut, close to family. I have found new friends and built community connections, forming a living web that supports and protects me.

Connections—family, friends, community—have been the key to my process of regaining my life following traumatic change. They create a network of support and also responsibility. Support groups are one important part of that network, providing support for the specific needs of survivors of trauma, cancer, limb loss, etc.

Over the next few years, I became more and more involved in amputee advocacy. Working together, my friend Herb (also an above-knee amputee) and I led efforts for new legislation in the State of Connecticut to protect health insurance coverage for prosthetics. We formed the Connecticut Amputee Network to organize grassroots support for the law and for limb loss education efforts. With strong backing from our local State Senators and Representatives, legislation passed in mid-2018 and became law in 2019. Advocacy for the limb loss community became a central activity of my new life.

After passage of the Connecticut State law, Amputee Coalition invited me and Herb to become Lead Advocates and to join other limb loss activists across the country to advocate for insurance protection at the federal level. In 2019 we participated in "Hill Day," visiting our Connecticut Representatives' and Senators' offices on Capitol Hill in Washington DC to discuss the need for a federal law to protect insurance coverage for prosthetics and to ask for support funding the National Limb Loss Resource Center. We were invited to speak at the Amputee Coalition 2019 Annual Conference and 2021 Virtual Volunteer Summit. Herb and I continue to work together to train certified amputee peer visitors and to educate healthcare workers about the effectiveness of peer visits and support groups in improving long-term health outcomes.

Reassessing Treatment

Looking back on my experience as a survivor of trauma and PICS, I can see where formal treatment options succeeded and where they fell short. Many of the key elements in my recovery and rehabilitation had been established long before my injury, yet some of these can be integrated into a multidisciplinary PICS treatment protocol.

1. Include in-patient peer visits.
2. Review home situation to ensure it can accommodate or be adapted for patient.
3. Provide psychological assessment for PTSD and PICS, including recommendations for treatment and scheduled follow-up. A full neuropsychological evaluation was helpful for me to understand posttraumatic changes to my mental capabilities.
4. Assess caretaker's anxiety and stress and provide referrals for support.

Forward!

Building new friendships, maintaining longtime relationships, caring for my physical health, and exploring a purpose I'm passionate about have been key to building a new self-identity. I'm able to use my personal experience to advocate and help people with limb loss regain their lives. In this sense, my disability has become a strength. The thing that I did not want to be recognized for has now become something about me that stands out—literally. I wear shorts and skirts no matter how often people notice or stare. My disability is a part of me now and I continue to live my live—not only *living with* my limb loss (and the accompanying trauma and PICS) but *thriving despite* it.

The shift from "living with" my disability to "thriving despite" it is a result of finding a purpose I'm passionate about that promotes positive change to help others living with limb loss. Amputee advocacy takes me outside of myself—my worries, desires, pain — to focus on helping others with similar challenges, putting my traumatic experience to good use supporting the limb loss community.

There are still setbacks. The process of learning to live with my disability, for me, is not over. My limb continues to change over time, causing the fit of my prosthesis to change. I still suffer from chronic (though well-managed) pain, and though in some ways I have become more capable and mobile, there remain things that I have not yet been able to relearn. Daily I see the mutilated skin on my residual limb, the scars on my sound leg that were sources of the skin grafts for my amputated limb, and the scar that runs from my sternum to my pelvis. No one easily accepts the permanent damage major trauma causes to their physical body, but by now I have accepted my prosthetic leg as part of me, part of my self-image, and am not ashamed to show it.

Reflection

As I write this, the COVID-19 pandemic is beginning to subside in the United States. During the pandemic, while we were encouraged to stay home and limit time spent in public places, I felt as if time paused while we all hibernated. Yet while we sheltered in place, nature moved forward outdoors.

Here in New England, springtime doesn't arrive suddenly or all at once. Instead, tiny steps lead to a burst of buds and blooms. Now, in May, I'm watching goldfinches turn from dull gray to bright yellow and the rose hedge transform from a thicket of sticks to a bouquet of chartreuse and pink. Spring is defined by the change from chill to warmth and from drabness to bright colors. Sometimes, in New England, the transition is subtle and we don't recognize we're in the midst of it until—all at once, it seems—we feel the summer sun on our faces and sizzling sand between our toes. Similarly, I can't identify the exact date that I was "recovered"—was it when I stopped using a cane? or when my nightmares ceased?

Rehabilitation after major trauma and recovery from PICS is a long winding road. Following injury, progression back to health and hope is a process of a thousand steps—and sometimes falling backwards before again moving forward—with each step building upon completion of the step before, always toward a new future. Looking back, I can identify the phases I've passed through to get to where I am now, from dying to thriving, though I did not see them at the time. Challenges continue, some symptoms of PTSD and PICS continue, but I am content and know that I will be able to *live with* and *thrive despite* the after-effects of trauma and limb loss.

Brenda Novak, JD
May 2021

REFERENCE

The framework I use, "moving from 'dying from' to 'living with' to 'thriving despite,'" to describe my recovery from major trauma was created by Celeste Watkins-Hayes in her 2019 book, *Remaking a Life: How Women Living with HIV/AIDS Confront Inequality*. I have used it here with her permission.

Preface

The seventy years since critical care became a specialty have been marked by vast technological advances shaping how we care for patients with critical illness or injury. New discoveries have informed our understanding of illness and have led to novel therapies for conditions ranging from infection to life-threatening hemorrhagic shock. Accordingly, an increasing number of patients survive their critical illness and define a unique group of patients known as "ICU survivors." Their struggles during recovery—as well as those of their loved ones—inspired us to craft this book as a guide and a touchstone. Since patient-and-family centered care is at the heart of team-based critical care, it is important to recognize the key role that loved ones play during convalescence, and the difficulties that they encounter. Our textbook targets patients, family members, but also primary care clinicians as these three often navigate recovery well outside of the ICU, and clinicians whose practice is principally confined to the hospital. We expect that this book will also be of interest to hospital-based providers, including hospitalists and ICU providers, who care for patients in the early phases of care but may be ill-equipped to provide anticipatory guidance about the journey to recovery.

We have arranged this book in three sections: (1) multiprofessional ICU team members and their roles and perspectives on ICU care, (2) innovative methods of promoting recovery, and finally (3) unique populations encountered in the ICU. Our goal is to help place all of the complex care that is required in the ICU into a framework that is readily understood, and to explore its impact on recovery. Within each chapter is a specific section dedicated to "Tips for Clinicians" that we hope will help further improve how care is rendered while including patients, loved ones, and primary care clinicians as part of a global team. Therefore, not all of the chapters are authored by healthcare professionals. In fact, this book opens with chapters from patients who describe their life-threatening illness, their journey to recovery, and the clinicians who helped them along the way. Each day, patients and family members just like them—and just like you—remind us of the joy found in caring for others.

Multidisciplinary Perspectives on ICU Care and Recovery

The Patient and Family Perspective

Colleen Kelly Alexander and Sean Alexander

Editors' Note

This book is meant to offer guidance on supporting patients and families through recovery from critical illness. Understanding and giving voice to the patient experience is at the heart of this work. The first chapter tells the story of a patient and her husband, starting with the injury that led to her critical illness. The story contains graphic details of the author's experience. We opted not to exclude these details, as they are central to the patient's narrative of injury, illness, and recovery. This chapter does not follow the format of the remaining chapters; it starts with the patient's experience, continues to the family experience, and concludes with considerations for recovery.

■ A PATIENT'S EXPERIENCE

Before the ICU

A year into living in Connecticut, I had begun to embrace my new work as a regional program manager for an international nonprofit organization. I had the honor of designing curriculum for elementary through college age students. The focus of my work was sharing the lives of various Nobel Peace Prize Laureates as real-world heroes and mentors showing that "ordinary" people can do extraordinary things when they have passion and conviction to create change, regardless of their origins or the challenges they face.

My main mode of transportation was bicycling. I used to live in Vermont and would cycle as often as I could instead of driving. I found cycling was not only a huge source of joy to me, but it was also a way I could be in harmony with nature. When you sit at a desk for most of the day, having the ability to exercise and be one with nature is such a gift. I kept cycling to and from work after the move to Connecticut. I would cycle up to 100 miles a day, then speak at night at area community centers and colleges. In Fall 2011, I had completed a 600-mile ride across New England and New York covering my work territory. My cycling was uneventful; throughout the entire trip that autumn, I did not even have a flat tire.

On October 8, 2011, I was called in for a work meeting—a 9.5-mile ride each way. The leaves were blissful and the weather was idyllic, with the sun high in the sky. As I rode back from work later, I thought about home—making dinner with my husband, taking a walk down to the water together bundled in fleece jackets, watching our Labrador swim. A large freight truck came toward me on a side street that crossed my route. I heard the truck downshift to come to a stop, but as I passed the side street, I heard the truck accelerate. As I was hit by the truck's front tires, I had enough time to think, "I'm going to die." My adrenaline kicked in.

I felt the weight of the truck knocking me down. My feet were clipped into my bike, and I could feel the bike getting tangled up under the chassis as I was ripped off the bike and run over again by the back set of tires. Once my body stopped rolling, the pain was unimaginable. I had felt a heavy crack inside of my body, and my lower back felt numb. My stomach and legs were on fire. I picked up my head to assess the damage and saw that all of my clothing had been shredded off. I saw the insides of my abdomen, that my right leg seemed unattached, and that the left was completely mangled.

I knew from my days as an EMT that if I screamed my chances of survival would be greater because it would preserve my blood pressure. I began screaming, as I was unable to move. Thankfully, a bystander saw the trauma and ran out to protect me from being run over again. The local ambulance was less than a mile away at a local event, allowing me to be transported without delay. I knew my time was probably brief as I could feel my heart struggling to pump and I could feel my body fighting to not pass out from shock. Still, I did not understand the magnitude of my injuries.

During transport, I remained aware and fighting. I screamed to let me live, to allow me to be a mother someday, to keep being a wife to the man I adore. I began losing consciousness on arrival to the hospital; I remember the double doors of the ambulance opening and hands reaching in, then my world went black. I did not have any experiences of seeing a divine being, or connecting with my family, or seeing rainbows and unicorns. I remember being warm, and completely powerful, energetic, and euphoric.

In the ICU

I do not have any memories of the beginning of my hospital stay. Dr. Kaplan told me later that I had screamed and cursed, then gone into shock and cardiac arrest. I awakened sometime later in the ICU after being in a coma, but then would lose memories for multiple hours or days. I would eventually regain awareness of being locked in my body with a machine breathing for me. The cycle of losing and regaining awareness and memory would continue for the next six weeks as I would go in and out of surgeries.

My memories of being in the ICU are much like a series of very bad nightmares. I was fully aware I was in a bed, able to hear, see, feel, smell, and taste. I was unable to make sense of anything happening around me. I saw light, shadows, darkness, and colors, but my brain was unable to process what I was seeing. I also heard voices but was unable to understand most words. I remember feeling my lungs inflate, I remember the sounds of the machines beeping, and the feelings of immense pain and fear that would occasionally dissipate with a warm touch or vocal tone. I remember being wheeled down long hallways and seeing what I thought were tunnel lights above me (I now understand I was just being wheeled to surgery). I remember one of the times laying under immense bright lights and things were extremely blurry; however, I could suddenly make sense of words. I felt painful pressure on my body and tried to move and tell them I was awake; I remember someone saying, "Her fingers are moving, she isn't fully out." Then I saw a shadow of a person lean over me and heard words. I then faded out only to awaken laying on my side trying to scream, but with nothing coming out. I felt like I was being gagged.

As unsettling as my waking experiences were, the nightmares truly began when I fell asleep. I remember fighting to not give into sleep. My dreams were incredibly vivid and violent. Most of my dreams were of being dehydrated and begging for water. I would often be in very hot environments where I was being sodomized, over and over again. I would later understand that they would increase my medications to allow dressing changes, causing me to drift in between awake and sleep. Given that some of my wound changes were rectal and vaginal, my mind interpreted wound care as being sexually assaulted.

■ A FAMILY MEMBER'S EXPERIENCE

Before the ICU

Every morning, I awoke to a snuggling embrace with Colleen. This norm has been an essential staple of our life together that recharges our souls as we begin each day. Before leaving for work, our lips touch, we exchange hugs and

I Love You's, and we start our days. I was employed as a United States Postal Service Rural Carrier Associate. (Unfortunately, this role did not require the adorable "face of the post office" hat, shirt, and short uniform, which was a letdown to Colleen.) I would go to work in our trusty and capable stripped-down sedan with a manual transmission, manual locks, and manual windows.

On October 8, 2011, I was pulling mail before getting on the road. My cell phone chimed; the display showed an unrecognizable number. Colleen and I had only lived in Connecticut for one year and I was unfamiliar with local area codes. Despite my usual reluctance to answer unknown numbers, I decided to pick up the phone. The gentleman on the other end of the line told me he was given my number from Colleen and that she was in an accident.

I knew she had been cycling to and from work that morning, so I asked if she was okay and about what happened. He explained that she had been hit by a truck and that she might have a broken leg. An ambulance had taken her to the hospital. He could not answer any more questions because he had to answer questions from the police. I left work and drove to the hospital. My brain was whirling with worst-case scenarios. I tried to reassure myself— "She's okay, it's just a broken leg. Just drive quickly and safely. Just a broken leg…"

I found parking and made my way into the unfamiliar hospital. I struggled to find the emergency department because of renovations, but eventually encountered a security officer. I asked about my wife, saying that she was brought in for a leg injury. He referenced his patient list and said, "She's not here. Are you sure you have the right hospital? Or maybe you arrived before her?" I tried asking again, explaining that Colleen had been hit by a truck. The officer turned to another staffer who had been listening to our conversation. She looked at him and softly mouthed the word, "Trauma." I could only muster, "What does that mean? Please explain." Neither could or would tell me more, instructing me to sit down and wait.

Seconds turned to minutes and minutes turned into hours. Every 45 to 60 minutes, a woman wearing business attire (I didn't then know her name or role) would bring me small snippets of information about Colleen. She could not, however, answer any of the questions I had. It seemed like her main concern was to keep me calm. I would find out later that she was the hospital chaplain assigned to my wife.

Many hours later, I was taken to a family lounge waiting area, still without answers. I was transferred to a smaller, more private area, then transferred back to the lounge, all without any idea of what was happening. About 6 or 7 hours after my arrival, I was taken to the hallway outside the lounge, where I met a very confident, stocky man. I asked how Colleen was; he told me "he's still working on her," "she's now in stable condition," "need to return and continue working on her." I said, "It's just a broken leg, right?" He told me stoically, "She was run over."

In the ICU

The doctors and nurses worked around the clock for 48 hours to get Colleen to a stable condition. The family lounge outside the ICU became my new home, but I still struggled to get a straight answer about what was happening with my wife. I attended each session of morning rounds to gather as much information as I could, as the nursing staff was reluctant to let me know how severe Colleen's condition was. My guess is that the staff didn't want me freaking out.

After several weeks of not working, I was encouraged to go back to work. This offered some sense of a normal life and some much-needed income. The daily routine was to attend rounds, go to work, shower at home, then return to the family lounge. I came to know how to support Colleen in her healing, including propping pillows on the outsides of her legs to lessen her movement, as she was very active despite being sedated. This was well-received by most of the nurses, but I vividly remember one exception. This nurse, who took care of Colleen on multiple occasions, had multiple issues including poor professionalism and a lack of care—on one occasion forgetting his scrubs and working in his casual clothes and on another being inattentive and allowing Colleen to endanger herself while in restraints. I had to ask that he never be assigned to her again, and I became much more vigilant in my interactions with the hospital staff. I found it unfortunate and concerning to encounter a staff member who was not fully invested in the care of such a vulnerable patient.

After the ICU

From Colleen: During the time in the ICU, I was completely vulnerable and at the will of the medical team. Even though my ICU experiences were traumatic, I give such thanks for the outcome of my life, as it is a testament to the care I was provided when I was unable to support myself in any way.

Considerations for recovery:

- Every patient is different; they may be strong willed, stubborn, scared, or anxious as they recover from critical illness.
- Every patient's healing journey is different.
- Patients may not initially understand the severity of their condition and may not be able to process information that may have been shared during the ICU stay.

- Meaningful recovery means something different to each patient. From Colleen: *"For me, as a former athlete I wanted to be back at races and moving as much as I could as soon as I could regardless of what that meant with respect to speed/ability or disability. I am so grateful that my surgeons and medical team were very honest with me about understanding my need to move for my emotional health."*
- Family members may need assistance in meeting the needs of patients who survive critical illness, including connections with social services.

Tips for Clinicians

1. **Allow the patient to be their own advocate** as much as possible.
2. **Be transparent with patients** about their own care plan. From Colleen: *"I am grateful that Dr. Kaplan was not only transparent with my care, he was also very straightforward and spoke to me not out of compassion so much, rather out of what was necessary for me to reach optimum healing in between each surgery."*
3. **Encourage patients to ask questions.** From Colleen: *"The better I understood what was happening or not happening with my body on my healing journey, the better able I was to take ownership and have a 'job' which was to be a steward of my own vessel and work WITH it to heal."*
4. **Realize that patients may have multiple emotions**, including fear, depression, anxiety, anger, and numbness. Acknowledge patients' feelings without ruminating with them.
5. **Acknowledge patient concerns promptly.** From Colleen: *"When a doctor is too busy to respond to patient concerns or even respond with suggestions on where to seek help, it will undermine emotional stability and interfere with physical healing."*
6. **Provide as much communication as possible** to family members about patients' care and potential future needs. From Sean: "Dr. Kaplan was very good about always being honest and never sugar-coating things. He always answered professionally and honestly even if the answer was not what I wanted to hear."

The Physician's Perspective

Randi N. Smith, Reka Somodi, and Lewis J. Kaplan

Patient Care Vignette

A 34-year-old woman, AB, was involved in a motor vehicle crash. She was transported by Emergency Medical Services (EMS) to a Level 1 trauma facility. Due to a very low blood pressure and obvious signs of abdominal injury, she was taken to the Operating Room (OR). After operative repair of multiple organ injuries using a damage control approach (fixing only life-threatening injuries), she was transported to the surgical ICU (SICU) for ongoing care. In the SICU she was cared for by a multiprofessional team led by a surgeon trained in surgical critical care. The damage control surgeon also has additional training in surgical critical care, and acted as the intensivist for nearly half of her SICU stay. After SICU admission, the surgeon updated her husband on what was found, what was done, what remained to be accomplished, and what was likely to happen over the next few days.

During her several weeks in the SICU, her husband participated in daily morning rounds as well as afternoon rounds. He had many questions that were regularly answered by the intensivist. The intensivist explained what other specialty surgeons including orthopedic, urologic, and gynecologic surgeons needed to do to help his wife. As a result of regular contact, the husband identified the initial surgeon as his wife's doctor—despite the surgeon's practice being one that functions as a team. Accordingly, even after SICU survival and hospital discharge the patient and her husband both maintained contact with the surgeon. They specifically solicited the surgeon's opinion about care-related decision-making. The durable contact with the surgeon-intensivist helped to identify that the patient demonstrated PICS. She was referred for cognitive and psychologic therapy with benefit.

■ ROLE OF THE PHYSICIAN IN THE ICU

Regardless of setting, the physician serves in a leadership role within the ICU. This is true in facilities where there is an intensivist as well as in the nearly 50% of US facilities that do not have an intensivist on staff. The physician is responsible for patient care as their top priority. Part of that responsibility is to coordinate care when there are other specialists involved in patient care. Regardless of setting (critical access vs community vs tertiary vs quaternary care center) there are three broadly different roles for physicians within the ICU that impact direct care decision-making as well as care coordination (Fig. 2-1). When there is no intensivist, the admitting physician also serves as the Attending of Record. In facilities where there is an intensivist in the ICU, the intensivist can serve as the Attending of Record—a process common within the medical ICU. Most medical ICUs function as "closed ICUs" where only the critical care team may write orders, render care decisions (in conjunction with the patient or family or surrogate), and embrace or reject consultant recommendations. Alternatively, the intensivist may serve as a consultant—a process more common in the surgical ICU. Most surgical ICUs function as collaborative ICUs where the operating surgeon remains the Attending of Record and the intensivist manages the critical care aspects of patient management (e.g., noninvasive or invasive mechanical ventilation, blood pressure–modulating medications, nutrition support, antibiotic selection, etc.). Moreover, the physician commonly spends time teaching, an undertaking that may be very much magnified when there are trainees

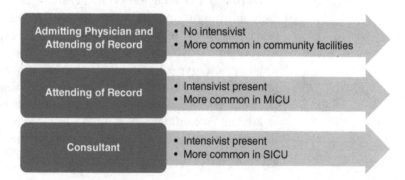

FIGURE 2-1 **The three types of physician roles in an ICU.**

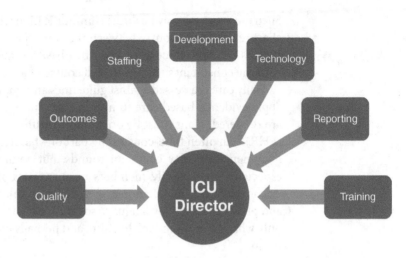

FIGURE 2-2 **ICU Director responsibilities.**

present, including students, residents, and fellows from a variety of parent disciplines. There are other more unique roles for physicians when they serve as the ICU Director.

Physicians may serve as the ICU Director and therefore shoulder an administrative role in addition to their bedside clinical care role (Fig. 2-2). Administrative roles routinely include physician staffing, credentialing, protocol and policy development and deployment, equipment sourcing, quality improvement, morbidity and mortality assessment, resource utilization analysis, as well as quality and outcome reporting. Additional roles may include budget creation, recruiting and training of Advanced Practice Providers (APP; Nurse Practitioners or Physician Assistants), as well as faculty and staff development. In teaching settings, the ICU Director may also serve as the Director of a Critical Care Medicine fellowship, or if not at the main teaching facility, the site director for that fellowship.

■ WHAT HAPPENS IN THE ICU FROM THE PERSPECTIVE OF THE PHYSICIAN

Regardless of setting, ICU care is complex and involves a number of individuals who bring unique specialty or subspecialty expertise to the care of the critically ill or injured patient. Throughout the day, care evolves within daily rounds as well as in a discontinuous fashion as consultants engage in patient evaluation and recommendation generation. This means that the physician must have a mechanism for keeping updated on consultant's assessments.

Such mechanisms may be direct communication with the consultant, repeated chart review, or discourse between the consultant and another team member such as the APP. Once informed, the physician must then decide what to do with the consultant's recommended course of action.

Daily care is assessed against guidelines and implementation tools that help apply evidence-based care to improve patient outcome. Once care decisions are rendered, plans must be documented within the electronic health record (EHR)—an often time-consuming part of what happens within the ICU. This documentation may occur on rounds, but commonly occurs after rounds especially when family members or surrogates also participate in rounds. Accordingly, the physician may spend a lot of time translating medical jargon and procedures into lay language so that the decision-maker understands not only what those things are, but also, and perhaps more importantly, what they mean.

Care activities and documentation are interwoven with a variety of scheduled as well as impromptu meetings and administrative activities throughout the day. In the afternoon, a repeat set of rounds is common to follow-up on the results of therapies started earlier in the day, diagnostic testing, consultant recommendations, or procedures. Care plans are then revised depending on how the patient responded. The evolution of care—or lack thereof—is important to track as the breadth of care will also need to be communicated with the physician who will assume care after the current intensivist's rotation is complete. In general, intensivists serve in the ICU for a week at a time, but other schedules may occur. Of course, when there is no intensivist, the admitting physician may share care responsibilities with others in their group (when there is a group); solo ownership of patient responsibility is becoming much less frequent over the last decade but may persist in critical access or smaller community facilities.

Daily assessments of organ injury or organ failure are a key part of the routine assessments that the physician must make regarding the patient's condition. For many organ failures there are specific technologies that may be used to support patients while they are trying to recover from the illness or injury that led to ICU admission. These technologies include non-invasive ventilation, invasive mechanical ventilation, dialysis (continuous or intermittent), and extracorporeal membrane oxygenation (ECMO). Some patients require a body cavity to be left open for a period of time—most commonly the abdomen—after life-threatening injury or emergency general surgery; this approach also has unique technologies that aid in management (see Chapter 21, Trauma). The decisions around initiation, continuation, and termination are shared across multiple team members from patients to family members to specialists all of which is coordinated by the intensivist. High-intensity care needs to be assessed in light of the patient's goals, values, and preferences to ensure that the patient receives goal-concordant care.

Determining goals of care, code status, and providing family or surrogate decision-makers updates are key elements that the physician must address. In many facilities, advanced practice providers (APPs) can help with many of these undertakings, but quite often palliative care medicine specialists are excellent partners (see Chapter 8, Palliative Care Perspective). Nonetheless, when family members or surrogate decision-makers cannot participate in daily rounds, family meetings are often scheduled to address all of these aspects of care. Most commonly scheduled in the afternoon, some meetings cannot occur in person due to distance from the healthcare facility, lack of transportation, or other constraints including child or elder care. Therefore, digital platforms help link the ICU physician with the other meeting participants. Digital platforms include those that became quite well-known during the SARS-CoV-2 pandemic such as ZOOM, Microsoft TEAMS, or Go-To-Meeting as well as others. Some proprietary platforms also exist, but are less widely available than smartphone, tablet, or computer applications such as Apple's FaceTime. Clearly, communication and care coordination are foundational aspects of what occurs within the ICU from the physician's perspective.

■ CONSIDERATIONS FOR RECOVERY

Since communication is a core aspect of what occurs in the ICU in addition to direct patient care, it should also inform aftercare. ICU care is generally complex, and may span weeks to months. Once the patient survives the ICU, their trajectory leads them to the acute care unit within the same facility, or transfer to another kind of facility such as a long-term acute care hospital (LTACH), a skilled nursing facility (SNF), or a rehabilitation facility. Movement to each of these different sites are underpinned by a transition in care. Within the same facility, there is often a hand-off that occurs in a direct physician-to-physician *and* nurse-to-nurse fashion accompanied by a transfer form that may or may not have a specific structure. Transfer to a different facility often occurs using a different approach.

Patient transfer to an LTACH for example occurs with a transfer form, a nurse-to-nurse but uncommonly a physician-to-physician hand-off, as well as a hospital stay encompassing discharge summary. The discharge summary may or may not be sent to the patient's primary care clinician (when one is present and identifiable); increasingly, that clinician is a nurse practitioner and not a physician. Moreover, the discharge summary is typically completed by an individual who has rendered care only outside of the ICU and is therefore only peripherally aware of the course of ICU care. This practice likely reduces the robustness of the information incorporated into the discharge summary that would describe events that occurred during the ICU stay. Some, but not all, facilities use a transfer form that describes the ICU stay when patients transfer to the acute care unit. Those forms help inform the content of the hospital stay discharge summary. Upon discharge from any of these secondary care sites, there is another discharge summary that may be sent to the referring physician from the acute care facility, and may or may not be sent to the primary care clinician. Communication with a primary care clinician is complicated by medical tourism where patients may travel from other states and sometimes other countries to pursue unique care at a specific complex care facility. Clearly, there are opportunities to help ensure that there is clear communication with the patient's primary care clinician.

One approach is to create an ICU-specific discharge summary that may be sent directly to the primary care clinician. Such a summary can also identify new diagnoses that are important for aftercare including whether the patient is at high risk for the post-intensive care syndrome. This same summary can be shared with secondary care sites to help guide assessment and care at that location. This is a relatively low-cost investment in ensuring effective communication. Another approach is to leverage the seemingly ubiquitous smartphone and its medical ID. If the patient or family member can unlock the phone, an ICU team member can enter new diagnoses and medications into the medical ID. While attractive, team members at other sites of care (including the primary care clinician's office) would need to do the same thing to ensure accuracy. Since medical IDs can be accessed without unlocking the device, they are used by Emergency Medical Services personnel during emergencies to identify key medical conditions, medications, and especially allergies. Therefore, accuracy is essential.

Finally, referring patients to a post-ICU clinic (when available) after discharge from a secondary care site helps reunite the patient and the family with a team attuned to ICU-related sequelae. This also provides another opportunity to link the ICU team with the primary care clinician in an updated fashion. The same digital platforms identified earlier can be used to facilitate team-based communication with the primary care clinician. This approach defines another essential role for the intensivist in ongoing patient care. Post-ICU clinics are increasingly prevalent across the United States and have demonstrated improved outcomes for patients, family members, as well as ICU staff (see Chapter 15, Post-ICU Clinics). Sometimes, a particular patient and family will develop a long-term and durable relationship with an ICU physician, but this is less common. When it occurs—as it has for one of this chapter's authors, LJK) it adds a uniquely rewarding dimension to the anchoring patient–physician relationship that blossoms outside the boundaries of the inpatient care facility.

Tips for Clinicians

1. There are many different models of physician involvement in direct patient care in the ICU. **Take the time to ensure that patients, families, surrogates, and staff clearly understand** the prevailing practice model.
2. Communication is a fundamental aspect of providing critical care and care coordination in particular, especially when there are consultants involved in complex care.
3. While medical phraseology facilitates healthcare professional communication, lay language is essential for patient and family or surrogate communication. **Explain not only what things are, but what they mean** in a granular way so that they can participate in shared decision-making in an informed fashion.
4. **Elicit goals of care, code status, as well as values and preferences** to ensure that goal-concordant care is provided. Some of these discussions may be challenging and may benefit from engaging partners such as palliative care medicine clinicians as partners.
5. Physicians with administrative responsibilities shoulder many obligations besides direct patient care. This is a nonintuitive skill set for many and a variety of medical professional organizations offer professional development courses and modules that aid in garnering the required administrative skills.
6. **A variety of opportunities exist to improve how ICU care is communicated across care transitions** within and outside of the acute care facility. There is no single best approach, but it is ideal to explore what solution will best work for the specific practice environment within which practice occurs.

KEY REFERENCES

Bakhru RN, Davidson JF, Bookstaver RE, et al. Implementation of an ICU recovery clinic at a tertiary care academic center. *Crit Care Explor.* 2019 Aug;1(8).

Buchman TG, Coopersmith CM, Meissen HW, et al. Innovative interdisciplinary strategies to address the intensivist shortage. *Crit Care Med.* 2017 Feb 1;45(2):298-304.

Cardwell K. Reducing medication errors and transitions of care. *Age Ageing.* 2020;49(4):537-579.

Haines KJ, Sevin CM, Hibbert E, et al. Key mechanisms by which post-ICU activities can improve in-ICU care: results of the international THRIVE collaboratives. *Intensive Care Med.* 2019;45(7):939-947.

Joffe AM, Pastores SM, Maerz LL, et al. Utilization and impact on fellowship training of non-physician advanced practice providers in intensive care units of academic medical centers: a survey of critical care program directors. *J Crit Care.* 2014;29(1):112-115.

Lane-Fall MB, Pascual JL, Massa S, et al. Developing a standard handoff process for operating room–to-ICU transitions: multidisciplinary clinician perspectives from the handoffs and transitions in critical care (HATRICC) study. *Jt Comm J Qual Patient Saf.* 2018;44(9):514-525.

Lopez KD, O'Rourke J, Lane-Fall MB, Abraham J. Improving handoffs using a systems framework and simulation. In: Deutsch ES, Perry SJ, Gurnaney HG, eds. *Comprehensive Healthcare Simulation: Improving Healthcare Systems.* Cham: Springer; 2021:73-76.

Müller M, Jürgens J, Redaèlli M, Klingberg K, Hautz WE, Stock S. Impact of the communication and patient hand-off tool SBAR on patient safety: a systematic review. *BMJ Open.* 2018;8(8):e022202.

Murphy DJ, Ogbu OC, Coopersmith CM. ICU director data: using data to assess value, inform local change, and relate to the external world. *Chest.* 2015;147(4):1168-1178.

Pastores SM, Kvetan V, Coopersmith CM, et al. Workforce, workload, and burnout among intensivists and advanced practice providers: a narrative review. *Crit Care Med.* 2019;47(4):550-557.

Pastores SM, Halpern NA, Oropello JM, Kvetan V. Intensivist workforce in the United States: the crisis is real, not imagined. *Am J Respir Crit Care Med.* 2015;191(6):718-719.

Penkoske PA, Buchman TG. The relationship between the surgeon and the intensivist in the surgical intensive care unit. *Surg Clin.* 2006;86(6):1351-1357.

Pronovost PJ, Thompson DA, Holzmueller CG, Dorman T, Morlock LL. The organization of intensive care unit physician services. *Crit Care Med.* 2007;35(10):2256-E11.

Siegal EM, Dressler DD, Dichter JR, et al. Training a hospitalist workforce to address the intensivist shortage in American hospitals: a position paper from the Society of Hospital Medicine and the Society of Critical Care Medicine. *Crit Care Med.* 2012;40(6):1952-1956.

Tully AP, Hammond DA, Li C, et al. Evaluation of medication errors at the transition of care from an ICU to non-ICU location. *Crit Care Med.* 2019;47(4):543-549.

Ward NS, Afessa B, Kleinpell R, et al. Intensivist/patient ratios in closed ICUs: a statement from the Society of Critical Care Medicine Taskforce on ICU Staffing. *Crit Care Med.* 2013;41(2):638-645.

The Advanced Practice Provider's Perspective

CHAPTER 3

Peter Sandor and Brandon Oto

> ## Patient Care Vignette
>
> A 64-year-old woman presents to the emergency department after a motor vehicle collision. She has bilateral pneumothoraxes and a grade IV liver laceration causing massive intra-abdominal hemorrhage. She is intubated and bilateral thoracostomy tubes are placed. The patient then undergoes emergent exploratory laparotomy, where the liver is packed, and the abdomen is left with a temporary closure device. Massive transfusion is performed, with nearly 10 liters of blood components given. She is brought intubated to the ICU for further stabilization, where a team of critical care physicians, advanced practice providers (APPs), and nurses assume responsibility for her care, managing respiratory failure, titrating medication infusions, correcting metabolic and coagulation abnormalities, and administering additional blood products.
>
> After 2 days, the patient returns to the operating room, but abdominal closure is impossible due to edema. She develops agitated delirium and her sedation regimen is modified for safety. She develops acute kidney injury requiring renal replacement therapy. The ICU APP inserts a temporary dialysis catheter, and continuous renal replacement therapy (CRRT) is initiated. Prophylactic anticoagulation is initially held due to ongoing bleeding, and on day 3, the bedside nurse notes swelling of the right leg; a deep venous thrombosis (DVT) of the right common femoral vein is diagnosed by ultrasound. The surgical service is concerned about recurrence of bleeding with anticoagulation, so an inferior vena cava (IVC) filter is placed. A registered dietitian estimates the patient's nutritional requirements and

enteral nutrition via feeding tube is initiated, first at a low dose, then cautiously advanced to provide full nutrition.

The next 2 weeks are marked by both clinical progress and setbacks. On her fourth surgery for serial exploration and washout, her midline abdominal incision is successfully closed. A heparin infusion is initiated for the DVT after her bleeding risk is deemed to be low. Unfortunately, she develops ventilator-associated pneumonia, and despite appropriate broad-spectrum antibiotic therapy, ventilator weaning proves to be difficult. The patient has no existing advanced directive, so the APP discusses the case with the patient's primary care provider and leads a multidisciplinary conversation with the patient's family to explore her wishes in the setting of critical illness. They agree on continuing with life-supportive measures, so percutaneous tracheostomy and percutaneous endoscopic gastrostomy (PEG) tubes are placed. Afterwards, sedation and ventilator support are more easily weaned, and she eventually tolerates spontaneous breathing through her tracheostomy with no sedation and minimal supplemental oxygen. Her CRRT is transitioned to intermittent hemodialysis. Physical and occupational therapists evaluate her and find her to be severely deconditioned, unable even to sit on the edge of the bed without assistance; a structured therapy plan is started, and she is recommended for placement in an acute inpatient rehabilitation facility.

She is transferred to a stepdown unit, where she is gradually liberated from more and more of the therapies initially required in the ICU. At one point the critical care team is consulted for a new borderline fever, and she is re-evaluated by the ICU APP and physician; she is again placed on a short course of antibiotics for possible pneumonia, but her respiratory status remains stable, and she does not require ICU readmission. Her renal function slowly improves, and with diuretic support, hemodialysis is successfully discontinued; her catheter is removed with a plan for close monitoring by the nephrology service. She is bridged from her heparin infusion to oral apixaban, and finally transferred to an acute rehab center for continued therapy and medical care.

■ ROLE OF THE ADVANCED PRACTICE PROVIDER IN THE ICU

The modern intensive care unit is a complex environment distinguished by its ability to provide the highest level of care to the most unstable and complicated patients. Although specific equipment and geographic co-location are useful tools to facilitate such care, the primary resource of an ICU is its specialized staff. This is illustrated by the ability of a skilled critical care team to care for patients even in unconventional settings, as seen in mass casualty incidents and the COVID-19 pandemic.

A variety of medical staff play key roles in the care of the critically ill, including critical care nurses (**Chapter 4**) who perform the bulk of bedside care; physical, occupational therapists and speech pathologists (**Chapter 7**) who administer skilled rehabilitation services; respiratory therapists (**Chapter 5**) who manage pulmonary interventions such as ventilators; pharmacists (**Chapter 6**); registered dietitians (**Chapter 11**); and others. The overall direction of care is typically guided by an intensivist, a physician who leads and directs the multidisciplinary team (**Chapter 2**).

Whether in a "closed" model where critically ill patients are admitted directly under the critical care service, an "open" model where other services act as the primary providers while the critical care team serves as consultants, or a hybrid model, the high-level supervision provided by an intensivist is typically supplemented by minute-to-minute care from other providers. These providers may include physician trainees such as residents and fellows, as well as advanced practice providers (APPs) such as physician assistants (PAs, also called *physician associates*) or nurse practitioners (NPs). These APPs direct diagnostic and therapeutic tasks, coordinate the numerous members of the care team, and perform bedside procedures, all in collaboration with the supervising intensivist.

The first physician assistant program was established in 1965 at Duke University, the first nurse practitioner program was created the same year at the University of Colorado, and both professions have grown in scope and numbers over the decades since. Historically, most critical care services were comprised exclusively of physicians and physician trainees. The addition of APPs to a critical care workforce evolved over recent decades in response to practical challenges such as physician shortages and work-hour restrictions for physician trainees. APPs now extend the coverage offered by house staff in many academic and community hospital ICUs and are found in a multitude of other settings. APPs have become a common feature in ICU staffing, and multiple studies have shown outcomes to be equivalent to those generated by resident-staffed teams. Although PA and NP training programs follow distinct educational philosophies, in a working critical care environment they function with similar scopes of practice and bedside roles. APP learning pathways may now also include formal PA and NP postgraduate critical care training programs for committed APPs seeking dedicated critical care specialty training.

APPs have proven to offer valuable benefits for patient care and ICU workflow that extend beyond merely adding staffing, particularly as the healthcare landscape has shifted to emphasize quality of care, cost reduction, and patient experience. The provision of consistently high-quality care in the modern ICU can be limited by the multiple roles and clinical responsibilities of physicians. For example, in many ICUs expert intensivists are unable to be physically present around the clock due to high patient volumes and limited availability. Trainees such as residents have a contrasting problem, often being available at the bedside, yet with limited experience and training in critical care. APPs bridge this gap by offering an extended, often continuous bedside presence by individuals who have focused training in caring for the critically ill.

By leveraging specialty training and a close collaborative relationship with an attending physician, APPs provide direct "eyes on, hands on" assistance for the management of unstable patients. This generally includes performing procedures, such as the insertion of central, peripheral, and arterial catheters, airway management, bronchoscopy, and bedside drainage of fluid for diagnostic or therapeutic purposes (e.g., paracentesis, thoracentesis, and lumbar puncture). APPs often have specialized training in managing mechanical ventilators, interpreting pulmonary artery catheter readings, and performing point-of-care ultrasound to obtain rapid diagnostic information for the care of critically ill patients. APPs may also provide out-of-ICU services such as staffing rapid response or cardiac arrest teams to deliver prompt evaluation, stabilization, and care escalation to acutely decompensating patients throughout the hospital. Finally, they can facilitate nonprocedural but equally complex tasks such as navigating family meetings regarding a patient's end-of-life plan, coordinating care between large inpatient teams, and monitoring the timeliness and adequacy of ongoing interventions.

Consistency of care is another benefit of APP presence. An ICU solely staffed by intensivists who are not continuously present and who are assisted by house staff who rotate on and off the team on a weekly to monthly basis may have difficulty maintaining continuity in ICU-level care practices (e.g., early mobilization for mechanically ventilated patients). Without such continuity, the ICU team may fail to adhere to standardized care plans and procedural guidelines or may encounter more prosaic challenges such as the operation, storage, and even location of specialty bedside equipment. Around-the-clock presence by a full-time critical care provider can mitigate these issues, as well as facilitate unit compliance with quality improvement initiatives and research protocols. As a result, rather than compromising the training environment for house staff in academic settings, APP presence has been shown to improve resident satisfaction and well-being. Bedside nurses also express better job satisfaction working with APPs due to improvements in efficiency and communication. The consistent presence and adherence to practice guidelines associated with APP staffing has been linked with lower rates of skin breakdown and catheter-associated urinary tract infections, shorter ICU and hospital lengths of stay, fewer ICU readmissions, and improved patient experiences.

In addition to PAs and NPs, a third type of APP is generally nonclinical but can serve a valuable adjunctive role in the multidisciplinary team. Clinical nurse specialists (CNS) combine clinical and preclinical training to optimize delivery of high-quality care; they implement quality improvement projects and practice guidelines, analyze and respond to outcome metrics, carry administrative responsibilities, educate nurses and other staff, resolve complex patient issues, and support evidence-based practice.

■ THE ADVANCED PRACTICE PROVIDER PERSPECTIVE ON ICU CARE

The working day of a critical care APP is dependent on their home unit's workflow and patient population. For example, in many surgical ICUs, the patient census is predominantly planned and unplanned postoperative admissions after complex surgeries and traumatic injuries, while medical ICUs are usually dominated by medically ill patients admitted from the emergency department, inpatient wards, or other hospitals.

Though patient populations may differ, many elements are common between institutions. The APP will typically start a shift by taking handoff on the patients for which they are responsible, ranging from one or two to over a dozen. They assess their patients by reviewing the patient medical record for updated signs and symptoms, recent events, diagnostic tests, and notes from other services, as well as physically examining the patient and conferring with the bedside team. They will then "round" on the entire patient panel, a collaborative process involving the intensivist, bedside nurse, and any other physicians or APPs on the service. During rounds, the team will make plans for the day, including medication changes, escalation or de-escalation of invasive interventions, and the possibility of transferring stable patients from the ICU to another ward under the auspices of a noncritical care service. Rounds may also be joined by representatives from the pharmacy, skilled therapy services, ICU management, and sometimes the patient's family, creating a truly multidisciplinary team.

After rounds, the APP's day usually involves implementing the discussed plan, performing necessary procedures, and documenting events in the medical record. New patients will be admitted as they arrive, and new problems involving existing patients will be addressed. Most APPs will generally remain physically present in the unit. At the end of their shift, they will sign out their patient census to staff covering the next shift, generally either another APP or a resident physician.

■ CONSIDERATIONS FOR RECOVERY

Seamless, well-coordinated, and well-communicated care is essential for any critically ill patient. However, this established continuity may be lost when patients leave the ICU and transfer to other services in the hospital and is particularly challenged in the transition to outpatient or other postacute settings. Most critical care departments do not offer direct outpatient services and are unable to follow patients after ICU discharge; this creates a necessary transition of care between provider teams after discharge. Any transition creates a potential for errors or omissions. This can result in a variety of challenges faced by patients during the transition to postacute care and even their needs in the long term. A complex ICU patient may receive treatment for a multitude of individual problems, but if communication and documentation are not excellent, these issues can be unintentionally omitted, and follow-up lost when they are transferred to other settings.

Some unique aspects of critical illness itself tend to manifest as prolonged or delayed problems. These include:

- **Persistent functional deficits:** There is growing awareness of the long-term consequences of critical illness and aggressive ICU care. Significant functional sequelae can persist for months or years after discharge, and in some cases may never resolve. This phenomenon has been dubbed the "post-intensive care syndrome" (PICS), and constitutes deficits in physical function (weakness, coordination), cognitive processing (memory, executive function, concentration), and psychological health (depression, anxiety, and post-traumatic stress disorder [PTSD]), all of which may be severe and life-altering. Without an understanding of PICS, downstream providers may be poorly equipped to manage or even acknowledge such symptoms. Some centers have implemented post-ICU clinics staffed by critical care personnel to help manage PICS and other complications after hospital discharge; however, such a service remains a relative rarity.

- **Delirium:** As many as 80% of ICU patients suffer from delirium of critical illness, an acute state of altered cognition and fluctuating attentiveness related to their underlying disease and/or chosen therapeutics. Patients with delirium may experience vivid visual hallucinations, paranoia, and delusions, often including perceptions of being attacked, persecuted, or placed into bizarre environments. These perceived realities can dominate memories of an ICU stay, often to the exclusion of actual events (of which some patients have little recall), resulting in psychological stress and other sequelae. There are no specific reliable treatments for delirium aside from supportive care and treatment of underlying pathophysiology (e.g., infection) that contributed to the delirium. For some unfortunate patients, delirium may persist even after precipitating causes are treated, and these patients may be discharged from the ICU to their next level of care in a delirious state.

- **Placing critical illness into broader context:** Many ICU admissions are the result of acute exacerbations of chronic diseases. Even a novel presenting complaint unrelated to previous diagnoses, such as a traumatic injury, will often be the starting point in a lengthy process of recovery and perhaps recurrent disease, especially in the patients with comorbid conditions. ICU care usually focuses on acute stabilization of physiological abnormalities with relatively little attention to the larger context in which they occur. The onus for such evaluation falls upon subsequent providers, who need to perform "big picture" tasks such as reconciling newly modified medication regimens, counseling patients on preventative measures to avoid future exacerbations, and discussing goals of care in patients approaching the end of their life.

Tips for Clinicians

A hospitalist service, primary care provider, or outpatient clinician evaluating a patient with a recent ICU stay should consider several points to provide effective care.

1. *Why did the patient become critically ill?* Although not all episodes of critical illness are avoidable, factors that predisposed patients to their acute problem should be evaluated. Any ICU admission, particularly recurrent admissions for related problems, should prompt a thoughtful assessment for factors contributing to disease exacerbations. Medication adjustments and other disease-modifying interventions, provision of skilled therapies, dietary changes, and other optimizations in the outpatient setting may reduce the chance of future ICU admissions, with their associated cost, risk, and morbidity. Advanced care planning for patients with serious, ongoing conditions is also prudent; a decision to decline future ICU admissions in favor of comfort-focused end-of-life care might be a reasonable course for certain patients.

2. *What follow up is needed?* Only in very rare situations will underlying conditions leading to critical illness completely resolve in the ICU. In most circumstances, once improvements are established and patients no longer require critical care services, they are transferred to less-acute settings and eventually discharged from the hospital. Disease states that improve until they no longer require critical care are not necessarily resolved, and effective management for any critical illness will require

additional management beyond the ICU phase. Specific considerations include the need to arrange follow-up with consultants (e.g., neurologists, urologists, rheumatologists), specific diagnostics for inadequately explained in-hospital findings (e.g., hypercoagulability assessment for recurrent thromboses), planning for future procedures (e.g., tracheostomy decannulation), and reassessment of the patient's social needs and resources. Incidental findings discovered on imaging may also need postdischarge evaluation and management. Often, these specific needs are brought to the attention of the APP during the patient's care.

3. *Is the current medication regimen appropriate?* Medication regimens are usually significantly altered during a hospital stay and often incompletely reconciled at discharge; subsequent providers may later encounter drugs that need to be resumed (such as home gout medications), modified (such as replacing inpatient nebulizer treatments with metered-dose inhalers), or discontinued (such as proton pump inhibitors used for stress ulcer prophylaxis, or antipsychotics used for sedation). Many drug therapies initiated in the ICU are not appropriate for long-term use and will require transition to another regimen better suited to patient long-term needs, tolerance, or even insurance coverage.

4. *How can the sequelae of critical illness be managed?* After an ICU stay, many patients will experience new challenges related to complications of their underlying illness, PICS, and iatrogenesis; support of these will fall to outpatient management, particularly primary care providers. The first step in caring for patients experiencing PICS symptoms is to acknowledge and validate them; many patients will not expect to experience weakness, cognitive changes, emotional lability, or other deficits many months after discharge, and should be counseled that this is a common phenomenon.

A multidisciplinary approach to rehabilitation is required, and primary care providers may need to coordinate multiple disciplines including physical therapy, occupational therapy, speech or cognitive therapies, wound care, and nursing support for newly acquired care adjuvants such as tracheostomies and stomas. Psychiatric issues may be addressed by counseling or pharmacologic therapies. Psychosocial problems may arise, such as challenges related to medical costs or loss of work, and solutions may be facilitated by social work consultation.

Finally, after a complex ICU stay, many patients simply need information, and long-term providers may be called upon to answer questions about their initial admission and course of care. Intensive care is confusing to laypeople, and amnesia or perceptual impairments related to illness may further limit accurate recall. Providers with an adequate understanding of the rudiments of critical care will be best equipped to answer questions and explain any aspects of a patient's ICU stay which continue to confuse them.

KEY REFERENCES

Dubaybo BA, Samson MK, Carlson RW. The role of physician-assistants in critical care units. *Chest.* 1991;99(1):89-91.

Gabbard ER, Klein D, Vollman K, Chamblee TB, Soltis LM, Zellinger M. Clinical nurse specialist: a critical member of the ICU team. *Crit Care Med.* 2021;49(6):e634-e641.

Kleinpell R, Grabenkort WR, Boyle WA 3rd, Vines DL, Olsen KM. The society of critical care medicine at 50 years: interprofessional practice in critical care: looking back and forging ahead. *Crit Care Med.* 2021. doi:10.1097/CCM.0000000000005276. Epub ahead of print. PMID: 34387239.

Needham DM, Davidson J, Cohen H, et al. Improving long-term outcomes after discharge from intensive care unit: report from a stakeholders' conference. *Crit Care Med.* 2012;40(2):502-509.

Wilcox ME, Girard TD, Hough CL. Delirium and long term cognition in critically ill patients. *BMJ.* 2021;373:n1007.

The Nurse's Perspective

Christa A. Schorr, Jamie L. Rubino, and Andrew Bergman

Patient Care Vignette

A 62-year-old male presents to the emergency department (ED) with fever, cough, and body aches for the past 3 days. He has three children and two young grandchildren, works full time in construction, enjoys sporting events and spending time with family. His family states that he was in his usual state of health until 3 days ago when he developed a productive cough, shortness of breath, and confusion. His past medical history includes insulin-dependent diabetes, hyperlipidemia, and hypertension. In the ED, he experienced increasing respiratory distress (difficulty breathing), desaturation to 88% on room air (low blood oxygen), and hypotension (low blood pressure, 82/50 mmHg). His chest X-ray showed bilateral lower lung field infiltrates consistent with pneumonia. He was poorly perfused and had signs of sepsis on examination as well as laboratory profiling. He demonstrated septic shock and acute respiratory failure due to pneumonia clearly establishing critical illness. He was intubated and placed on mechanical ventilation. He required fluid resuscitation, empiric antibiotics to treat pneumonia, as well as a vasopressor to support his blood pressure. Invasive monitoring devices were required to guide care.

This patient was admitted to the ICU for critical care. After 24 hours, his lung function worsened, requiring substantial increases in support from the ventilator. Accordingly, he was diagnosed with acute respiratory distress syndrome (ARDS), a condition that may follow many kinds of infections. ARDS is characterized by difficulty clearing carbon dioxide (a waste product) and onloading oxygen across an increasingly stiff lung. In order to help improve gas exchange, he required deep sedation and neuromuscular blockade by continuous infusion, as well as prone position therapy (while on the ventilator he is rolled from his back to his chest, the prone position). This meant that his family could no longer see his face for 16 hours of the day while he was prone, and received no feedback from him indicating that he knew that they had come to visit, hold his hand, and speak to him. The family is distraught having never experienced critical illness with any other family members and is worried that something has gone terribly wrong.

■ THE BEDSIDE CRITICAL CARE NURSE'S ROLE IN THE ICU

The bedside critical care nurse (CCN) is a vital team member to initially explain what is happening, address their questions, and develop a patient- and family-centered bond with this patient's loved ones. This chapter provides insight into the nurse's role in caring for a critically ill patient and their family toward recovery. When one thinks about caring, one may envision the nurse holding a patient's hand, helping during a procedure, engaging in bedside titration of infusing medications, monitoring life-sustaining equipment, or serving as a point of contact for family. Besides all of these functions, the nurse coordinates care, provides support, and maintains a safe environment for healing and recovery.

■ CARE COORDINATION

The critical care nurse's (CCN) role in care coordination relies on understanding the patient's condition, providing ongoing patient assessment, administering therapies, and caring for the patient's overall well-being during critical illness. Each patient encounter—before, during, and after ICU team rounds—allows the nurse to evaluate how the patient is progressing toward healing and recovery, intervene when appropriate, and engage in team-based care when additional expertise is required. In addition to the nurse at the bedside, advanced practice providers (APPs), including nurse practitioners (NP) as well as physician assistants (PA), may help provide care in the ICU contributing to care continuity, improved quality and safety, and patient satisfaction. Moreover, nurses regularly interface with families at the bedside, by phone, or increasingly, digital platforms such as FaceTime, Teams, or ZOOM.

■ FAMILY SUPPORT

After admission, the CCN is often the first member of the ICU team to have contact with family members. Thus, the CCN is in a unique position to help build a supportive relationship. Families can be overwhelmed due to the physical and emotional distress associated with a critically ill loved one.

When family needs are met, family members or significant others are better equipped to handle the stressors of critical illness. CCNs blend the technological components of nursing with advocacy for the needs of patients and families in the ICU. Some of these actions include reassuring, explaining, comforting, holding a patient's hand, sitting with the family, and empathizing with the patient and family over a diagnosis or the progression of care.

■ PATIENT SAFETY

ICU nurses are vital in promoting patient safety. Critically ill patients require nursing care delivered in a timely manner by knowledgeable nurses with essential skills since the ICU is a complex care area with substantial potential for life-threatening events. CCNs administer medications and treatments that may be life sustaining, while continuously assessing and evaluating the patient's response to those therapies. In addition, the CCN ensures patient safety by monitoring for and helping prevent adverse events such as pressure ulcers, falls, and hospital-acquired infections related to care devices.

■ ENACTING AND TRACKING THE PLAN OF CARE

Throughout the 24-hour day the CCN collaborates with other members of the admitting and ICU teams, consultants (when engaged), physical therapy, occupational therapy, pastoral care, social work/transitional care, as well as case management. The CCN work as a core member of the team to help ensure that patient needs are met and that resources are aligned along a path toward recovery for both the patient and the family. Interdisciplinary collaboration among healthcare providers is a core component of a well-functioning patient safety culture with higher-level collaboration being linked to improved quality and better outcomes.

■ AN ICU TIMELINE FROM THE PERSPECTIVE OF THE CRITICAL CARE NURSE

The start of every ICU shift for the CCN is preplanned and commences with nurse-to-nurse shift report (aka: nurse-to-nurse handoff; Fig. 4-1). Shift report is an exchange of patient information, which includes technical information regarding every aspect of care from ventilator settings to medications to consultants to family contact. Essential elements are shared between the off-going CCN and the incoming CCN so that a consistent plan is supported by regular information sharing. Often, shift report occurs at the bedside, but other models exist. The typical ICU nursing assignment is two patients to one nurse, but can convert to one-to-one depending on increases in illness or care needs.

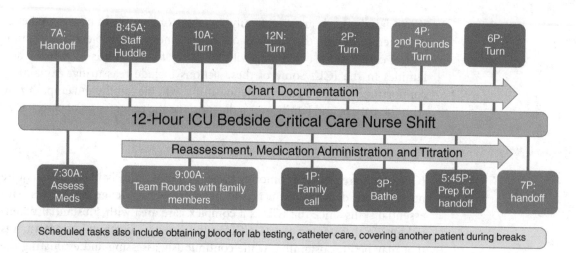

FIGURE 4-1. A 12-Hour Daytime Shift. This graphic depicts key events in a typical 12-hour ICU nursing shift. Assess = patient assessment; Meds = medications to be delivered or titrated; Turn = patient repositioning to relived pressure and prevent pressure ulceration.

Following report, the CCN completes a head-to-toe physical assessment of this patient and the CCN's second patient. The dynamics of this assessment and associated documentation can vary greatly from patient to patient depending on the patient's condition and needs. In this patient's case, he is sedated, receiving a vasopressor and is invasively mechanically ventilated (tube across his vocal cords as opposed to noninvasive ventilation using a face mask). Following the assessment, the oncoming nurse initiates a complex and comprehensive document that details the specifics of that assessment for each patient in the electronic health record (EHR). Documentation continues throughout the shift and records care that is provided, the patient's response, as well as new information relevant to care. For example, every 2 hours a pain assessment is performed. If the patient is experiencing pain, analgesic medication is administered and the response to treatment is documented at that time in the EHR. Similarly, scheduled evaluations occur for other organ systems from the brain to the kidneys.

The documentation process can be time consuming due to illness complexity; other patients may require much more straightforward documentation if they are less ill. Nonetheless, documentation is important and occurs throughout the 12-hour shift regardless of transportation to radiology, procedures performed at the bedside, consultant evaluations, or calls from the laboratory with a critical value. All the while, the CCN also fields phone calls from family members, speaks with patient visitors, and when awake and engaged in their own care, the patient. As the CCN has planned breaktime to attend to personal needs including nutrition, the immediate aspects of care are also shared with a "covering" nurse during breaks. In order to make this process more seamless, some ICUs use a shift change "huddle" where patients with escalating or unique needs are discussed as a group. This way, the entire ICU CCN team helps ensure safety.

Medication administration and evaluation of continuous infusions occur throughout the 12-hour shift. Safe-and-effective medication administration is aided by the CCNs knowledge of medication side effects, as well as how they interface with the patient's organ such as the heart or the kidney. While some ICUs are supported by a pharmacist specifically trained for ICU care, many are not, and instead substantially rely on the bedside CCN. Titration (regular adjustment to achieve the desired effect) of medications that affect blood pressure, awareness, and pain control consumes a lot of bedside time and require specific expertise to be done safely—all of which must also be documented.

In many ICUs a bar code scanning safety system is in place that allows the patient bracelet bar code to interface with the EHR to ensure the right patient receives the right medication at the right time. This is an added step that supports safety in a complex care environment and benefits the patient. Given the multiple interwoven tasks that care for both the patient and the family, CCNs often work in a high-stress environment. Indeed, caring for critically ill patients is associated with an increase in CCN physical, emotional, and intellectual workload. The common sequence of events over the course of a 12-hour shift presented in Fig. 4-1 illustrates how the CCN interfaces with the rest of the team caring for the patient as well as the family. Different ICUs have different typical times for the events detailed in Fig. 4-1, but they all have the following commonalities: nursing handoff, direct patient care, team-based rounds, reassessment, titration of care, coverage of other patients while another nurse goes on break, responding to admissions and emergencies within the ICU, and patient and family communication. Some ICUs designate a nurse to respond outside of the ICU for cardiac arrest care or as part of a Rapid Response Team. Therefore, depending on when families visit, the "usual" nurse may not be at the bedside, but another CCN is immediately available for care.

■ CONSIDERATIONS FOR RECOVERY

Family Members on Rounds

Patient and family engagement is a high priority in optimizing critical illness outcomes. The patient's family is welcome to attend and participate in daily rounds. This key event helps families to understand the complexity of care, as well as the daily goals. Often, family members have additional information to contribute to rounds, and can readily participate in shared decision-making. Most studies of families on rounds demonstrate benefit for the patient, the family, and the bedside nurse. Moreover, the common practice of a "family meeting" for information sharing and decision-making may become infrequent as the desired information has already been shared during rounds. Rounding Intensivists must be cognizant of the need to translate technical medical language into easily understood terms. Especially with life-threatening critical illness, family members who participate in rounds may experience anxiety or anger. Conversations with family require sensitivity and compassion due to a need to communicate difficult and complex information. Often family members need time to process the reality of their loved one's condition and the new information provided. Since the time available to round on each patient is finite, the CCN often addresses family emotional needs as well as informational needs after the team move on to the next patient. More information about families on rounds is available in **Chapter 16**.

Prevention Activities

During routine ICU care, the CCN engages in several prevention activities designed to reduce harm. These include routine turning and repositioning of patients to avoid pressure ulcers, regular assessment/cleaning/redressing of catheters that cross the skin, and assessing for conditions that increase the risk of falling when being moved out of bed, during toileting, or during ambulation. Catheters come in a variety of types and have unique needs, all of which require care from the CCN. Some enter veins to enable medication administration, others enter the GI track to support nutrition, and other enter spaces where there is infection so that it can be drained. These are but a few of the types of catheters the CCN must address. In particular, those that enter veins are prone to infection—an event that is substantially reduced by excellent CCN care. Moving patients out of bed to the chair when they cannot move themselves helps patients in a host of ways including reducing the likelihood of pneumonia, improving their alertness, and encouraging them to participate in their own care. When patients are strong enough to walk around, they routinely do so with the aid of a physical therapist as well as the CCN. Therefore, the CCN is at the heart of preventing harmful events from occurring, and in this way, the CCN fully supports progress toward recovery. Every action that reduces the amount of time a patient needs to spend in the ICU improves their overall outcome. Many ICUs use a structured approach to moving patients toward liberation from their ICU stay called the ICU Liberation Bundle.

ICU Liberation Bundle

To improve patient safety and quality of care, the Society of Critical Care Medicine (SCCM) published the Clinical Practice Guideline for the Management of Pain, Agitation, Delirium, Immobility and Sleep Disruption in Adult patients in the Intensive Care Unit—the PADIS Guideline—in 2018. To help implement the PADIS Guideline, a linked set of practices was developed that is termed "a bundle." Guidelines discover the evidence that supports particular practices, and bundles help clinicians implement beneficial interventions. Bundles are ideally designed so that the more elements are applied, the greater the benefit to the patient. One such bundle, previously termed the A-2-F, or ABCDEF, bundle is now known as the ICU Liberation Bundle. This bundle is designed to help clinical teams to do six things that help reduce the amount of time a patient spends on the ventilator or in the ICU.

The bundle consists of six alphabet-letter-based elements (Fig. 4-2): **A**ssess, prevent, and manage pain; **B**oth spontaneous awakening trial (SAT) and spontaneous breathing trial (SBT); **C**hoice of sedation and analgesia; **D**elirium monitoring and management; **E**arly mobility and exercise; **F**amily engagement and empowerment. The ICU Liberation Bundle can be delivered in totality or partially throughout a patient's ICU course by an interprofessional team daily and can be utilized on every patient (who passes a safety screen). Application of the ICU Liberation Bundle promotes keeping patients awake, engaged, and active in their recovery, which results in the patient's independence and the capacity to share any unmet needs. It also reduces the amount of time spent on the ventilator, the incidence of delirium, and is associated with improved survival as well. As a result of decreasing medication that are sedating when using the ICU Liberation Bundle, patients are more awake and engaged but will also report more pain. Therefore, the CCN has a vital role in ensuring that pain is addressed so that it is tolerable by the patient and does not impede their road to recovery; a goal of zero pain is often not achievable especially after surgery, rendering a tolerable level of pain a more appropriate goal. Both pharmacologic (i.e., multiple modality medications) and nonpharmacologic approaches (i.e., repositioning, music, relaxation therapy, hot or cold packs) to pain should be used in tandem.

The specifics of each element of the bundle work together to benefit patients. Some of them are quite technical and are beyond the scope of this work. However, it is important to note that the bundle also provides a daily checklist of activities for the team that shapes how care is delivered, and asks whether certain aspects of care need to be continued (mechanical ventilation), or if others need to be started (getting out of bed). Nonetheless, a vital element of the bundle is the family. Including families on rounds is an excellent way to engage and empower families. To that end some ICUs have family members help with certain activities such as stretches, passive range of motion to prevent stiffness, bathing, and more. Perhaps most importantly, having family members understand what care is being delivered—and why—helps them prepare for how to best support their loved one during recovery. Often a journal

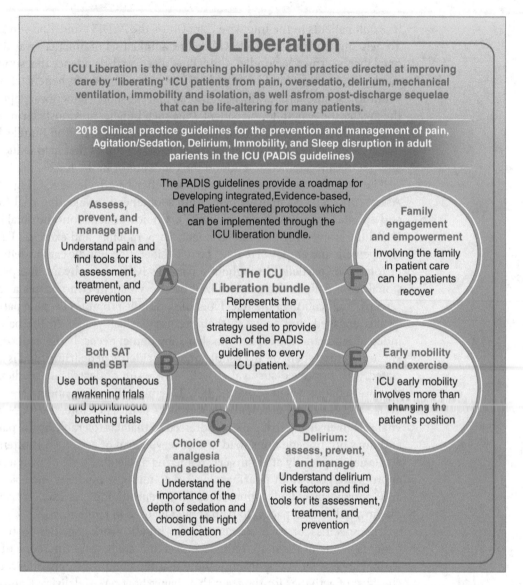

FIGURE 4-2. ICU Liberation Bundle. Reproduced with permission from the Society of Critical Care Medicine.

helps them to monitor who visited, what happened, and also enables them to fill in gaps in the patient's memory about what happened. It is common for patients not to recall large portions of their ICU stay if they are profoundly ill. The CCN and the family often work together to have a robust set of journal entries to support patient recovery after ICU discharge and return home. Some patients do not go directly home from the hospital, but instead pursue one of the following three routes: (1) ICU to floor to rehabilitation facility, (2) ICU to Long Term Acute Care Hospital to rehabilitation facility to home, or (3) ICU to floor to skilled nursing facility to rehabilitation facility to home. Other variations exist, and journals, just like CCNs, help make transitions of care easier for patients and families. ICU survivorship is a celebrated event but may come with recovery challenges for patients and families alike.

PICS and PICS-F

Life-threatening critical illness takes a profound toll on patients and families alike. From the patient perspective, cognitive difficulties, weakness, and disordered psychosocial dynamics characterize the post-intensive care syndrome (PICS). Patients may not think clearly or rapidly or may seem to have difficulty reaching a sound decision. Accordingly, regulating their own medication may be challenging and unsafe. They may be globally weak and tire rapidly even during activities of daily living, let alone physical therapy designed to help restore strength or endurance. Previously independent people may be quite dependent on family members when they initially return home. Driving may be quite unsafe for a period of time. How they interact with family, friends, and even pets may be different from how they behaved before becoming ill. They may be withdrawn, easy to anger, or seem to have little joy when engaging in previously pleasurable activities. These are typical signs of PICS, but not the only ones. Therefore, when returning for an outpatient office visit, you may be asked questions about the patient, even though they can speak for themself. This is so that during the evaluation, a perspective other than the patient's can be obtained, as they may not realize any of the difficulties detected by other caregivers such as family.

Family members appear to serve as uncompensated caregivers when their loved one demonstrates PICS. The impact on the family has also been well-characterized and may include anxiety, depression, the need to leave gainful employment, decreased joy, and anger. This is termed PICS-F and represents an opportunity for rescue. Both PICS patients and PICS-F family members may find help within post-ICU clinics and post-ICU support groups. Initially uncommon, post-ICU clinics are now more commonly available and bring a multiprofessional team to the clinic to care for patients—and often family members—during the aftermath of surviving life-threatening critical illness. Many of those clinics also offer support groups akin to those for cancer survivors, heart surgery patients, and those on a weight-loss journey including bariatric surgery. The post-ICU clinic and the post-ICU support group also have roles for the CCN to help during recovery outside of the ICU. Therefore, the CCN may be integrally involved from acute care through the recovery process.

■ **TABLE 4-1.   Critical Care Nurse Contributions Toward Patient Recovery**

Patient Aim	Nurse Contribution Toward Patient Recovery
Return to previous functional capacity:	
Resolve current critical illness diagnosis	Collaborate with the multiprofessional team; provide ordered therapy, enact plan of care, and evaluate patient's response to management
Prevent adverse events:	
• Prevent pressure ulcers	Turn patient every 2 hours, place safety materials in high-pressure areas (i.e., assessment during prone positioning)
• Prevent falls	Complete a falls risk assessment; utilize equipment to facilitate mobility; seek support from other ICU staff when necessary
• Prevent hospital-acquired infections	Assess wounds, invasive devices; remove devices when feasible; turn patient frequently; keep the head of the bed elevated when possible; increase patient mobility
Implement the ICU Liberation Bundle:	
• Prevent and relieve pain	Assess pain, provide pharmacologic and nonpharmacologic methods of pain relief (if pain is present) and prior to procedures
• Liberate from mechanical ventilation	Assess readiness for being liberated from the ventilator
• Avoid oversedation	Complete frequent assessments; titrate sedatives and analgesics to a manageable pain level and anxiety relief
• Prevent/reduce delirium	Complete frequent assessments for delirium, promote sleep, and avoid medications that trigger delirium
• Increase mobility and exercise	Collaborate with physical therapy to increase mobility
Moving toward recovery:	
• Regain previous cognitive function	Support patient in exercise; engage patient in conversation; reorient as needed; create a board with pictures of patient and family; help families complete a journal
• Reduce stress, anxiety, depression	Provide emotional support and encouragement; suggest consulting a behavioral health clinician as needed; administer medications for anxiety, depression as necessary
• Limit effects of PICS and PICS-F	Perform functional assessment on ICU admission and at each transition of care; communicate often with family
• Post-ICU recovery in a safe environment with resources for medication, food, and housing (when going directly to home)	Evaluate socioeconomic needs and required resources with the ICU team; engage social work or similar team as needed
• Discharge from the ICU	Evaluate support system with patient and family prior to ICU discharge
• Understand recovery from critical illness and risk factors for clinical decompensation	Provide education regarding the patients care plan; encourage follow-up with a clinician after discharge, especially for those who survive life-threatening critical illness

Weinhouse GL. Reproduced with permission from Weinhouse GL. Delirium and sleep disturbances in the intensive care unit: can we do better? Curr Opin Anaesthesiol. 2014;27(4):403-408.

Tips for Clinicians

1. **Consider that family members may have had variable experiences** with ICU staff during the critical care admission. They may have unmet informational or emotional needs that can be elicited during post-ICU visits.
2. **Remember that ICU patients are cared for by multidisciplinary teams.** Seek out care and recovery insights from all the members of the ICU and inpatient teams if possible.
3. **Assess and record the patient's functional status after hospital discharge,** considering that this may have changed significantly as compared to their functional status at the time of admission.
4. **Monitor for PICS and PICS-F** and provide education and resources to patients and families.

KEY REFERENCES

Al Ma'mari Q, Sharour LA, Al Omari O. Fatigue, burnout, work environment, workload and perceived patient safety culture among critical care nurses. *Br J Nurs*. 2020;29(1):28-34.

Allen SR, Pascual J, Martin N, et al. A novel method of optimizing patient-and family-centered care in the ICU. *J Trauma Acute Care Surg*. 2017;82(3):582-586.

Barnes-Daly MA, Phillips G, Ely EW. Improving hospital survival and reducing brain dysfunction at seven California community hospitals: implementing PAD guidelines via the ABCDEF bundle in 6,064 patients. *Crit Care Med*. 2017;45(2):171-178.

Barr J, Fraser GL, Puntillo K, et al. Clinical practice guidelines for the management of pain, agitation, and delirium in adult patients in the intensive care unit. *Crit Care Med*. 2013;41(1):263-306.

Cao V, Tan LD, Horn F, et al. Patient-centered structured interdisciplinary bedside rounds in the medical ICU. *Crit Care Med*. 2018;46(1):85-92.

Davidson JE, Aslakson RA, Long AC, et al. Guidelines for family-centered care in the neonatal, pediatric, and adult ICU. *Critical Care Med*. 2017;45(1):103-128.

Davidson JE, Jones C, Bienvenu OJ. Family response to critical illness: postintensive care syndrome-family. *Crit Care Med*. 2012;40(2):618-624.

Devlin JW, Skrobik Y, Gélinas C, et al. Clinical practice guidelines for the prevention and management of pain, agitation/sedation, delirium, immobility, and sleep disruption in adult patients in the ICU. *Crit Care Med*. 2018;46(9):e825-e873.

Elliott D, Davidson JE, Harvey MA, et al. Exploring the scope of post-intensive care syndrome therapy and care: engagement of non-critical care providers and survivors in a second stakeholders meeting. *Crit Care Med*. 2014;42(12):2518-2526.

Harvey MA, Davidson JE. Postintensive care syndrome: right care, right now ... and later. *Crit Care Med*. 2016;44(2):381-385.

Herridge MS, Tansey CM, Matté A, et al. Functional disability 5 years after acute respiratory distress syndrome. *N Engl J Med*. 2011;364(14):1293-1304.

Inoue S, Hatakeyama J, Kondo Y, et al. Post-intensive care syndrome: its pathophysiology, prevention, and future directions. *Acute Med Surg*. 2019;6(3):233-246.

Kleinpell RM, Grabenkort WR, Kapu AN, et al. Nurse practitioners and physician assistants in acute and critical care: a concise review of the literature and data 2008-2018. *Crit Care Med*. 2019;47(10):1442-1449.

Kress JP, Hall JB. ICU-acquired weakness and recovery from critical illness. *N Engl J Med*. 2014;370(17):1626-1635.

Lane D, Ferri M, Lemaire J, et al. A systematic review of evidence-informed practices for patient care rounds in the ICU. *Crit Care Med*. 2013;41(8):2015-2029.

Lautrette A, Darmon M, Megarbane B, et al. A communication strategy and brochure for relatives of patients dying in the ICU. *N Engl J Med*. 2007;356(5):469-478.

Ludmir J, Netzer G. Family-centered care in the intensive care unit—what does best practice tell us? *Semin Respir Crit Care Med*. 2019;40(5):648-654.

Mikkelsen ME, Still M, Anderson BJ, et al. Society of Critical Care Medicine's international consensus conference on prediction and identification of long-term impairments after critical illness. *Crit Care Med*. 2020;48(11):1670-1679.

Oliver D, Healey F, Haines TP. Preventing falls and fall-related injuries in hospitals. *Clin Geriatr Med*. 2010;26(4):645-692.

Poon EG, Keohane CA, Yoon CS, et al. Effect of bar-code technology on the safety of medication administration. *N Engl J Med*. 2010;362(18):1698-1707.

Pun BT, Balas MC, Barnes-Daly MA, et al. Caring for critically ill patients with the ABCDEF bundle: results of the ICU liberation collaborative in over 15,000 adults. *Crit Care Med*. 2019;47(1):3-14.

Schweickert WD, Pohlman MC, Pohlman AS, et al. Early physical and occupational therapy in mechanically ventilated, critically ill patients: a randomised controlled trial. *Lancet*. 2009;373(9678):1874-1882.

Selph RB, Shiang J, Engelberg R, et al. Empathy and life support decisions in intensive care units. *J Gen Intern Med*. 2008;23(9):1311-1317.

Stollings JL, Devlin JW, Lin JC, Pun BT, Byrum D, Barr J. Best practices for conducting interprofessional team rounds to facilitate performance of the ICU liberation (ABCDEF) bundle. *Crit Care Med*. 2020;48(4):562-570.

The Respiratory Therapist's Perspective

J. Christian Brown, Ashley M. Thompson, Jason Hansen, Philip Efron, and Jessica E. Taylor

Patient Care Vignette

A 68-year-old obese male, 40-pack-year smoker, with a history of hypertension, chronic obstructive pulmonary disease (COPD), and coronary artery disease presents to the emergency department with 3 days of progressively worsening abdominal pain, nausea, and vomiting. On arrival he has low blood pressure, a high heart rate, low oxygen saturation, and he is breathing quite quickly. He has a distended abdomen that was diffusely tender suggesting infection and inflammation. He has an IV placed and receives intravenous fluids and supplemental oxygen by face mask. Laboratory testing reveals evidence of infection as well as impaired kidney function that is new. A CT scan demonstrates much more than normal fluid in his pelvis as well as gas outside of the bowel indicating intestinal perforation and the need for an urgent operation to which he agrees.

He is started on broad-spectrum antibiotics and undergoes an urgent exploratory laparotomy to remove the perforated section of colon and create a colostomy, as the highly contaminated abdomen made a single stage operating unsafe. He did well in the OR and had the breathing tube removed at the end of the operation. He is transferred directly to the ICU where he develops difficulty breathing and recurrent low oxygen saturation that does not improve despite the ICU team's best efforts. Therefore, he has the breathing tube replaced to support oxygenation and removal of carbon dioxide. His chest X-rays and arterial blood gasses indicate that he has developed acute respiratory distress syndrome (ARDS)—a serious and life-threatening condition that may occur after severe infection or injury—and requires intensive care and frequent ventilator adjustments as well as secretion clearance from the breathing tube by a registered respiratory therapist (RRT).

■ INTRODUCTION

Breathing is fundamental to life, and many acute illnesses threaten life by compromising respiratory function. Respiratory failure requiring support beyond supplemental oxygen via conventional nasal cannula is sufficient to justify ICU admission in many hospitals. In this chapter, we discuss critical illness and recovery from the perspective of a registered respiratory therapist (RRT) and other ICU clinicians who support the respiratory system.

■ RESPIRATORY SUPPORT APPROACHES

Critical illness may compromise respiratory function directly, as with pneumonia or respiratory muscle failure, or indirectly, as when sepsis and metabolic acidosis dramatically increase the body's drive to breathe. When a patient cannot continue to support the work required to maintain normal oxygen levels or to eliminate carbon dioxide, respiratory support is required.

Most patients with respiratory insufficiency or respiratory failure will first be supported with supplemental oxygen provided using nasal prongs or a face mask. When additional support is needed, noninvasive ventilation (NIV; ventilation support without a breathing tube) is often pursued. NIV approaches have been more widely known in the wake of the SARS-CoV-2 pandemic. These approaches include continuous positive airway pressure (CPAP), bilevel positive airway pressure (BiPAP), and high-flow nasal cannula oxygen ($HFNCO_2$). Unlike supplemental oxygen through nasal prongs, NIV requires a specialized provider—usually an RRT—to deploy and adjust. In conjunction with other supportive therapies—such as controlling the source of infection as in the patient care vignette above—NIV may meet the patient's respiratory needs and can help avoid invasive mechanical ventilation with a breathing tube.

When NIV is insufficient or when NIV is contraindicated (as with active vomiting, unconsciousness, or recent esophageal surgery), invasive mechanical ventilation requiring a breathing tube and a ventilator can support respiratory function. As with NIV, a specialized clinician (again, usually an RRT) is required in most facilities to start ventilation, to adjust settings and alarms, to perform pulmonary toileting procedures (e.g., clearing secretions, performing chest physiotherapy), and to administer inhaled medications.

The most severe form of acute respiratory failure, acute respiratory distress syndrome (ARDS), affects about 1 in 10 critically ill or injured patients.

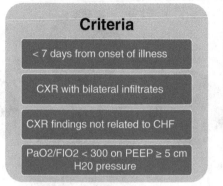
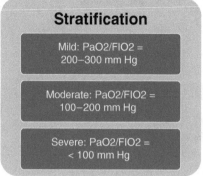

FIGURE 5-1. **Berlin Criteria for Acute Respiratory Distress Syndrome (ARDS) Diagnosis and illness severity.**

Standardized criteria help healthcare professionals diagnose ARDS (Fig. 5-1). Prolonged ICU length of stay, increased death rate, and decreased quality of life in survivors are common in patients with ARDS. Importantly, a standardized approach to ARDS management is key in helping patients to survive their ARDS and ICU stay. Such protocols leverage the RRT as an essential member of the ICU team and include using small-sized breaths (i.e., low tidal volume ventilation) and prone positioning (positioning the patient on their stomach to improve oxygenation).

ROLE OF THE RESPIRATORY THERAPIST IN THE ICU

The role of an RRT can vary greatly from setting to setting, including work performed in hospitals or even on aeromedical flight teams. The scope of respiratory care is broad (Fig. 5-2) and includes both supportive and therapeutic measures. In the rural setting, the RRT may be the only person with the skill set to place a breathing tube (i.e., intubate) or place a blood pressure monitoring catheter in a patient's artery if the physician is not in the hospital, especially at night. In a large teaching facility, the RRT may not be credentialed to independently perform procedures outside of managing respiratory therapy devices. Even in these situations, RRTs also have an active role in educating health professions trainees (e.g., residents, fellows) on respiratory device management, lung function assessment, and lung hygiene.

A typical day for an RRT in the ICU can bring many challenges. The RRT may have multiple ICU patients for whom they help provide care; 9-12 critically ill patients is a common RRT assignment. In some facilities, the RRT may also be expected to cover and manage patients on non-ICU acute care units.

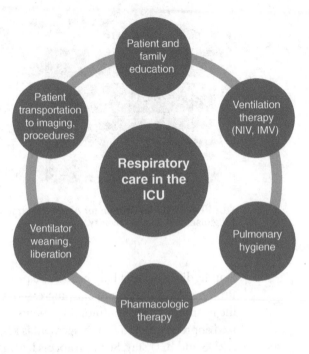

FIGURE 5-2. Key Registered Respiratory Therapist (RRT) Roles in the ICU. ICU: intensive care unit; IMV: invasive mechanical ventilation; NIV: noninvasive ventilation.

This approach is more common in community facilities that may care for less complex patients than those cared for at quaternary referral centers. Critical care RRT care typically involves repeated rounds of patients and their respiratory system needs throughout an 8- or 12-hour shift. Such needs span from supplemental O_2 to inhalers to pulmonary toilet to ventilator adjustments. The RRT is responsible for ensuring that ordered settings for NIV and invasive mechanical ventilation match what is on the device. More importantly, they are frontline clinicians who assess whether those settings are working well for a specific patient. Many facilities have protocols that empower the RRT to reduce the amount of ventilator support while patients are doing well to help move them toward no longer needing the breathing tube. This process is called ventilator liberation. If patients are not doing well, then the RRT is often critical in suggesting how to better match what the patient's lung needs by altering the ventilator settings (also called the ventilator prescription).

Respiratory therapy also involves assisting in procedures such as bronchoscopy—a procedure akin to endoscopy of the GI track, but instead uses a much smaller scope to pass through the breathing tube to assess the airways from the inside. Bronchoscopy is used for both diagnostic (e.g., obtaining specimens for microbiologic testing) and therapeutic (e.g., clearing thick secretions) purposes. In addition, patients in the ICU often need to travel outside of the ICU. The RRT is involved in the transport of patients who require NIV or invasive mechanical ventilation during those trips. Patients travel to and from the operating room and imaging suites with great frequency, especially from surgical ICUs.

During physical therapy, the RRT plays an important role in ensuring that the patient's respiratory system demands during therapy are met. Patients awake and alert enough to participate in physical therapy, especially mobilization and walking in the ICU, also benefit from RRT aid. Even patients who require invasive mechanical ventilation can be ambulated within the ICU but may require temporary increase in mechanical ventilatory support. Since respiratory gasses may provide insight into metabolism, in some centers, RRTs may perform those assessments using a metabolic cart. The data that the RRT acquires helps inform the nutritional prescription so that it can be ideally adjusted to support normal metabolism. In addition, RRTs respond to medical emergencies such as "codes" and rapid response team activations to help provide respiratory support. Therefore, a typical day in the ICU for an RRT may be quite varied, requiring a broad range of knowledge and unique skills that reflect the specific environment and patients within which the RRT works.

■ UNIQUE THERAPIES AND THE RRT

Many therapies in which the RRT engages can be delivered throughout the acute care facility as well as in other locations such as rehab hospitals, skilled nursing facilities, and long-term acute care hospitals. These therapies include inhalers, supplemental O_2, and CPAP for conditions such as obstructive sleep apnea. In fact, many of these therapies are used by lay people at home! However, other therapies are much more specialized and are restricted (in general) to acute care facilities, and principally to the ICU or specialized monitored care units. These include NIV (mentioned earlier), invasive mechanical ventilation adjusted to provide lung protection (an essential part of ARDS management), recruitment maneuvers (sometimes needed to reverse collapse of parts of the lung), and prone position therapy (also helpful in lung recruitment and managing oxygenation). Prone position therapy became familiar to many during the SARS-CoV-2 pandemic. Turning an intubated patient from the supine to the prone position requires coordination to ensure safety. Commonly, the RRT is responsible for ensuring that the breathing tube does not become dislodged during the turn and that there is appropriate padding to avoid undue pressure on the patient's face. It is clear that the RRT serves in many capacities, with some being more complex than others. Relatedly, lung protective ventilation is complex and involves the ventilator prescription and its evaluation using pressures, gas flow waveforms, and derived indices that describe many aspects of lung inflation and deflation during the respiratory cycle. The prime monitor of all of these parameters is the RRT, who then interfaces with the ICU team (physician, nurse practitioner, physician assistant, bedside critical care nurse) to facilitate team-based evaluation and ventilator adjustment to meet the patient's needs. This kind of therapy is not limited to a specific shift or time of day, but instead occurs in a continuous fashion.

Some of the adjustments to the ventilator prescription are accompanied by very specific kinds of inhalation therapy that is quite different from the inhalers patients use at home for chronic obstructive pulmonary disease (COPD) or asthma, for example. Two inhalation therapies are inhaled nitric oxide and inhaled epoprostenol. These two agents, adjusted by the RRT, help with both oxygenation, especially for those with ARDS, and other more chronic conditions that may impair lung blood flow. These therapies underscore that the RRT must also be well versed in the pharmacology that impacts lung function and how a variety of therapeutic agents interface with support devices such as the mechanical ventilator.

As patients improve, the support provided by the ventilator is gradually decreased. This process is termed "weaning." When the amount of support is quite minimal—and overcomes only the work imposed by the breathing tube and the ventilator tubing—the patient is ready to be evaluated for tube removal (i.e. liberation). This entire process is overseen by the RRT, often along an institutional protocol; more difficult patients benefit from an individualized approach that is set by the ICU team. If after evaluation, the patient is determined to be ready to breathe without the ventilator or the breathing tube, it is the RRT most commonly who suctions away secretions within the tube and then removes it. Liberation is followed by an assessment of the ability to breathe independently as well as speak clearly and fluently while being able to clear oral secretions. These assessments are also done by the RRT in conjunction with the bedside critical care nurse in many institutions. Teaching institutions may involve trainees or fellows who have completed their training in a parent discipline and are then undergoing specialized education in critical care medicine in this process as well. Therefore, the RRT is integral to the spectrum of respiratory care throughout a patient's acute care hospitalization, and especially during their ICU care.

■ CONSIDERATIONS FOR PATIENT RECOVERY

While the influence of RRTs is most acutely identified during a patient's ICU stay, their influence commonly permeates ongoing care on the acute care unit.

Perhaps most importantly, and quite relevant for those with ARDS, lung recovery takes much longer than the inpatient total hospital length of stay. Specific patient as well as family education and training that helps support recovery through the convalescent period contributes in a meaningful way to excellent outcomes. New inhaler use, methods of pulmonary toilet, incentive spirometer use, and, for some, tracheostomy care extend for weeks to months after hospital discharge. Family members who become uncompensated care-givers specifically benefit from bedside instruction given by the RRT. That training complements what is also taught by the bedside critical care nurse. However, patients who are transferred from outlying facilities into tertiary or quaternary care facilities may find themselves quite remote from readily accessible support agencies and individuals. Therefore, RRT and critical care nurse education and training become essential elements of recovery. As facilities continue to incorporate telehealth into their armamentarium, patients with new or complex pulmonary care regimens may be ideal candidates for postdischarge outreach using a digital platform to link patients, family members, and RRTs or critical care nurses with them on a scheduled or impromptu basis during recovery at home. Equally important is the appropriate cessation of prescribed therapies that are no longer needed. Complex care patients may benefit from participation in a post-ICU clinic that attends to patients using a multiprofessional approach that includes an RRT and a pharmacist alike.

Tips for Clinicians

1. RRTs are integral to the care of the critically ill or injured patients in the ICU and after ICU discharge. **Maintain a low threshold for referring patients** who continue to demonstrate respiratory system compromise to pulmonary clinics or outpatient RRTs.
2. Patient and family education and training provided by RRTs as well as bedside critical care nurses often facilitate recovery during convalescence. **Ask patients and families about their experiences with respiratory care** during their ICU admission and elicit questions about ongoing respiratory support.
3. **Consider referring complex pulmonary care patients to a post-ICU clinic** that cares for patients in a multiprofessional fashion to evaluate progress, guide rehabilitation, adjust current therapy, and discontinue unnecessary medications.
4. For patients who were receiving NIV prior to admission (e.g., continuous positive airway pressure [CPAP] or bilevel positive airway pressure [BiPAP]), their **therapy may need to be reassessed after ICU admission**.

For example, body weight changes can affect NIV mask fit, emotional disturbances like posttraumatic stress disorder may affect mask tolerance, and new medications such as sedating antipsychotic medications (e.g., quetiapine, risperidone) may change the quality of the patient's sleep.

5. In training facilities (e.g., academic hospitals), **incorporate RRTs into the educational curriculum** for trainees, including fellows.

KEY REFERENCES

Becker EA, Hoerr CA, Wiles KS, et al. Utilizing respiratory therapists to reduce costs of care. *Respir Care*. 2018;63(1):102-117.

Bellani G, Laffey JG, Pham T, Fan E. The LUNG SAFE study: a presentation of the prevalence of ARDS according to the Berlin Definition!. *Crit Care*. 2016;20(1):1-2.

Ervin JN, Kahn JM, Cohen TR, Weingart LR. Teamwork in the intensive care unit. *Am Psychol*. 2018;73(4):468.

Goligher EC, Hodgson CL, Adhikari NK, et al. Lung recruitment maneuvers for adult patients with acute respiratory distress syndrome. A systematic review and meta-analysis. *Ann Am Thorac Soc*. 2017;14(Suppl 4):S304-S311.

Grieco DL, Menga LS, Raggi V, et al. Physiological comparison of high-flow nasal cannula and helmet noninvasive ventilation in acute hypoxemic respiratory failure. *Am J Respir Crit Care Med*. 2020;201(3):303-312.

Guérin C, Albert RK, Beitler J, et al. Prone position in ARDS patients: why, when, how and for whom. *Intensive Care Med*. 2020;40(12).2385-2396.

Karthika M, Wong D, Nair SG, et al. Lung ultrasound: the emerging role of respiratory therapists. *Respir Care*. 2019;64(2):217-229.

Levy SD, Alladina JW, Hibbert KA, et al. High-flow oxygen therapy and other inhaled therapies in intensive care units. *Lancet*. 2016;387(10030):1867-1878.

Modrykamien AM, Stoller JK. The scientific basis for protocol-directed respiratory care. *Respir Care*. 2013;58(10):1662-1668.

Ng JA, Miccile LA, Iracheta C, et al. Prone positioning of patients with acute respiratory distress syndrome related to COVID-19: a rehabilitation-based prone team. *Phys Ther*. 2020;100(10):1737-1745.

Pack S, Hahn PY, Stoller JK, Mummadi SR. Respiratory therapist-managed arterial catheter insertion and maintenance program: experience in a non-teaching community hospital. *Respir Care*. 2017;62(12):1520-1524.

Srinivasan SR. Tele-ICU in the age of COVID-19: built for this challenge. *J Nutr Health Aging*. 2020;24(5):536-537.

Villar J, Blanco J, Kacmarek RM. Current incidence and outcome of the acute respiratory distress syndrome. *Curr Opin Crit Care*. 2016;22(1):1-6.

Weiss TT, Cerda F, Scott JB, et al. Prone positioning for patients intubated for severe acute respiratory distress syndrome (ARDS) secondary to COVID-19: a retrospective observational cohort study. *Br J Anaesth*. 2021;126(1):48-55.

The Pharmacist's Perspective

Amy L. Dzierba and Jeffrey F. Barletta

Patient Care Vignette

A 76-year-old woman presents to the emergency department (ED) with confusion, lethargy, fever, cough, and shortness of breath. Her symptoms have progressively worsened over the past 3 days, during which time she has been using acetaminophen (Tylenol) and over-the-counter antihistamines. Her medical history is significant for epilepsy (though she has been seizure-free for 20 years), hypertension, coronary artery disease, diabetes mellitus, hypothyroidism, and end-stage renal disease. She undergoes hemodialysis three times weekly.

In the ED, she had low blood pressure that did not respond to intravenous fluid. She also had a low oxygen saturation that only slightly improved with 100% oxygen. A chest X-ray shows pneumonia. Shortly thereafter, she was working so hard to breathe that she required a breathing tube to be placed and she was started on mechanical ventilation. Her blood pressure fell further, and she required an infusion of a vasopressor to raise her blood pressure to a safe level. Given pneumonia, she was also administered broad-spectrum antibiotics. ICU care was required for septic shock related to pneumonia.

The ICU pharmacist helps the admitting team with the medication reconciliation process, obtaining the patient's medication list from her outpatient pharmacy. The patient's home medications include divalproex, levothyroxine, metformin, metoprolol, lisinopril, furosemide, rosuvastatin, calcium acetate, ferrous sulfate, and a daily multivitamin. The patient's home medications are not initially re-ordered, as each one needs to be considered in light of septic shock. The ICU pharmacist ensures that medications that may decrease her blood pressure such as metoprolol, lisinopril, and furosemide are not initially resumed. Her new medications, aside from antibiotics and a vasopressor, include intravenous fluid, a sedative infusion, a gastric acid–reducing agent for stress ulcer prophylaxis, subcutaneous unfractionated heparin for deep venous thrombosis prophylaxis, and a chlorhexidine rinse for oral care. She also has Tylenol and an as-needed dose of an analgesic for pain management.

Pharmacotherapy in critically ill patients is complex as it addresses multiple comorbidities, preexisting medication regimens, and the interactions of both of these elements with critical illness pathophysiology and management. The hypothetical case above highlights these considerations. For example, some of the patient's medications will benefit her ongoing care (e.g., divalproex, levothyroxine) while some may be detrimental (e.g., furosemide, lisinopril, metoprolol). Some conditions like diabetes mellitus may be appropriately treated with existing therapy but may not be suitable for administration in the ICU (e.g., metformin). Furthermore, the use of extracorporeal therapies presents additional challenges particularly as the mode of therapy changes from the outpatient setting to one more fitting for critical illness (e.g., intermittent hemodialysis to continuous renal replacement therapy). Finally, the potential for drug interactions exists which the clinician must consider when choosing a new medication in the hospital to avoid under- or overdosing the patient. Some medications will reduce the rate at which another medication is cleared, leading to an inadvertent increase in one agent. That increased concentration may cause complications ranging from seizure to kidney injury to cardiac arrhythmia. Thus, the pharmacist plays a key safety role in the ICU.

With patients admitted to the ICU typically receiving more than 30 different medications throughout their admission, critical care clinicians are faced with multiple important medication-related decisions each day. Even when the correct medication is chosen, a dose or route of administration that is not optimal can result in an adverse outcome. Furthermore, failure to appropriately integrate past medication use with ongoing medical indications across the continuum of care can markedly impact drug-related outcomes and long-term recovery. This chapter will highlight the role of the pharmacist in the provision of multiprofessional care for critically ill and injured patients and discuss implications for the ongoing care of critical illness survivors.

■ ROLE OF THE PHARMACIST

As the medication specialists on the multidisciplinary ICU team, pharmacists are uniquely positioned to contribute to the care of critically ill patients.

The critical care pharmacist's responsibilities include, but are not limited to, prospective medication management, medication reconciliation, education, answering drug information questions, and daily evaluation for safe and effective medication use. ICU pharmacists also maintain vigilance for interactions between changing physiology (e.g., acute kidney injury that changes how many drugs are cleared) and medication dosage and timing. Specialized critical care pharmacists' involvement in patient care is associated with better patient outcomes, more rapid achievement of therapeutic goals, improved quality and safety, and enhanced organizational performance.

Critical care pharmacists undergo extensive training focused on the safe and effective use of medications in patients with critical illness. In the United States, all graduates from an accredited college of pharmacy receive a Doctor of Pharmacy degree. While there is no standardized postgraduation pathway to train pharmacists providing critical care pharmacotherapy, the conventional approach is a general residency in pharmacy (postgraduate year 1) followed by a residency in critical care (postgraduate year 2). Specialized training in research can be sought through either a 2-year fellowship or an alternative degree (e.g., Masters, PhD). Critical care pharmacy is recognized as a specialty area by the Board of Pharmacy Specialties for which board certification is offered.

■ THE PHARMACISTS' APPROACH

Like other ICU clinicians, critical care pharmacists use a systems-based approach when reviewing patient data to tailor a treatment plan. Pharmacists place a special focus on the identification of drug-related problems and pharmacotherapy (Table 6-1). For example, critical review of a patient's medical record will frequently identify duplications in drug therapy (e.g., multiple opioid orders such as fentanyl and hydromorphone), unnecessary or ineffective medications (e.g., bronchodilator therapy without an indication), and opposing medications (e.g., metoprolol and norepinephrine). In addition, drug–drug interactions or adverse effects will be identified which often necessitates a dose adjustment or an alternative treatment plan. Finally, pharmacists proactively evaluate for opportunities where indications for drug therapy exist, but no medication is being provided.

Several factors complicate providing drug therapy in the ICU. First, drug-dosing regimens are typically derived from studies conducted on non-ICU patients or healthy volunteers. Critically ill patients, however, suffer from a variety of physiologic changes that alter pharmacokinetic or pharmacodynamic elements including volume status, protein binding, perfusion, and

■ **TABLE 6-1. Classification of Drug-Related Problems and ICU-Specific Examples**

Drug-Related Problem	Example
Medication used with no medical indication	Famotidine for stress ulcer prophylaxis in a patient considered low risk for clinically important bleeding
Medical conditions exist with no medication prescribed	Insulin for a patient with hyperglycemia
Medication prescribed inappropriately for a particular condition	Pantoprazole 40 mg daily prescribed for a patient with an acute upper GI bleed
A better alternative exists based on clinical evidence (efficacy/safety)	Oral vancomycin in place of metronidazole in a patient with *Clostridium difficile* infection
A more cost-effective alternative exists	Low-molecular-weight heparin versus unfractionated heparin for venous thromboembolism prophylaxis
Inappropriate medication dose	Meropenem 1 gram every 8 hours in a patient with septic shock and estimated creatinine clearance >130 mL/min
Inappropriate route or method of administration	Enteral administration of phenytoin in a patient receiving continuous tube feeds
Therapeutic duplication	Intravenous morphine and intravenous fentanyl for treatment of severe pain
Medications with conflicting effects or prescribing cascades	Addition of metoprolol in a patient with tachycardia but also receiving norepinephrine
Severe allergies	Piperacillin/tazobactam for empiric therapy in a septic patient when anaphylaxis to penicillin is documented
Presence of or potential for adverse drug events	Vancomycin for methicillin-resistant *Staphylococcus aureus* pneumonia in a patient with acute kidney injury where renal function is deemed recoverable
Presence of or potential for clinically significant drug–drug, drug–disease, drug–nutrient, or drug–laboratory interactions	Additive risk for QTc prolongation with the addition of methadone to a patient receiving quetiapine and a fluoroquinolone

end-organ function which have considerable effect on bioavailability, volume of distribution, and clearance. The application of "standard" dosing regimens could lead to unintended therapeutic failures or toxicities. As a result, it is common for nonstandard doses (i.e., those that vary from the product labeling) to be used. In addition, pharmacodynamic changes that could lead to increased sensitivity to drug effect may be related to altered drug receptor density or affinity. It is important to note that many of these pharmacokinetic and pharmacodynamic changes subside as patients progress across the continuum of care and recovery, further complicating the selection of an appropriate medication regimen. Pharmacists must remain alert for these changes and nimble in drug-dosing recommendations to achieve desired therapeutic goals.

Pharmacists adjust drug-dosing regimens to reduce the potential for under- or overdosing. In the initial phase of critical illness, the intravenous route may be preferred because it provides 100% bioavailability and eliminates absorption delays. Transition to enteral delivery is usually considered when the patient has stabilized, and enteral access is available. The enteral route reduces drug cost, eliminates additional fluid burden, and reduces infection risk. If a patient is unable to swallow, safe and effective delivery of certain drugs may be restricted depending on the availability of a commercially available liquid oral formulation or the ability to be crushed or compounded as an oral liquid.

Given the frequency of renal and/or hepatic impairment in critically ill patients, ICU pharmacists frequently provide dosing recommendations to prevent drug accumulation and subsequent adverse reactions, including drug-associated acute kidney injury and drug-induced liver injury. Some patients, including those who have sustained injury or neurologic disease, may present with augmented renal clearance leading to subtherapeutic drug concentrations and treatment failure. While many changes in organ function are driven by events that precede ICU admission, some organ injuries may be related to medications. Pharmacists play a key role in identifying potential culprits of medication-induced organ injury and formulating strategies to reduce injury potential through knowledge of drug mechanism of action, toxicity potential, and strategies for reversibility.

Specific populations within the ICU may also present unique challenges to drug dosing because of additional pharmacokinetic aberrations. These special populations include patients with extremes in weight, pregnancy, trauma, and thermal injury, and patients on specialized therapies such as continuous renal replacement therapy and extracorporeal membrane oxygenation. Each of these patient populations pose pharmacokinetic and physiologic challenges with variable levels of evidence to help guide clinicians in drug dosing. An individualized approach is necessary to optimize outcomes. Therapeutic drug monitoring, where available, can be particularly useful. Many institutions have ceded the ability to order laboratory-based drug concentration monitoring to pharmacists to ensure appropriateness and to link the data with expert evaluation.

■ CONSIDERATIONS FOR RECOVERY

Medication Reconciliation

Accurate medication reconciliation is an integral component of key transitions of care for an ICU patient. The stepwise medication reconciliation process provides a systematic assessment of all medications performed by pharmacists and other healthcare clinicians. Pharmacists are equipped with the knowledge to establish and maintain the medication reconciliation process to promote continuity of care, potentially reduce medication errors, and minimize adverse effects. The medication reconciliation process includes assessing which medications for chronic conditions should be continued (e.g., hypothyroid drugs), what medication adjustments should be made to reduce toxicity (e.g., dose reduction of beta-lactam antimicrobials in acute kidney injury), or what medications should be temporarily held (e.g., beta-blockers while on vasopressors with beta-agonist activity) depending on the clinical scenario (Fig. 6-1). While in the ICU, a patient will likely have several new medications initiated which should be evaluated for continuation as the therapeutic indication may be no longer present upon ICU discharge; acid suppressive agents and oral antipsychotics are often continued inappropriately

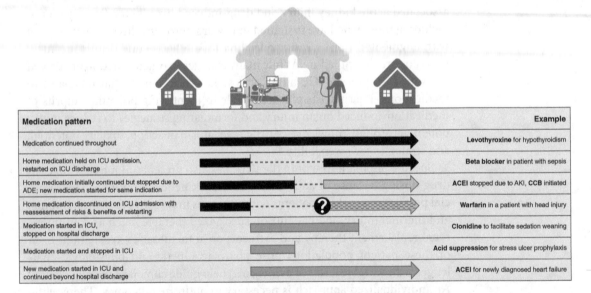

FIGURE 6-1. Medication Reconciliation and the Continuum of Care. This graphic demonstrates key aspects of medication management along the course of critical illness or injury and how medication reconciliation detects opportunities for improved safety or efficacy as well as decreased medication use. ACEI = angiotensin-converting enzyme inhibitor; AKI = acute kidney injury; ADE = adverse drug event; CCB = calcium channel blocker; SUP = stress ulcer prophylaxis. ? = clinical decision-point that must weight benefits against risks and incorporate therapeutic drug monitoring into the decision-making process.

after ICU discharge. Finally, upon ICU discharge, any medications that were adjusted or held should be re-evaluated for continuation (same drug and dose) or modification (different regimen or adjusted dose).

Medication Safety

Medication errors and adverse drug events are more likely to occur in the setting of critical care due to the patient's rapidly changing physiology and the need to acutely respond to threats to life or organ function. Critical care pharmacists help improve patient safety through a variety of daily workflow activities including: (1) auditing medication use followed by feedback to support clinician education, (2) minimizing the use of unnecessary medications, (3) developing and updating computerized physician order entry and clinical decision support systems, (4) creating guidelines, pathways, and protocols that improve medication use or monitoring, and (5) participating in medication reconciliation. The safety profile of medications administered to patients recovering from critical illness may change during recovery. Therefore, all medications, doses, and routes of administration should be reconsidered upon discharge from the ICU and again upon discharge from the hospital. The first primary care visit should include attention to medication changes and an assessment of the new regimen's appropriateness for the patient.

Anticoagulation

An increasing number of options for anticoagulation present challenges for clinicians to consider when developing a regimen for ICU survivors. Special populations of patients exist that require an altered dosing anticoagulation approach to optimize efficacy and safety (e.g., patients with BMI $\geq$40 kg/m^2, patients with acute kidney injury or chronic kidney disease). The expanding number of medications that interact with anticoagulants requires constant attention and familiarity. Finally, reversal strategies have become more complicated with the availability of newer agents (e.g., direct thrombin inhibitors, anti-Xa inhibitors), thereby requiring expert guidance when selecting rescue or reversal therapy in the setting of major bleeding such as after injury.

Infectious Diseases

Many ICU patients will be diagnosed with infections that are community- or hospital-acquired. While antibiotic treatment courses may be completed in the ICU or inpatient setting, a small number of patients may need prolonged oral or parenteral antimicrobial therapy. Long-term monitoring for toxicity (e.g., weekly creatine kinase levels for daptomycin therapy) may be needed.

Where infectious disease transition teams exist, these services help maintain continuity of antimicrobial therapy and appropriate diagnostic testing (e.g., repeat blood cultures) and monitoring.

ICU Recovery Clinics

Pharmacists are active in post-intensive care recovery clinics, a care setting that is growing in availability as the recovery needs of critical care survivors are increasingly recognized. Specific functions of the pharmacist in this setting include performing a full medication review, medication reconciliation, patient interview, counseling, assessment of adverse effects, drug interaction assessment, and medication regimen compliance. Relatedly, pharmacists may also participate in an opioid de-escalation program for patients who require opioid-based analgesic programs after critical illness or injury. Often, pharmacists identify medications from the ICU that were inappropriately continued after discharge. The most common medications discontinued include gastric acid suppressive agents, corticosteroids, bronchodilators, and antimicrobials. Therefore, pharmacists serve as key members of the ICU team with penetrance into multiple aspects of recovery after ICU survival.

Tips for Clinicians

1. **Evaluate medication regimens** and de-prescribe specific agents when indicated. Some medications that are initiated in the ICU may no longer be indicated once critical illness resolves. Common medications started in the ICU that may no longer be indicated upon transfer to a non-ICU setting include gastric acid suppressive agents (for stress ulcer prophylaxis), antipsychotics (for delirium), opioids (for acute pain), and clonidine (for sedation weaning).
2. **Reconcile medications for chronic diseases** that may have been held upon ICU admission.
3. **Individualize drug doses** for ICU patients because of the pharmacokinetic variability that exists in this population. Doses therefore may be different than what is listed in reference texts.
4. **Transition from intravenous to oral medication use** may be considered as critical illness resolves provided bioavailability is adequate, an appropriate dosing formulation exists, and interactions with enteral nutrition are negligible or manageable.
5. **Adjust drug doses for organ function** and the use of extracorporeal therapies. These regimens should be reassessed with changes in organ function or when extracorporeal therapies are initiated or discontinued.

6. **Use caution with medications that have a narrow therapeutic window**, particularly those that cause respiratory depression, alter mental status, or reduce blood pressure, when patients are transferred to a setting where monitoring may be less intense (i.e., ICU to an acute care unit).

7. **Avoid prescribing cascades** (i.e., prescribing a new medication to treat an adverse effect of another).

8. **Evaluate for therapeutic duplication or substitution upon hospital discharge.** Home medications may be adjusted or substituted in the hospital according to the institution's preferred formulary agent (e.g., atorvastatin instead of simvastatin).

KEY REFERENCES

Abdul-Aziz MH, Alffenaar JC, Bassetti M, et al. Antimicrobial therapeutic drug monitoring in critically ill adult patients: a Position Paper. *Intensive Care Med*. 2020;46:1127-1153.

Adie SK, Thompson AN, Konerman MC, et al. Impact of a pharmacist in an interdisciplinary post-cardiac intensive care unit clinic. *Heart Lung*. 2022;52:48-51.

Alhameed AF, Khansa SA, Hasan H, et al. Bridging the gap between theory and practice; the active role of inpatient pharmacists in therapeutic drug monitoring. *Pharmacy*. 2019;7(1):20.

Borthwick M. The role of the pharmacist in the intensive care unit. *J Intensive Care Soc*. 2019;20(2):161-164.

Heck CC, Tichy EM, Vonderheyde R, et al. Optimizing pharmacist-driven protocols and documentation of interventions using clinical decision support systems. *Am J Health Syst Pharm*. 2020;77(11):830-834.

Kane-Gill SL, Dasta JF, Buckley MS, et al. Clinical practice guideline: safe medication use in the ICU. *Crit Care Med*. 2017;45:e877-e915.

Lee H, Ryu K, Sohn Y, et al. Impact on patient outcomes of pharmacist participation in multidisciplinary critical care teams: a systematic review and meta-analysis. *Crit Care Med*. 2019;47(9):1243-1250.

MacTavish P, Quasim T, Shaw M, et al. Impact of a pharmacist intervention at an intensive care rehabilitation clinic. *BMJ Open Quality*. 2019;8(3):e000580.

Mohammad RA, Betthauser KD, Korona RB, et al. Clinical pharmacist services within intensive care unit recovery clinics: an opinion of the critical care practice and research network of the American College of Clinical Pharmacy. *J Am Col Clin Pharm*. 2020;3(7):1369-1379.

Sherwin J, Heath T, Watt K. Pharmacokinetics and dosing of anti-infective drugs in patients on extracorporeal membrane oxygenation: a review of the current literature. *Clin Ther*. 2016;38(9):1976-1994.

Smith BS, Yogaratnam D, Levasseur-Franklin KE, et al. Introduction to drug pharmacokinetics in the critically ill patient. *Chest*. 2012;141:1327-1336.

Stollings JL, Bloom SL, Wang L, et al. Critical care pharmacists and medication management in an ICU recovery center. *Ann Pharmacother*. 2018;52:713-723.

The Therapy Team's Perspective— Physical Therapist, Occupational Therapist, and Speech-Language Therapist

Linda Mackay-Morgan, Annalise N. Slicer, and Mary Elizabeth Bouchard

Patient Care Vignette

A 25-year-old man named KD was injured in a high-speed motorcycle collision. He was wearing a helmet that the Emergency Medical Services personnel removed. He was initially unresponsive at the scene but started to awaken during ambulance transport to the nearest hospital, a trauma center. KD arrived in the Emergency Department confused and with difficulty breathing. A breathing tube was placed and he was evaluated for injuries. Multiple displaced rib fractures, lung injuries, a pelvis fracture, a liver injury, and a wrist fracture were found. He needed to have chest tubes to evacuate air that had leaked out of his lungs, his wrist was splinted, and he was transferred to the ICU for ongoing care.

As a result of KD's injuries, his hospital care was complex and involved multiple operations. Therefore, the planned initial Physical Therapy and Occupational Therapy (PT/OT) sessions were delayed while he underwent multiple trips to the operating room. Initial PT/OT evaluations were performed more than 10 days into KD's hospital stay. PT/OT clinicians remained engaged in his care throughout the ICU stay, working on range of motion and strength despite he being intubated and mechanically ventilated. He slowly recovered from his injuries and was able to be weaned from mechanical ventilation. With removal of his breathing tube and de-escalation of acute care interventions, the KD's rehabilitation needs expanded.

In addition to PT/OT care, KD was also evaluated for ongoing nutrition support needs. During most of his hospital stay, he received nutrition via a feeding tube placed in his mouth (an orogastric tube). When the breathing tube was removed, the orogastric tube was also removed. The clinical team wanted to assess whether he could safely swallow food. A speech and language pathologist (SLP) assessed KD's ability to swallow in a coordinated fashion. The SLP determined that he had some dysfunction including aspiration of thin liquids. He needed a modified diet so that he could safely swallow. The SLP prescribed a full liquid diet with thickened liquids and daily swallowing exercises. The clinical team worked with the SLP and the dietitian to provide foods that met these textural requirements while still being palatable to KD.

Following a 64-day admission, KD was discharged to an acute inpatient rehabilitation facility. He remained in an inpatient program until his discharge home 2 months later. He received outpatient therapy for several months focusing on endurance and strength to facilitate independence with activities of daily living and his eventual ability to return to work as an auto mechanic. His rehabilitation was key in returning to work as he also financially supports his elderly parents.

■ INTRODUCTION

Active and aggressive rehabilitative services are vital contributors to critical illness recovery. The tools, technologies, and protocols used in therapy continue to evolve, but early and continued interventions are key. Prospective studies consistently demonstrate the benefits of rehabilitative services for acutely ill patients, including patients who are intubated and mechanically ventilated. Indeed, therapy can be initiated at almost any time in the recovery arc, provided that the patient is stable enough for participation in therapy assessments and interventions. Early rehabilitative efforts help recovery momentum and may help with both weaning from the ventilator and avoiding delirium.

Given the profound physical impairments experienced by many critical illness survivors, continuing active physical therapy after surviving the ICU is also important. This chapter describes different therapeutic modalities that can support critical illness recovery and the various settings (e.g., inpatient, outpatient, at home) in which therapy can be provided. In general, the goal of therapy is to restore premorbid functioning. Therefore, these therapies should generally be offered as long as the patient continues to improve.

■ THERAPEUTIC MODALITIES

The primary rehabilitative therapies involved in the assessment and treatment of individuals recovering from critical illness are physical therapy, occupational therapy, and speech and swallowing therapy. Each of these therapies is delivered by clinicians specifically trained in their particular kind of therapy. Other relevant rehabilitative disciplines include physiatry (rehabilitation medicine), neuropsychology (recovery of normal brain function), and audiology (hearing). We will first describe therapy in the intensive care unit, as post-ICU rehabilitative care is more likely to be successful if therapy starts while the patient is still in the ICU.

The initiation of any rehabilitative therapy in the ICU is contingent on patient stability—especially as it relates to heart rate, blood pressure, breathing, and cognitive ability. Once a patient is stable to participate, rehabilitative therapists should be rapidly engaged. Of note, a patient's ability to actively participate in therapy sessions is desirable but is not a prerequisite for all types of intervention. For example, a patient on bedrest may not be able to participate in physical therapy but could be evaluated by a Speech and Language Pathologist (SLP) for swallowing safety. Despite earlier concerns, support devices like a ventilator, or support therapies like blood pressure supporting medications (vasopressors) are not absolute contraindications to therapy. Even patients who require mechanical ventricular support devices, and some patients on extracorporeal membrane oxygenation (ECMO), may participate in physical therapy including walking! Virtually all patients with critical illness can benefit from rehabilitative interventions while receiving care in the ICU.

The most frequently encountered rehabilitative discipline in critical care is physical therapy. Physical therapy is designed to improve strength, endurance, and mobility to help prevent ICU-associated complications, shorten time spent on a mechanical ventilator, and reduce the likelihood of unanticipated ICU readmission. The physical therapist (PT) introduces early mobilization and helps patients to progress from simple repositioning and passive bed activities to those requiring active patient participation, ultimately including ambulation. The PT initially identifies areas of weakness or limited motion to target therapies and improve function. An important byproduct of active therapy is cognitive stimulation that may help reduce delirium. Family members who are present also benefit from education regarding exercises—including those that improve range-of-motion—that may need to be continued at home. In this way, the PT also helps family or loved ones find a role in supporting recovery.

Occupational therapy is often delivered alongside PT. The primary focus of occupational therapy is on the activities of daily living (ADLs), or those essential actions and tasks required for personal care, such as hygiene, dressing, toileting, and eating. While PT addresses large muscle group movements (thigh muscles to stand), occupational therapist (OT) addresses smaller muscle group movement and control (hand movements to manipulate a fork). Therefore, the PT and the OT both help with endurance and strengthening, but with slightly different targets. The PT might use a rolling walker as an assistive device, and the OT might use hand or foot splints to maintain a "position of function" for those who have been at bedrest for a while and have joint stiffening. Often, activities supported by the OT may progress more rapidly than those addressed by the PT. For example, patients in the ICU may manage their own hygiene while remaining unable to walk more than 50 feet without using a walker. Interventions to mitigate sensory overstimulation as well as reduce external stimuli that can contribute to patients' agitation are within the scope of OT practice as well. With patients on ventilators, the OT can introduce relaxation techniques that do not use medications but can reduce patient stress and anxiety, especially during weaning. As for the PT, patient and family education is an important role for the OT.

The role of the SLP is additionally collaborative. Oropharyngeal dysphagia—difficulties in swallowing and speech—is a primary area of focus for the SLP in the ICU. The presence of dysphagia is linked to an increased risk of aspiration and aspiration-induced pneumonia; both increase ICU mortality. Dysphagia is present in up to 62% of critically ill or injured patients. The SLP assesses for and treats dysphagia and therefore helps patients to swallow, control secretions, and speak. In addition to a physical examination, assessment tools may include a Modified Barium Swallow (MBS—a radiology examination performed when the patient swallows thin barium) or Fiberoptic Endoscopic Evaluation of Swallowing (FEES—an endoscopic examination using a very small scope placed through a nostril).

Acute dysphagia treatment can include an oral hygiene program, strengthening exercises (oral, pharyngeal, laryngeal), specific swallow strategies, and diet modification. Patient communication is a key area of concern in the ICU, and the SLP focuses on leveraging effective means of communication. These can range from low-technology aids (picture boards, erasable writing boards) to high-technology communication systems (eye-gaze, electronic tablets, text-to-speech programs). Patients who have required a tracheostomy may be suitable for a "speaking valve" that helps them to speak even while the tracheostomy remains in place. Regaining speech—or a reasonable substitute—immeasurably helps address key patient needs during critical illness care and recovery. Patients can clearly share their thoughts, concerns, and needs while clinicians can have an effective way of assessing mental status, orientation, and more. Like their PT and OT counterparts, patient and family education is embedded in SLP patient care.

■ THERAPY IN THE ICU: CONSIDERATIONS AND BARRIERS RELEVANT TO RECOVERY

Even when the patient is able to participate in physical therapy and occupational therapy, delivering that care may be met with challenges both patient-driven and system-related. Depending on the specifics of a patient's critical illness or injury, or their mental state, patients may be unwilling to engage in therapy. Sleeplessness, depression, pain, withdrawal syndromes, or pre-illness or pre-injury psychiatric conditions may lead patients to decline participating in therapy. System challenges include the number of available therapists based on health or illness (shortages during the early part of the COVID pandemic were common), as well as the total patient load for the number of employed therapists. As a result, therapy may not occur, or may occur for less time per day, or fewer times per week than desired. If therapy is not initiated in the ICU or if therapy is inconsistently delivered, post-ICU recovery may suffer due to ICU-acquired weakness, muscle atrophy, and reduced joint mobility.

SLP interventions around swallowing and speaking that benefit ICU patients may also be derailed by patient and system factors. Patients with serious brain injuries or facial injuries may not be able to engage early in their course. Delirium, withdrawal syndromes, and preexisting psychiatric illness may also impede SLP interventions. SLP availability may be subject to the same constraints as those that impact PT and OT availability. Nonetheless, dietary advancement is often guided by SLP input and helps inform the decision to pursue—or forgo—feeding tube placement. Given that a single aspiration event can cause respiratory compromise, induce a fear of meals, and threaten nutrition, SLPs maintain vigilance for signs of aspiration in patients with, or at high risk for, dysphagia. After ICU discharge, the SLP can provide ongoing therapy to help patients who have not yet resumed their usual dietary intake.

■ CONSIDERATIONS FOR RECOVERY

Given the frequency of physical and cognitive impairments following critical illness, ICU survivors are likely to have therapy needs that exceed their time in a healthcare facility. Outpatient rehabilitation specialists such as

PTs, OTs, SLPs, and physiatrists may be helpful in establishing recovery programs that may be continued at home. Post-ICU clinics (Chapter 15) may also be helpful in assessing patients' needs and developing a rehabilitation regimen, especially when those clinics include PT/OT and SLP clinicians. Most patients, however, will likely have their needs addressed by primary care clinicians with support from family caregivers and friends. To encourage success for survivors with post-ICU functional impairments, patients and families benefit from education on the available pathways to pursue maximal recovery.

Impairments in ADLs, walking, breathing, strength, endurance, and comfort occur in up to 70% of survivors after critical illness. These acquired disabilities and conditions may last months, or in some cases, years. These impairments may also include the need for assistance in bathing, dressing, grooming, and other household tasks. Survivors and families may need to modify aspects of their lifestyle or incorporate assistive devices into their daily routine. An activity such as grocery shopping is much more difficult if a rolling walker is required for mobility. As a result, survivors have less independence, less community involvement, difficulties getting to healthcare appointments, and difficulty returning to work. Difficulty returning to work because of an inability to drive may further compound emotional and cognitive impairments and threaten well-being. Up to one-third of survivors of critical illness or injury are unable to safely return to driving one year after discharge from the ICU. Clearly, both PT and OT clinicians play key roles in helping patients return to normal. Despite the best efforts of therapists, progress may be limited by mental health issues. Therefore, screening for depression and anxiety should be performed while screening for postdischarge physical impairments.

Tips for Clinicians

1. For patients who have been discharged from the ICU, **assess the degree to which the patient's mobility and ability have changed** with respect to completing their activities of daily living (ADLs) as compared to their pre-hospital baseline. If deficits persist, referral to PT and/or OT services is appropriate.
2. **Ask the patient whether they have recently had difficulty swallowing** during their first discharge visit. Ask specifically about thin liquids such as water, compared to solid foods. Ask family caregivers about the patient's swallowing if possible. If signs of dysphagia are reported, refer the patient to an SLP for therapy and rehabilitation.

3. If therapy is needed, **help the patient and family determine the best site of care** for the patient. Inpatient physical therapy is potentially costly and requires that the patient be able to tolerate multiple hours per day of therapy services. Therapy services can sometimes be effectively delivered in the outpatient setting, or the patient's home, and typically utilizes a reduced intensity compared to an inpatient program.

4. Referrals to physical therapy, occupational therapy, and speech and language pathologists should be accompanied by the assessments performed in the hospital when possible. **Maintain a low threshold for establishing direct contact with the inpatient therapist.**

5. **Reassure patients** that the results of therapy take time and may span months to years to recover to the greatest extent possible.

6. Online resources about post-ICU therapy vary in quality and the degree to which they are updated. **Access reputable sources to help guide therapy decisions.** A good resource is the guidelines produced by professional organizations of physical and occupational therapists and speech and language pathologists.

KEY REFERENCES

Álvarez EA, Garrido MA, Tobar EA, et al. Occupational therapy for delirium management in elderly patients without mechanical ventilation in an intensive care unit: a pilot randomized clinical trial. *J Crit Care.* 2017;37:85-90.

Connolly B, Salisbury L, O'Neill B, et al. Exercise rehabilitation following intensive care unit discharge for recovery from critical illness. *Cochrane Database Syst Rev.* 2015;(6).

Hongo T, Yamamoto R, Liu K, et al. Association between timing of speech and language therapy initiation and outcomes among post-extubation dysphagia patients: a multicenter retrospective cohort study. *Crit Care.* 2022;26(1):98.

Hopkins RO, Miller RR, Rodriguez L, et al. Physical therapy on the wards after early physical activity and mobility in the intensive care unit. *Phys Ther.* 2012;92(12):1518-1523.

Khan BA, Lasiter S, Boustani MA. Critical care recovery center: an innovative collaborative care model for ICU survivors. *Am J Nurs.* 2015;115(3):24-31.

Ko Y, Cho YH, Park YH, et al. Feasibility and safety of early physical therapy and active mobilization for patients on extracorporeal membrane oxygenation. *ASAIO J.* 2015; 61(5):564-568.

McRae J, Montgomery E, Garstang Z, Cleary E. The role of speech and language therapists in the intensive care unit. *J Intensive Care Soc.* 2020;21(4):344-348.

Merati AL. In-office evaluation of swallowing: FEES, pharyngeal squeeze maneuver, and FEESST. *Otolaryngol Clin North Am.* 2013;46(1):31-39.

Sedighimehr N, Fathi J, Hadi N, et al. Rehabilitation, a necessity in hospitalized and discharged people infected with COVID-19: a narrative review. *Phys Ther Rev.* 2021;26(3): 202-210.

van Der Schaaf M, Beelen A, Dongelmans DA, Vroom MB, Nollet F. Functional status after intensive care: a challenge for rehabilitation professionals to improve outcome. *J Rehab Med*. 2009;41;360-366.

Walsh TS, Salisbury LG, Merriweather JL, et al. Increased hospital-based physical rehabilitation and information provision after intensive care unit discharge: the RECOVER randomized clinical trial. *JAMA Intern Med*. 2015;175(6):901-910.

Weinreich M, Herman J, Dickason S, et al. Occupational therapy in the intensive care unit: a systematic review. *Occup Ther Health Care*. 2017;31(3):205-213.

The Palliative Care Perspective

Rebecca Anna Gersten, Courtney Wagner, Bradley J. Heyward, and Anand S. Iyer

> *More and more ICU teams have come to value the role that palliative care can play in the critical care setting and to understand that it is not only for when a patient is dying.* Wes Ely, *Every Deep-Drawn Breath*

Patient Care Vignette

Ms. Jones is a 31-year-old female who collapsed at work after significant coughing. For weeks she experienced progressive breathlessness, finger ulcers, and joint pain. When the ambulance arrived, she was profoundly hypoxemic and was immediately intubated, connected to a portable ventilator, and transported to the local hospital. After initial evaluation in the Emergency Department, she was admitted to the ICU where she was treated with high-dose steroids and invasive ventilator support for a newly diagnosed severe lung disease. Her lung function was so poor that she was rapidly evaluated for extracorporeal membrane oxygenation (ECMO) rescue as a bridge to life-saving lung transplantation. However, as the sole provider for three young children (who were now being cared for by a neighbor) with recurrent housing and food instability and a limited support system, the medical and surgical teams viewed her as a poor candidate. Therefore, a long ICU course to try to improve her lung function was anticipated.

In the ICU, she felt trapped in her body and was unable to effectively communicate due to the endotracheal tube, medications for pain and anxiety, and the use of safety restraints so that she did not dislodge critical life support devices. Because ECMO rescue was not offered, the ICU team consulted Palliative Care Medicine (PCM), who helped address her needs in conjunction with the ICU team. Importantly, as she was recovering and could be more engaged, the PCM team also helped address emotional and spiritual aspects of her recovery. After being able to breathe on her own, she shared her concerns with the PCM team. If she became critically ill again in the future, she could not imagine going through another ICU stay again, but found it too anxiety provoking and stressful to discuss care planning while she was still in the hospital, even though she was outside of the ICU. After leaving the ICU, she suffered from intractable cough, severe dyspnea (shortness of breath), anxiety, posttraumatic stress disorder (PTSD), and persistent hypoxemia needing supplemental oxygen. She required rehabilitation for critical illness myopathy and polyneuropathy (weakness) acquired during her critical illness. She needed to file for disability as she could not meet the physical and cognitive demands of her job. Finally, regular outpatient follow-up for her new serious respiratory illness and complicated care transitions along her long road to recovery defined a new course for her daily life that impacted her children as well (Fig. 8-1).

This chapter focuses on the role of palliative care in the intensive care unit (ICU), with a special emphasis on how proactively integrating principles of palliative care can promote patient and family well-being and facilitate post-discharge recovery. Critically ill patients frequently experience delirium and immobility, which can have substantial long-term detrimental impacts on post-ICU quality of life and function. Meanwhile, families also experience significant distress as they navigate critical illness alongside their loved ones. Palliative Care Medicine (PCM) clinicians are often pigeonholed within a narrow scope in the ICU—goals of care discussions, conflict management, and end-of-life care. However, PCM provides a broad range of care outside the ICU and the acute care facility including symptom management and aiding in adjustments when patients experience major changes in their life circumstances. Palliative care is ideally proactively initiated within ICU care and then continues through discharge into convalescence to help ensure that the goals, values, and preferences of patients and their families are prioritized through survivorship. Drawing upon the authors' experiences in nursing, medicine, palliative care, and pulmonary and critical care medicine, we illustrate the palliative care perspective from critical illness to recovery.

■ THE ROLE OF THE PALLIATIVE CARE MEDICINE (PCM) TEAM MEMBER IN THE ICU

Palliative Care Medicine is a clinical specialty and can be conceptualized as an overarching approach to care that can be incorporated into routine practice by

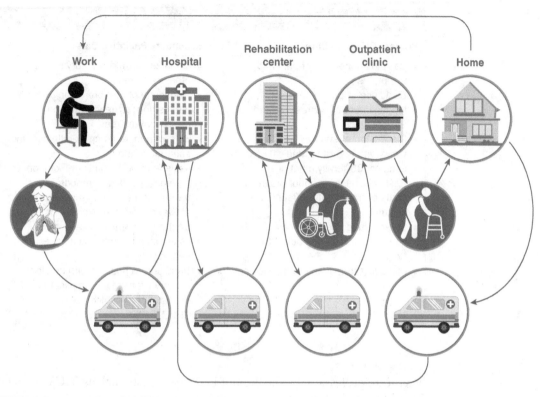

FIGURE 8-1. Care Transitions in Serious or Critical Illness. Patients with serious illness often experience compli-cated transitions of care across the continuum. Patients and families are frequently unprepared for the complexities of these transitions.

any clinician who treats people with a serious illness. The overarching goals of palliative care in the ICU are to assess and alleviate the physical, psychological, social, and spiritual dimensions of suffering and to understand and facilitate patient and family goals, values, and preferences for care. Palliative care has evolved as a model of healthcare focused on quality of life during serious or critical illness. PCM builds on the foundations of hospice, which is focused on the end of life, and extends those principles across the trajectory of serious ill-ness from its onset. While hospice care focuses on individuals with life-limiting illness—generally less than 6 months—palliative care is appropriate at any stage of a serious illness. Moreover, palliative care is beneficial when provided in concert with treatment pursuing a curative or life-prolonging intent across all major clinical conditions from cancer to heart failure to traumatic brain injury.

Palliative care can be delivered in two principal forms: primary or sec-ondary palliative care (Table 8-1). *Primary* palliative care is delivered by

■ **TABLE 8-1. Differences in Primary and Secondary Palliative Care Skills**

Primary Palliative Care	Secondary Palliative Care
• Basic management of pain and symptoms	• Management of refractory pain or other symptoms
• Basic use of pain relievers	• Management of more complex depression, anxiety, grief, and existential distress
• Management of depression and anxiety	• Help with more complex religious and spiritual suffering
• Discussion of spiritual and religious views with regard to medical care	• Assistance with conflict resolution regarding goals or methods of treatment, i.e., within families, between staff and families, among treatment teams
• Leading ICU family meetings	
• Basic discussions about prognosis, goals of treatment, suffering, code status	• Assistance in addressing cases of near futility
• Coordinating specialist care	• Transition to hospice with no clear primary clinician or complicated discharge to hospice care
• Managing transitions out of the hospital	
• Managing transitions to hospice care	

healthcare professionals who are not PCM specialists such as ICU clinicians fellowship trained in critical care medicine. Secondary palliative care, on the other hand, is delivered by fellowship trained (generally one additional year) and certified specialist PCM clinicians. Secondary palliative care is typically provided by an interdisciplinary team of physicians, nurse practitioners, nurses, social workers, spiritual care professionals, and others such as music therapists, child life specialists, physical therapists, and community health workers. In clinical settings, secondary palliative care is often provided in palliative care inpatient units and ambulatory clinics. As shown in Fig. 8-2, a "mixed approach" has been proposed by Curtis and colleagues where palliative care spans a continuum from primary to secondary palliative care, seamlessly blending the skills of ICU clinicians with integrated specialist palliative care teams to improve patient- and family-centered outcomes. PCM clinicians are typically involved in the ICU within the following four broad areas: (1) complex symptom management; (2) discerning "goals of care" for interventions and procedures near the end of life; and (3) facilitating providing comfort care (addressing pain, anxiety, and comfort through the dying process while removing life support devices and therapies); and (4) helping resolve conflicts that arise between patients, families, and care teams often centered around end-of-life issues.

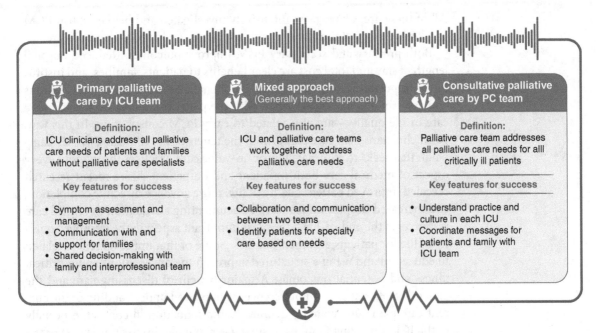

FIGURE 8-2. The Spectrum of Primary and Palliative Care. This figure by Curtis et al. (From *Intensive Care Medicine 2021*) illustrates the spectrum of palliative care in the ICU from primary to secondary and a mixed approach that blends the strengths of each.

■ WHAT HAPPENS IN THE ICU FROM THE PCM PERSPECTIVE?

Major critical care societies have embraced the integration of palliative care in the ICU, and its uptake has been increasing over the last 20 years. Palliative care provides multidimensional and interprofessional treatment for the patient and their family during and after critical illness. Domains of palliative care that have been defined by patients, their families, and experts include: (1) management of distress from physical, psychological, and spiritual symptoms; (2) engaging in sensitive and timely communication about patient and family goals of care; (3) alignment of interventions with the goals, values, and preferences of patients and their families; (4) attention to family needs and concerns; and (5) support for clinicians. The National Consensus Guidelines for Quality Palliative Care defines eight domains of palliative care which easily map to the care needs of patients and their families in the ICU: (1) structure and process of care; (2) physical aspects of care; (3) psychiatric and psychological aspects of care; (4) social aspects of care; (5) spiritual, religious, and existential aspects of care; (6) cultural aspects of care; (7) care of the patient nearing the end-of-life; and (8) ethical and legal aspects of care.

All of these areas have been intensively investigated and help establish PCM as a key member of the team providing patient- and family-centered care.

Both primary and secondary PCM improve outcomes. Reduced hospital length of stay and total cost are clear benefits to patients, families, and institutions. Importantly, reduced use of "nonbeneficial therapies"—interventions and assessments that do not align with the patient's goals or do not improve care or life quality—are also related to early PCM consultation. In this way, PCM clinicians help care conform to the tenets of the Choosing Wisely campaign that seeks to eliminate low or no-value care practices throughout every aspect of medical care both inpatient and outpatient. More recent research revealed improved patient quality of life, more advance directive completion, and increased hospice utilization all documenting a reduction in critical care resources at the end-of-life—the most important aspect in the improved quality of life for patients and their families. Some of that improvement is related to education and using a structured approach to conversations about critical illness and potential outcomes. A major benefit of discussing care and the patient's goals, values, and preferences is improved understanding of the current care plan, anticipated outcomes, and a reduction in conflict, especially in the ICU. Engaging families or surrogates in daily discussions is part of the ICU Liberation approach to care that benefits from early PCM consultation for those with critical illness or injury (Fig. 8-3). This approach is a bundle-based way of approaching daily ICU care that seeks to help patients become liberated from a breathing machine, off sedatives, and out of the ICU more rapidly while reducing delirium, weakness, and the occurrence of the Post-Intensive Care Syndrome (PICS) and the Post-Intensive Care Syndrome-Family (PICS-F). Unsurprisingly, family members are key members of the ICU team in using this approach.

PICS is a well-characterized syndrome that impacts survivors of critical illness. It has three major components: cognitive dysfunction, weakness, and psychosocial dysfunction. Those suffering from PICS have difficulty thinking clearly and rapidly and are generally globally weak. Furthermore, their interaction with friends or family is different compared to that before they became ill, and maintaining relationships suffers as a result. Often, they are distant, unengaged, and no longer find joy in activities that were previously important to them. Ongoing interactions with a member of the PCM team may detect PICS and guide survivors into rehabilitation as well as support groups. Moreover, PICS can impact family members as well. Increasingly, family members serve as uncompensated caregivers helping their loved one during convalescence. Providing medical care at home (e.g., wound care, ostomy appliance management, tracheostomy suctioning) can be anxiety provoking, and depressing, but can also reinforce PTSD-like symptoms that are related to specific events that

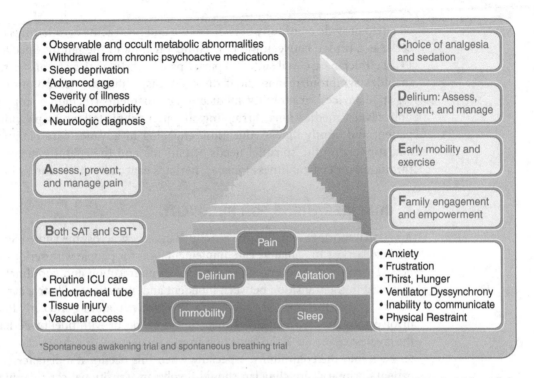

- Observable and occult metabolic abnormalities
- Withdrawal from chronic psychoactive medications
- Sleep deprivation
- Advanced age
- Severity of illness
- Medical comorbidity
- Neurologic diagnosis

Choice of analgesia and sedation

Delirium: Assess, prevent, and manage

Early mobility and exercise

Family engagement and empowerment

Assess, prevent, and manage pain

Both SAT and SBT*

- Routine ICU care
- Endotracheal tube
- Tissue injury
- Vascular access

Pain

Delirium   Agitation

Immobility   Sleep

- Anxiety
- Frustration
- Thirst, Hunger
- Ventilator Dyssynchrony
- Inability to communicate
- Physical Restraint

*Spontaneous awakening trial and spontaneous breathing trial

FIGURE 8-3. A Conceptual Model of the ICU Liberation Bundle as Upstream Palliative Care to Address Pain, Agitation, Delirium, Immobility, and Sleep Issues. This conceptual model demonstrates how proactive palliative care in the ICU through the ICU Liberation Bundle could help to prevent pain, agitation, and delirium and improve patient- and family-centered outcomes.

occurred in the ICU. Counseling and support groups can help family members to manage fears, address concerns, and preserve the wellness of all affected. PCM clinicians take care of the patient and the family during recovery and family members should feel free to share their observations and concerns during visits whether in person or by digital virtual platform.

■ WHAT HAPPENS AFTER THE ICU FROM THE PALLIATIVE CARE PERSPECTIVE?

Patients with critical illness or injury frequently move between care settings such as a long-term acute care hospital, a rehabilitation hospital, or a skilled nursing facility before returning home. These transitions are often associated with new or worsening symptoms and can be accompanied by gaps in communication between acute care clinicians and family members. Communication failure is more likely when the patient is new to the facility and there is no relationship yet established with the family. PCM teams can help provide continuity between acute and post-acute care settings and serve as a bridge between the new clinical team and the family. Specialist PCM clinicians are well suited to participate in the logistics of transfer that includes symptom management during transportation, incorporation of assistive devices for mobility, medication adjustments (including stopping unnecessary medications), arranging outpatient clinic follow-up, providing patient and family illness education, engaging in advance care planning, and supporting the spiritual needs of patients and their family members through their critical illness journey, perhaps especially at the end of life.

■ CONSIDERATIONS FOR RECOVERY

A national shortage of palliative care clinicians access across the United States are key barriers to palliaitve care implementation for people with serious illness. There are also several other gaps in communication and coordination that exist in the transition between inpatient and outpatient palliative care as well as hospice that impede quality care. Preemptive planning and early PCM involvement are key in ensuring that transitions occur with fidelity. Perhaps the greatest challenge is the transition from a quaternary or tertiary care center back into the community, especially when this occurs at a distance. The patient's primary care clinician should involve in transitional care planning, particularly when palliative care is required. When PCM clinicians are not present within the community, virtual care may be key. Those who do not have smart phone, computer, or tablet access may be able to participate via a primary care clinician's office, or via a home health agencies' device during home health visits. Inequity in PCM access remains a major hurdle in delivering quality care across regions with divergent socioeconomic strata. Furthermore, professional guidelines on the integration of palliative principles into specialist care are difficult to implement in resource-limited settings and across the continuum of care. While less than ideal, in the absence of PCM services educational resources exist for a variety of clinicians, and may prove useful to bridge the gap. (See Table 8-2). Geographic distance, transportation issues, and lack of access to palliative care specialists limit integration of quality palliative and end-of-life care for patients and their families in certain settings.

Nonetheless, in resource replete spaces, there are many models of interweaving palliative care into post-ICU outpatient care. Most patients return to their primary care clinicians, and to a lesser extent subspecialists, for care after surviving critical illness or injury. Direct engagement with PCM clinicians during or after office visits can serve as a link between patients, families, and palliative care without requiring another transportation event and office visit. Increasingly, survivors of critical illness are being cared for in post-ICU

■ **TABLE 8-2. Primary Palliative Care Training Programs for Clinicians**

Communication Tools or Training Programs	Description
Serious Illness Conversation Guide	Guide and tools to help ensure care aligns with goals, values, and preferences of patients through Ariadne Labs
Oncotalk	Program for oncology fellows to learn and practice primary palliative care skills under supervision
Center to Advance Palliative Care	National organization dedicated to increasing availability of quality healthcare for patients living with serious illnesses. Provides tools and training for health professionals in communication skills, pain and symptom management, and other primary palliative care basics
VitalTalk	Training organization for health professionals to advance communication skills, using simulated patients with multiple tools available even without training. Useful free phone application with various resources
The Conversation Project	Built for the public to help people talk about their wishes for care through the end of life with tools, guides, and other resources that may be helpful for patients and families
Five Wishes	Initially a workbook to help with advance care planning but has expanded to offer more tools and resources for patients, families, and organizations
The African American Spiritual and Ethical Guide to End-of-Life Care—What Y'all Gon' Do with Me?	Interactive guide and workshop geared toward patients who are African American built to address historical, cultural, and spiritual factors that can influence decisions
UCLA 3 Wishes	Program that promotes the inherent dignity of dying persons and their families by eliciting and implementing meaningful wishes at the end of life
AACN: American Association of Critical Care Nurses	Three-part webinar series on "Palliative Care in the ICU" covering the role of nurses in primary palliative care and communication skills between the nurse, provider, patient, and family

clinics, generally but not exclusively housed within the auspices of a teaching facility. As shown in Fig. 8-4, post-ICU clinics are a unique way to meet the specific needs of patients after critical illness and are typically staffed by ICU clinicians and rehabilitation specialists. A multiprofessional post-ICU clinic also includes pharmacists, social workers, case managers, and advanced practice providers. Most post-ICU clinics provide physical assessment, global needs assessment, cognitive assessment, ICU debriefing, behavioral health referral, and communication with primary care, all of which are essential elements that support a palliative care focus as well. Therefore, a post-ICU clinic may provide an ideal space in which to ensure that multidimensional palliative care can be delivered for the appropriate patient in a team-based fashion.

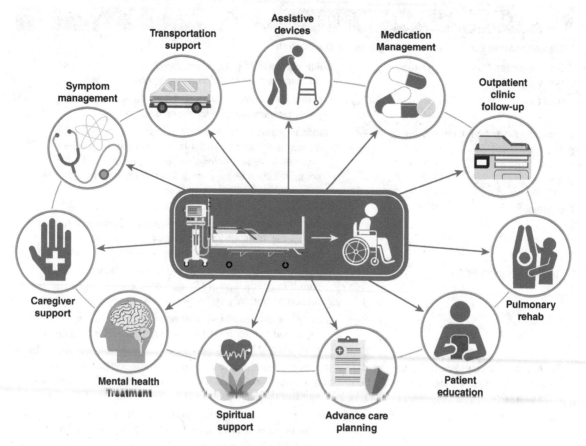

FIGURE 8-4. Domains of Palliative Care in a Post-ICU Clinic. There are several domains of palliative care that can be addressed in a post-ICU clinic model.

Tips for Clinicians

1. **Have discussions with patients and family caregivers about their values** while accounting for attitudes regarding burden of treatment and possible outcomes shortly after ICU admission.

2. Palliative care clinicians provide much more than end-of-life care, goals of care clarification, and conflict management; **consider consulting palliative care to help with symptom management and psychosocial support in the setting of new, life-changing illness.**

3. **Understand the difference between primary and secondary palliative care** (Table 8-1). Many different types of clinicians, including primary care providers and ICU providers, can readily provide

primary palliative care. Fellowship-trained PCM clinicians are expert at providing *secondary* palliative care.

4. **Involve PCM clinicians early.** Early involvement of PCM clinicians helps with transition planning and provides another way of rendering patient- and family-centered care that also improves outcomes including quality of life.

KEY REFERENCES

Aslakson RA, Curtis JR, Nelson JE. The changing role of palliative care in the ICU. *Crit Care Med.* 2014;42(11):2418-2428.

Brown SM, Bose S, Banner-Goodspeed V, et al. Approaches to addressing post–intensive care syndrome among intensive care unit survivors. A narrative review. *Ann ATS.* 2019; 16(8):947-956.

Chaaban S, McCormick J, Gleason D, McFarlin JM. Palliative care for the interstitial lung disease patient a must and not just a need. *Am J Hosp Palliat Care.* Published online August 19, 2021:104990912110402.

Curtis JR, Higginson IJ, White DB. Integrating palliative care into the ICU: a lasting and developing legacy. *Intensive Care Med.* Published online May 16, 2022:s00134-022-06729-7.

Danesh V, Boehm LM, Eaton TL, et al. Characteristics of post-ICU and post-COVID recovery clinics in 29 U.S. health systems. *Crit Care Explor.* 2022;4(3):e0658.

Davidson JE, Powers K, Hedayat KM, et al. Clinical practice guidelines for support of the family in the patient-centered intensive care unit: American College of Critical Care Medicine Task Force 2004–2005. *Crit Care Med.* 2007;35(2):605-622.

Ely W. *Every Deep-Drawn Breath.* New York, NY: Scribner; 2021.

Ferrell BR, Twaddle ML, Melnick A, Meier DE. National consensus project clinical practice guidelines for quality palliative care guidelines, 4th edition. *J Palliat Med.* 2018; 21(12):1684-1689.

Iyer AS, Sullivan DR, Lindell KO, Reinke LF. The role of palliative care in COPD. *Chest.* 2022;161(5):1250-1262.

Kayser JB, Kaplan LJ. Conflict management in the ICU. *Crit Care Med.* 2020;48(9):1349-1357.

Mayr FB, Plowman JL, Blakowski S, Sell-Shemansky K, Young JM, Yende S. Feasibility of a home-based palliative care intervention for elderly multimorbid survivors of critical illness. *Am J Crit Care.* 2021;30(1):e12-e31.

National Hospice and Palliative Care Organization Facts and Figures. Published online 2020. Accessed June 21, 2022. https://www.nhpco.org/hospice-facts-figures/.

Pun BT, Balas MC, Barnes-Daly MA, et al. Caring for critically ill patients with the ABCDEF bundle: results of the ICU liberation collaborative in over 15,000 adults. *Crit Care Med.* 2019;47(1):3.

Quinn KL, Bell CM. Pandemic health consequences: grasping the long COVID tail. *PLoS Med.* 2022;19(1):e1003891.

Saunders S, Killackey T, Kurahashi A, et al. Palliative care transitions from acute care to community-based care—a systematic review. *J Pain Symptom Manage.* 2019;58(4):721-734.e1.

Serrano P, Kheir YNP, Wang S, Khan S, Scheunemann L, Khan B. Aging and postintensive care syndrome—family: a critical need for geriatric psychiatry. *Am J Geriatr Psychiatry.* 2019;27(4):446-454.

White DB, Angus DC, Shields AM, et al. A randomized trial of a family-support intervention in intensive care units. *N Engl J Med.* 2018;378(25):2365-2375.

Zimmermann C, Mathews J. Palliative care is the umbrella, not the rain—a metaphor to guide conversations in advanced cancer. *JAMA Oncol.* 2022;8(5):681.

Spiritual and Pastoral Care Perspective

Christine C. Toevs

Patient Care Vignette

Mr. Jordan, a 64-year-old male with underlying lung disease, was admitted to the Intensive Care Unit (ICU) with the flu. He required respiratory support from a mechanical ventilator. For the first few days he was sedated and not able to interact with the ICU care team or his family. As he improved, the sedation was decreased, and he became more awake. Although he still required multiple medical interventions and was still quite ill, the care team began to encourage participation with physical therapy and sitting in a chair every day. He was then helped to walk using a walker, all while still attached to the ventilator. The care team provided a variety of communication devices for him to interact with his family since he was unable to talk. After several more days of intense medical therapy, he was removed from the life-support machines and could finally talk with his family. He was then transferred to the inpatient rehabilitation ward for 3 weeks of therapy to help him recover and return home.

During his time in the ICU and in rehab, Mr. Jordan's family noticed that he seemed depressed and withdrawn. He seemed anxious, especially when he was attached to the life-support machines. They thought he was concerned about possibly dying. The care team thought he was trying to "put on a good face" for the family when they visited, but otherwise he was difficult to engage in recovery efforts. The family said he did not attend church but asked for a visit from the hospital chaplain. The chaplain visited regularly and met with the patient and his family, both in the ICU and on the rehabilitation ward. Mr. Jordan developed a supportive relationship with the chaplain, and thought about returning to his church once he was discharged home. When he finally returned home, Mr. Jordan was encouraged by his family to attend church and include a spiritual component throughout his ongoing recovery.

ROLE OF THE CHAPLAIN AND SPIRITUAL SERVICES IN THE ICU

Most major medical centers have a dedicated chaplaincy (pastoral care) service. The chaplains are non-denominational and will meet with patients and families of many religious faiths. If there is not a hospital chaplain, often there are volunteer chaplains within the community who will provide spiritual services at the hospital. Patients and families can ask their pastor/priest/spiritual guide to come to the hospital and provide support. The "why" questions can be distressful for patient and family alike (i.e., *Why did this happen to me? Why has this occurred now?*). The care team does not have answers to the "why" questions, and neither does the chaplain. However, the chaplain can help the patient and family explore these questions during their journey through critical illness and during recovery (Fig. 9-1). For patients with a

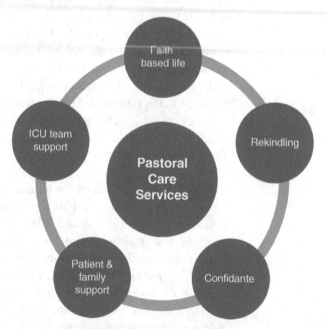

FIGURE 9-1. Key Aspects of Pastoral Care in the ICU. This graphic demonstrates five key aspects of pastoral care within the ICU. Note that support is provided for patients, families, and critical care team members.

faith-based existence, pastoral care within the ICU is an extension of their usual life before developing critical illness or sustaining critical injury. For others, pastoral care serves as a kind of renewal or rekindling of prior practice. Moreover, such services provide support through an individual not involved in medical or surgical decision-making; this individual may also serve as a confidante. Finally, the chaplaincy also supports the critical care team members during difficult experiences and during periods of religious observance.

■ WHAT HAPPENS IN THE ICU FROM THE PERSPECTIVE OF THE CHAPLAIN OR PASTORAL CARE SERVICE

The ICU is a place that focuses on physical recovery and may neglect the other components of being human, including the emotional and spiritual aspects of life. Physical recovery and surviving the acute phase of illness to leave the ICU is considered a success in medicine. However, many patients suffer from anxiety, depression, and stress during their hospital course as well as posttraumatic stress disorder (PTSD) once they have returned home. The medications used to treat pain and sedate ICU patients can lead to confusion and delirium. Patients often feel they are in a most unusual, neither sleeping nor waking dream state; they may also hallucinate. Patients often lose sense of time and will report that they remember none of their ICU stay, or will recall small, distorted glimpses of events. This loss of time, memory, and perceptions can cause great distress for the patient and the family. The emotional and spiritual distress can last for an extended period—potentially months to years—after an ICU stay.

Patients often have concerns about the well-being of their family, who they see as upset, crying, and talking in hushed tones around them. The care team will often talk about the patient in front of the patient and family, rather than talk to the patient (who may be sedated), creating the impression the care team is ignoring the patient. If the patient is the primary financial support for the family, the patient may have anxiety about providing for them while they are sick. If the family relies on the patient as the "glue" that holds the family together, seeing them in this weakened state can be very traumatic. The patient may be dealing with the reality of their potential death, and the impact that will have on others. All these concerns and more are seen every day by the care team in an ICU setting, driving the need for deliberate patient and family support. To that end, no single support technique works for everyone, cementing the need for multiple avenues of support, and pastoral care fills a unique role to meet that need.

Each care team member plays a different role in the emotional and spiritual support of the patient and family. The ICU physician (intensivist), who leads the team, will meet the patient and family, answer questions about the plan of care and prognosis, expected recovery, and provides information regarding the completeness of care. If the patient is steadily recovering, that will be shared in a reassuring way. When patients are doing poorly—despite maximal care—the intensivist must also inform family members or other decision-makers of a poor prognosis. These conversations are quite challenging for everyone, including the intensivist. Intensivists are often supported by Advanced Practice Providers (APP; Nurse Practitioners or Physician Assistants) who also address acute medical and surgical care (see Chapter 3). The Intensivist tends to focus on the physical components of the medical or surgical plan and relies on other members of the team to help with the psychosocial concerns.

The bedside nurse, who spends the most time with the patient, often provides most of the emotional support to the patient and family. The ICU pharmacist will help guide medication changes to safely manage patient discomfort and help reduce delirium and confusion. The social worker or case manager provides information on financial resources and emotional support. All members of the care team are critical to the treatment and recovery of the patient. However, very few, if any, focus on the spiritual aspect of the patient and family, thus the important role of the chaplain in patient care.

The chaplain often spends considerable time with patients and family members learning about their emotional and spiritual needs. Importantly, the latter occurs regardless of the specific faith practiced by the patient and family—or if they are not currently practicing or have never practiced. Spiritual needs may blossom in the face of critical illness, and especially around grave diagnosis such as metastatic cancer, or at the end of life after injury. For patients who cannot speak due to care devices such as a breathing tube connecting them to a ventilator, there are pictorial guides that may be used to help learn about and support spiritual care in the ICU. The chaplain helps address all of these aspects of care. Quite often, patients (if they can participate) and families (if the patient cannot participate) desire to pray at the bedside. The chaplain helps facilitate this and will welcome critical care team members who wish to participate.

On occasion, and primarily for those with a pre-hospitalization faith-based life, a member of the religious community who leads the place of devotion that the patient attends will come to the bedside to guide prayer. The chaplain commonly helps facilitate those events. Specific faith-based or spiritual needs required at the end-of-life needs may necessitate engagement from spiritual and religious leaders outside hospital-based chaplains, especially within specific faiths. Since many patients transition from an acute care facility to one that provides more long-term care or acute rehabilitation services, ongoing spiritual care is also facilitated by the chaplaincy support services at the next facility along the patient's journey to recovery.

When there is conflict regarding how care is to be delivered, or what care is to be pursued, that conflict routinely impacts the critical care team members as well. Unanticipated diagnoses, complex cancer care, and end-of-life issues, in particular, trigger conflict between the patient and the care team, the patient and their family, the family and the care team, as well as between different care teams. Moral distress is common and is quite difficult to manage during a busy shift while caring for critically ill or injured patients. These observations apply to every team member, not just the intensivist, the bedside nurse, or the APP. Chaplains often leverage break times to help support distressed team members. It is a common observation that the person who is routinely met with a smile and wished well upon entry into the high acuity ICU is the chaplain. Naturally, chaplains support one another but they each also pursue comfort, guidance, and aid within their individual faith-based pursuits.

■ SPECIAL CONSIDERATIONS

Jehovah's Witness Patients and Blood Transfusion

Occasionally a patient will arrive to the hospital *in extremis*, unable to communicate, and without family present. Standard medical and surgical treatments are provided in the absence of a directive to avoid specific ones including cardiopulmonary resuscitation or blood component transfusion. Occasionally, the patient will be a Jehovah's Witness, who if asked, would refuse all blood transfusions. Until the patient regains consciousness, or the family arrives and shares the patient's spiritual beliefs, the care team is obligated to provide usual care. Once the team understands the patient's preferences, care can be aligned with the patient's beliefs. Nonetheless, Jehovah's Witness patients who received emergency blood transfusions may experience great distress. Care team members may similarly experience distress once they learn about the patient's beliefs. Discussions that provide full disclosure are commonly undertaken so that everyone is clear about what has occurred and why.

The care team will meet with the patient and family and reassure them they did not intend to violate the patient's spiritual beliefs, but that they did not know the beliefs at the time they needed to provide emergency care. Moreover, the standard of care was to transfuse blood products to save the patient's life—an obligation that the care team was legally required to meet. Then the care team will address the limitations of blood products as some Jehovah's Witness believers will accept products that are not red blood cells such as plasma, platelets, albumin, and erythropoietin—a protein-based hormonal stimulator of red blood cell production. The leaders of their denomination often come to the hospital to work with the care team in providing direction for further treatments, discuss the blood products that were given, and recognize the patient was unable to participate in their care at the time, and that the patient did not request the transfused blood components. The chaplain often serves as a liaison for the care team with the church leaders. Further discussions with the patient and the family about salvation and heaven are handled by the church leaders.

Culturally and Religiously Sensitive Care

In diverse ethnic cultures, religious beliefs are intimately linked to cultural beliefs. As international migration and travel continues to increase—especially for medical tourism—interactions within an ICU with individuals and family members raised in a non-Western culture are increasingly common. These aspects are important to recognize as the ethical principles that guide their decision-making and thoughts about specific aspects of care may be quite different from the four traditional pillars of Western ethics. These four pillars are autonomy, beneficence, justice, and non-maleficence. Chaplains are specifically trained to recognize and be facile at helping ICU clinicians navigate non-Western ethics. As such, chaplains are a key resource especially as discussions address goals of care and end-of-life issues. In this way, the chaplaincy often works synergistically with members of the Palliative Care Medicine team (see Palliative Care Medicine chapter 8). Depending on language capabilities, the use of a medical interpreter may be required to fully understand a patient's and family's goals, values, and preferences (see Limited English Proficiency chapter 24).

■ CONSIDERATIONS FOR RECOVERY

Patients will often experience suffering and spiritual distress after a brush with death. The uncertainty of outcome in the ICU, the anxiety about responsibilities, concerns for the family, and prolonged recovery all contribute to emotional distress of the patient and the family. When spirituality is of value to the patient, identifying and supporting that aspect is a key component of complete recovery. Although the patient may have physically recovered physically, the psychosocial, emotional, and spiritual component of convalescence can last months to years. Involving spiritual care services in the hospital, usually in the form of a chaplain, will provide important support for the patient and family—but may also support the care team. When pastoral care has measurably impacted critical illness or injury care, ongoing spirituality may be particularly impactful following home repatriation.

Tips for Clinicians

1. **Recognize** that the treatment and care of a patient and family involves **an emotional and spiritual component**.
2. **Ask patients and families if they have a spiritual belief system** and how best to support them.
3. **Offer spiritual support** through the hospital's chaplaincy service or the patients' outside spiritual support structure. Encourage spiritual support individuals to visit early and regularly during the course of critical illness or injury regardless of anticipated outcome.
4. **Spiritual support should be encouraged as a matter of routine** for critically ill or injured patients, and not principally reserved for the end of life.
5. **Recognize that patients may have spiritual distress** after an ICU stay especially when death was a prominent possibility.
6. When spiritual aid has been of value during ICU care, **it is appropriate to encourage patients to embrace spiritual care** as part of their recovery. Encouraging a spiritual journey and fellowship can be an important part of outpatient treatment and recovery.
7. **If you are comfortable, offer to pray with the patient and family**, or if the family asks, join in their prayer. Even standing silently at the bedside while the family prays is helpful to the patient and family as your presence is commonly viewed as supportive. Moreover, this action becomes the converse of having the family join the ICU team—you become a member of their team as well.

KEY REFERENCES

Balboni TA, Paulk ME, Balboni MJ, et al. Provision of spiritual care to patients with advanced cancer: associations with medical care and quality of life near death. *J Clin Oncol.* 2010;28(3):445.

Berning JN, Poor AD, Buckley SM, et al. A novel picture guide to improve spiritual care and reduce anxiety in mechanically ventilated adults in the intensive care unit. *Ann Am Thorac Soc.* 2016;13(8):1333-1342.

Gijsberts MJ, Liefbroer AI, Otten R, Olsman E. Spiritual care in palliative care: a systematic review of the recent European literature. *Med Sci.* 2019;7(2):25.

Hennessy N, Neenan K, Brady V, et al. End of life in acute hospital setting—a systematic review of families' experience of spiritual care. *J Clin Nurs.* 2020;29(7-8):1041-1052.

Ho JQ, Nguyen CD, Lopes R, et al. Spiritual care in the intensive care unit: a narrative review. *J Intensive Care Med.* 2018;33(5):279-287.

Hope AA, Munro CL. Sacramental moments: presence as spiritual care in the intensive care unit. *Am J Crit Care.* 2022;31(4):261-263.

Johnson JR, Engelberg RA, Nielsen EL, et al. The Association of Spiritual Care Providers' activities with family members' satisfaction with care after a death in the ICU. *Crit Care Med*. 2014;42(9):1991.

Labuschagne D, Torke A, Grossoehme D, et al. Chaplaincy care in the MICU: describing the spiritual care provided to MICU patients and families at the end of life. *Am J Hosp Palliat Med*. 2020;37(12):1037-1044.

Massey K, Barnes MJ, Villines D, et al. What do I do? Developing a taxonomy of chaplaincy activities and interventions for spiritual care in intensive care unit palliative care. *BMC Palliat Care*. 2015;14(1):1-8.

Simeone IM, Berning JN, Hua M, et al. Training chaplains to provide communication-board-guided spiritual care for intensive care unit patients. *J Palliat Med*. 2021;24(2):218-225.

Wall RJ, Engelberg RA, Gries CJ, et al. Spiritual care of families in the intensive care unit. *Crit Care Med*. 2007;35(4):1084-1090.

Willemse S, Smeets W, Van Leeuwen E, et al. Spiritual care in the ICU: perspectives of Dutch intensivists, ICU nurses, and spiritual caregivers. *J Relig Health*. 2018;57(2):583-595.

CHAPTER 10

Wound Care Specialist Perspective

Aron Wahrman

Patient Care Vignette

A 67-year-old woman was admitted for an elective aortic valve replacement. Operation was uneventful and she was admitted to the ICU having been extubated in the Operating Room. She did well and was transferred to the acute care floor on day 2. A Rapid Response Team was activated due to shortness of breath and low oxygen saturation. She was readmitted to the ICU where she was found to have pneumonia. She required intubation and invasive mechanical ventilation, and then developed septic shock. She needed temporary dialysis for salt and water overload while her kidneys recovered. She survived the long ICU course (2 months) but developed pressure ulcers along her buttocks, heels, and the back of her head. Local wound care including a wound care specialist addressed her wounds and they were starting to heal when she was transferred to an acute rehabilitation facility. The wounds are painful and interfere with her ability to participate in rehabilitation as completely as she and her family would like.

▉ ROLE OF THE WOUND CARE SPECIALIST IN THE ICU

Wound care specialists (WCSs) are unique clinicians who are brought to the bedside by a clinical team to aid in preventing, managing, and following both acute and chronic wounds. In the ICU, acute wounds are the more common problem to be addressed. WCSs may be specifically trained nurses, advanced practice providers (more commonly nurse practitioners than physician assistants), but quite commonly include surgeons trained in plastic and reconstructive surgery (aka. plastic surgeon). For certain wounds, surgeons will need to operate to clear infected or dead tissue, a process termed *debridement*.

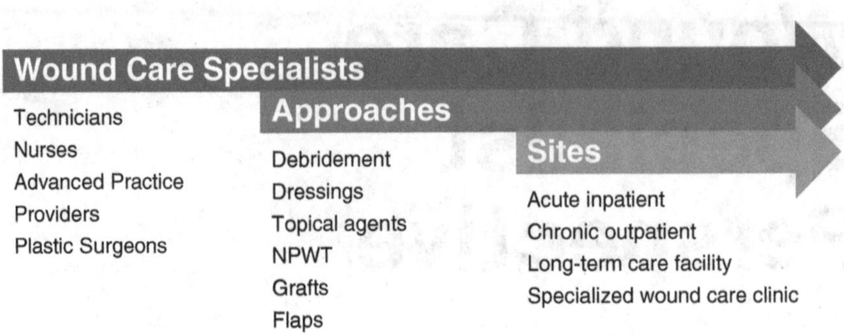

Wound Care Specialists

Technicians
Nurses
Advanced Practice
Providers
Plastic Surgeons

Approaches

Debridement
Dressings
Topical agents
NPWT
Grafts
Flaps

Sites

Acute inpatient
Chronic outpatient
Long-term care facility
Specialized wound care clinic

FIGURE 10-1. **Wound Care Specialists and Types of Care Provided.**

In some facilities, there is a wound care team that involves all of these kinds of WCSs. These team members help assess wounds, determine how they arose, prescribe and deliver therapies to address wounds, and regularly participate in quality initiatives to help decrease the likelihood of acute wounds from developing. Examples of such initiatives include deploying pressure relief mattresses and specialty beds for certain patient populations, evaluating the impact of long Operating Room (OR) times on pressure ulcers in those with clinically severe obesity, and recommending best practices for hospital teams to reduce wounds related to how devices are secured to patients (e.g., indwelling bladder catheter, aka "Foley" catheter). Therefore, the WCS is an integral member of the ICU team with roles that extend to the acute care floor and outpatient care since wounds may persist beyond the patient's ICU and hospital stay (Fig. 10-1).

■ WHAT HAPPENS IN THE ICU FROM THE PERSPECTIVE OF THE WOUND CARE SPECIALIST?

The surgical ICU presents a particular set of challenges with respect to wounds. Wounds encountered in the ICU range from the acute wounds of injury, burns, incisional wounds related to the elective procedures, to the wounds that arise due to complications of care. The latter are particularly troubling for patients and family members as they are unanticipated—even if their presence is not particularly surprising to the bedside clinician. For instance, a patient with a surgical site infection after colon resection occurs with a non-zero frequency—a complication that is infrequent (<2%) but difficult to completely eliminate. When that infection surfaces, it is a surprise for the patient and the family and generates tremendous concern. Moreover, daily wound care serves as a regular reminder that "something is not right." The WCS plays a key role in addressing not only wound management, but also patient and family concerns. In this way, the WCS integrates with the rest of the ICU team to support patient- and family-centered care.

When patients have critical illness or injury, the ICU is the best hospital location to provide care. Nonetheless, the kinds of care that are required are often invasive, cross skin barriers, and increase the risk of infection. Advanced therapies such as extracorporeal membrane oxygenation, or an open body cavity (abdomen or chest), may preclude the usual measures that help prevent pressure ulceration (e.g., frequent repositioning for pressure relief). Sometimes, the disease process increases the risk of wounds such as those that have prominent diarrhea (e.g., *Clostridium difficile* infection) and need a catheter and bag management system to control stool flow. This therapeutic device is known as a fecal management system but may lead to buttock and perianal skin maceration, infection, and ulceration. Nonetheless, it is better than not having such a system with regard to skin care. Much less commonly, such as with certain kinds of infections (e.g., "flesh-eating" bacterial infections of the buttocks and perineum), fecal diversion with a temporary colostomy may be ideal. Other therapies such as concomitant external beam radiation therapy for certain cancers, such as those of the head and neck region, also damages skin and makes it vulnerable to minor stress or injury that healthy skin would otherwise tolerate. Indeed, wounds are injuries and impact the human body's largest organ—the skin. The skin provides barrier function and has key roles in protective sensation, thermoregulation, and excretion of salt and water. Therefore, while not all wounds are avoidable, there is a significant emphasis on trying to do so, and a WCS is an essential part of that approach. When wounds are identified, care is designed to support the well-defined healing process.

Healing of the skin, in an otherwise healthy individual, follows a predictable chain of events but always occurs with an increase in metabolic demand; healing requires energy and relies on having appropriate nutrition as well as optimal vitamin supplementation (especially Vitamin C). There are three phases of wound healing: inflammation, proliferation, and remodeling. Inflammation brings cells to the wound to help address infection and increase local blood flow. This is a helpful process that is supported by either systemic or local antibiotics if there is infection. Proliferation is the phase when the wound starts to fill in and may also begin to contract. The wound looks smaller and may look quite red at its base as blood vessels continue to increase—an adaptive process as wound repair requires oxygen and nutrients for growing cells. Remodeling occurs once the wound is closed and benefits from topical protectants that maintain skin moisture and provide UV protection as well (if there is to be sun exposure). During this phase, redness begins to fade, and the healing wound may be more pale than surrounding uninjured skin. It is important to recognize that the first two processes occur much more rapidly than remodeling—a process that can continue for up to 2 years.

These processes are often inapparent when wounds are closed quite rapidly after they are created. This occurs after a simple laceration, or during an elective operation (primary closure). Some wounds may be left open for a few days to determine if they are clean enough to close; sutures are often placed but not tied in this circumstance (delayed primary closure). Other wounds are left to fill themselves in and close over a much longer period of time (secondary closure); healthy people often close a wound from the edge toward the center by about 1 mm per day. Some wounds that are left open (especially those that were heavily contaminated or infected, or those that had some dead tissue that was removed and is now clean) may be closed using a graft or a flap. This method of closure reduces the metabolic demand on the wound and the patient and may achieve immediate wound closure. Not everyone is suitable for this approach depending on their medical conditions, available tissue (muscle, fat, and skin), or nutrition. The customization of wound care using the wide array of approaches and products requires a clinician well-versed in their use to most rapidly help wounds to heal. The WCS is also ideally suited to help address preexisting wounds using those same approaches and products. Of course, some wounds need to be prepared to benefit from those products, and a surgical approach may be required.

Mentioned above, debridement is the removal of dead, badly scarred, infected, or poorly perfused (inadequate blood supply) tissue in the OR, or applying specific enzymes to wounds, or by using a variety of dressings that help in this process. The goal is to create a clean wound that is healthy and can then begin to heal on its own or be helpful to heal using a surgical approach to wound closure. An interesting combination of the surgical and the enzymatic approaches can involve the use of medical-grade maggots—an approach termed *biosurgery*. Maggots only consume dead tissue and always leave a healthy base behind. While helpful in wound care, patients and families (as well as ICU clinicians) may be uncomfortable at the prospect! The maggots are sterile and cannot reproduce. A wide variety of other kinds of dressings are more commonly used and worthwhile exploring.

■ DRESSINGS (FIG. 10-1)

In general, moist environments are good for wounds. Even the act of removing a dressing is fraught with potential injury if newly grown skin is stuck to a dried-out dressing (specifically allowing the dressing to dry out is useful for debridement but not for healing). Dressings can be simply categorized in the following fashion:

1. Gauze dressing: A simple dressing that can hold topical agents in place, and provides a breathable barrier over the top of wounds; generally, it requires some adhesive tape or wrap to keep it in place.

2. Adhesive semipermeable barrier: Retains moisture and can be coupled with a topical agent that is held in place by the dressing.
3. Foam dressing: Some absorptive capacity for low-volume drainage wounds.
4. Alginate dressing: Absorbs moisture to reduce fluid and protein losses; absorbs more fluid than simple gauze dressings; often contain antimicrobial silver ions.
5. Negative pressure wound therapy (See device-based therapies): A dressing that requires an external powered device to generate continuous negative pressure across a wound; manages large volume drainage and must be applied to only a clean wound; device also has battery power to support mobility; generally, it is applied by a clinician rather than the patient or uncompensated caregiver like a family member.
6. Collagen products and decellularized scaffolds: These are most commonly applied as a cover for chronic ulcers; may help attract specific cells needed for wound healing; many come from mammals (humans, pigs, sheep, etc.) but can also come from fish (cod).

Dressings often keep topical agents in place which also help with wound care and healing. They may start to be used in the ICU and may continue through discharge. These may be conveniently grouped as follows:

1. Salt and water (0.9% NSS solution) simply provides moisture and is often used as an initial moisture providing solution that is allowed to desiccate to aid in debridement.
2. Dilute bleach solution (Dakin's solution) is a topical solution that helps control bacteria, especially *Pseudomonas* (bacteria that turns dressings green).
3. Hydrocolloid gel: This thick gel helps maintain wound moisture to aid in healing.
4. Platelet-derived growth factor: The only FDA-approved topical containing a known cytokine in isolated form involved in wound healing; its best use may be in rescue for diabetic foot ulcers that have failed other therapies.
5. Collagenase: This enzyme helps with wound debridement using an enzyme that breaks down collagen.

■ DEVICE-BASED THERAPIES

Negative Pressure Wound Therapy (NPWT)

Open wounds heal on applying negative pressure across the wound surface(s). Originally identified as vacuum-assisted closure (i.e., a wound "VAC"), the variety of devices are broadly categorized as NPWT devices (Fig. 10-1). Negative pressure across a wound surface increases blood flow, decreases bacteria, and decreases inflammatory molecules, all of which increase the rate of healing and closure. That pressure is applied across a sponge placed in the wound and then covered by an adhesive barrier that is attached to the suction device. The dressing is then changed every other, or every third, day as opposed to daily or more frequently. This approach reduces pain and resource use and is well-received by patients and families. Devices may be quite small or much larger depending on the volume of drainage. Modifications of these devices are plentiful and include intermittent or continuous suction, as well as the ability to irrigate wounds with a variety of substances.

Hyperbaric Oxygen (HBO)

While oxygen is required for the vast majority of living organisms, very high concentrations of oxygen may be toxic to bacteria. This is the premise behind using hyperbaric oxygen (HBO) therapy. The only way to reach very high oxygen concentration in tissues is to deliver that oxygen under pressure. Indeed, HBO is delivered in a "dive" chamber in order to increase the pressure above atmospheric pressure. HBO is generally used for certain difficult to treat infections (e.g., some soft tissue infections as well as osteomyelitis, a bone infection) and to help in wound healing when there may be inadequate but not absent blood flow. There is some data that HBO can help increase the density of local small blood vessels as a means of supporting wound repair. HBO may be used for critically ill patients but does come with risks related to transport out of the ICU, as well as risks related to the pressure—risks that are similar to those from scuba diving including the "bends," eardrum rupture, visual changes, and lung injury. Naturally, since compression is a slow process to reach the desired pressure, so too is decompression to avoid complications with too rapid pressure decreases. HBO is not the standard therapy, but may be beneficial for specific patient populations. Not all centers can provide HBO and reimbursement may be insurer dependent. HBO may be more ideally aligned with the management of chronic wounds, and therefore, outpatient HBO may follow initial inpatient therapy.

■ CHRONIC WOUNDS

Wounds, particularly chronic wounds, represent a tremendous financial and psychological burden beyond the individual patient and those engaged in patient care (clinicians and family members). Upward of 2% of the population in the developed world will at some point be afflicted with a chronic wound. In the United States this accounts for roughly 6.5 million people at an estimated cost of about $25 billion. Such wounds are increasingly common related to increased life-span coupled with comorbid conditions such as diabetes and cancer that are also on the rise. Chronic wounds lead to hospitalizations and other acute sequelae such as sepsis and limb loss. Early recognition of risk factors, team-based approaches to care, evidence based care regimens, and management of co-morbid conditions are each essential to reducing the incidence of chronic wounds and the cost of their care. In all cases, whether traditional wound care or advanced products, one cannot over emphasize the concurrent management of diabetic (glycemic) control, adequate nutrition, cessation in any nicotine use (especially inhaled tobacco products), and optimization of blood inflow and outflow. Clearly, the WCS is only one team member needed in the comprehensive care of patients with acute or chronic wounds (Fig. 10-1).

■ CONSIDERATIONS FOR RECOVERY

Acute wound care may be initiated in the ICU but may extend into convalescence (Fig. 10-1). It is essential to note that the therapy initiated during a critical care episode often needs periodic adjustment as the wound evolves toward healing, or devolves toward expansion or infection. This requires repeated evaluation by a WCS, some of which can be accomplished using telehealth instead of in-person visits. This approach has been popularized during the SARS-CoV-2 pandemic when in-person care was derailed. As complex care is often regionalized to tertiary or quaternary centers, patients may receive their initial care far from where they live. Convalescent care in an acute rehabilitation facility, or skilled nursing facility that is close to their home, places them remote from those engaged in their critical care. Telehealth can bridge that gap for the patient and the family, and ideally also embraces the primary care clinician.

Having an integrated team-based approach to wound care helps navigate some of the social determinants of health that include home-based nursing evaluation, durable medical equipment, transportation, and wound care supplies, and helps reflect access to care as well as the financial underpinning to secure that care. Furthermore, telehealth approaches help bolster patient and family comfort with care that they are providing, as well as the security that flows from engaging in scheduled re-evaluation. Finally, it also provides an opportunity to determine when an in-person visit is truly required. One of the reasons for in-person care relates to the capabilities of a fully resourced wound care clinic including equipment, specialty dressings, and skilled wound care technicians who work with a WCS.

On occasion, wounds develop during convalescence that expose implanted medical devices (aka. prosthetic devices). Such devices may include vascular access devices (e.g., a "port" for nutritional therapy or chemotherapy), nonbiologic mesh used for hernia repair, hardware placed for fracture fixation, and pacemakers. This is a complex kind of wound that generally requires inpatient evaluation and care. Most commonly, the device needs to be removed to control infection with later reimplantation of the device. Surgical therapy may also require a local rearrangement flap to bring healthy tissue to the wound site, but may also require an advanced microsurgical flap to be created. Regardless of the approach, initial care is best accomplished as an inpatient. Infections of devices implanted in the vascular space are true emergencies to address.

Nutrition therapy is essential and should deliver more protein that individuals need at baseline to support wound repair. Routine vitamin supplementation including a multivitamin, B-complex, thiamine, folate, and zinc should be coupled with vitamin C. Individuals with problematic absorption of iron or B12 should also receive supplementation. Importantly, each of these has some impact on red blood cell production and in turn supports oxygen uptake, carriage, and delivery. Consultation with a registered dietitian may be particularly helpful in constructing an appropriate regimen, especially when the patient has baseline organ failure (e.g., hepatic, pulmonary, endocrine, or renal).

Tips for Clinicians

1. Wound care may begin in the ICU but often carries over into convalescence. **Assess ICU survivors' wound care needs early in the ICU recovery period** and ensure that patients and families have sufficient support to care for wounds.
2. Patients with advanced age, multiple comorbidities, malnutrition, and tobacco use are at high risk for developing acute and chronic wounds. **Monitor wound progression over time** (photographs can be useful for this) and consult plastic surgeons, wound care specialists, and/or nutritionists as needed to ensure timely healing.
3. A wound care specialist team, as well as a wound care clinic, is ideally suited for acute care, but may also interface with patients, families, and primary care clinicians during outpatient recovery. **Maintain a low threshold for consulting outpatient wound care specialists** for complex, worsening, or nonhealing wounds.
4. Wound care may be quite costly and challenging when patients are repatriated to their home communities from a tertiary or quaternary care center. **Telehealth resources may help bridge service gaps** in a financially responsible manner that also supports patient- and family-centered care.

KEY REFERENCES

Agarwal P, Kukrele R, Sharma D. Vacuum assisted closure (VAC)/negative pressure wound therapy (NPWT) for difficult wounds: a review. *J Clin Ortho Trauma*. 2019;10(5):845-848.

Chanussot-Deprez C, Contreras-Ruiz J. Telemedicine in wound care: a review. *Adv Skin Wound Care*. 2013;26(2):78-82.

Hajhosseini B, Kuehlmann BA, Bonham CA, Kamperman KJ, Gurtner GC. Hyperbaric oxygen therapy: descriptive review of the technology and current application in chronic wounds. *Plast Reconstr Surg Glob Open*. 2020;8(9):e3136.

Han G, Ceilly R. Chronic wound healing; a review of current management and treatments. *Adv Ther*. 2017;344:599-610.

Huang C, Leavitt T, Bayer LR, Orgill DP. Effect of negative pressure wound therapy on wound healing. *Curr Prob Surg*. 2014;51(7):301-331.

Jones C, Rothermel A, Mackay D. Evidence based medicine: wound management. *J Plastic Reconstruct Surg*. 2017;140(1):201e-216e.

Kim PJ, Evans KK, Steinberg JS, Pollard ME, Attinger CE. Critical elements to building an effective wound care center. *J Vasc Surg*. 2013;57(6):1703-1709.

Memar MY, Yekani M, Alizadeh N, Baghi HB. Hyperbaric oxygen therapy: antimicrobial mechanisms and clinical application for infections. *Biomed Pharmacother*. 2019; 109:440-447.

Nazarko L. Choosing the correct wound care dressing: an overview. *J Comm Nurs*. 2018; 32(5):45.

Nuutila K, Eriksson E. Moist wound healing with commonly available dressings. *Adv Wound Care*. 2021;10(12):685-698.

Rohrich RJ. The "soft-tissue wound management: current applications of negative pressure wound therapy with instillation" supplement. *J Plast Reconstr Surg*. 2021;147(1S-1):1S-2S.

Tavakoli S, Klar AS. Bioengineered skin substitutes: advances and future trends. *Appl Sci*. 2021;11(4):1493.

Zhang AY, Meine JG. Flaps and grafts reconstruction. *Dermatologic Clin*. 2011;29(2):217-230.

The Nutritionist's Perspective

Kim Sabino and Julie Fuller

Patient Care Vignette

A 70-year-old man, BT, presented to the emergency department with acute onset abdominal pain, vomiting, tachycardia, hypotension, and an increased white blood cell count. Past medical and surgical history were notable for type 1 diabetes mellitus, hypertension, and total knee and hip replacements. His admission weight was 70 kg with a height of 71 inches (BMI 21.5 kg/m^2). His weight was stable, and he had a normal appetite until the day prior to admission. Imaging was suggestive of diverticulitis with an uncontained perforation. BT was taken to the operating room for an emergent exploratory laparotomy and underwent a sigmoid colectomy with end colostomy. He was admitted to the ICU due to septic shock, and the need for mechanical ventilation and a continuous vasopressor infusion to maintain an adequate blood pressure. With source control and appropriate antibiotic therapy, BT's clinical condition rapidly improved.

After having his breathing tube removed, BT was advanced to a diet that included oral nutrition supplements (ONS) appropriate for a patient with diabetes by postoperative day (POD) 2. On POD 4, BT reported poor appetite and was taking less than 25% of his estimated nutritional needs. He related his poor appetite to feeling full earlier than usual (early satiety) and fatigue. To maximize menu options, BT's diet was liberalized to a regular diet. Alternative ONS were explored, and his family agreed to bring in food from home. By POD 7 his oral intake increased to about 50% of estimated needs from meals and ONS. At this point he had lost ~3.6 kg (~5% body weight) since admission. Given his persistent suboptimal intake and weight loss, the patient met criteria for supplemental enteral nutrition (EN). He agreed to nasogastric small-bore feeding tube placement. Nocturnal EN was initiated to provide ~70% of his estimated caloric needs to supplement his oral nutrition. Despite these maneuvers, BT's oral intake did not improve. A more durable feeding tube would be of benefit and his surgeon planned on placing a gastrostomy tube (a feeding tube that crosses the abdominal wall to directly enter the stomach).

While awaiting time in the operating room (OR), BT's wound opened and drained both pus and what seemed to be stool. BT's wound fell apart due to infection related to a fistula that formed from his colon to the surgical closure. His skin was opened by removing the skin staples and the wound was packed with moistened gauze with plans for regular dressing changes. Relatedly, gastrostomy tube placement was deferred in the setting of acute infection. Since the fistula seemed to be low output, the surgical team pursued nonoperative management of the fistula with continuation of EN and oral diet. Many low-output fistulas will close on their own if their output is low and nutrition is excellent. Unfortunately, the fistula output progressively increased and became a high-output fistula. At that point in time, reoperating would be quite challenging due to adhesions that normally form, increasing the risk of unintentional intestinal injury. Therefore, EN and oral diet were both discontinued to try to decrease fistula flow. To meet BT's nutritional needs, he was started on parenteral nutrition (PN; also called total parenteral nutrition or TPN), an intravenous approach that would meet his nutritional needs. Despite PN, he sustained a further ~2.5 kg weight loss. His strength and endurance progressively deteriorated as he developed progressive malnutrition.

His PN prescription was adjusted to meet his protein needs to support healing. As his strength began to improve, BT's condition was appropriate for considering transfer to an inpatient rehabilitation center to further improve strength and endurance. He was discharged on PN with a plan to await either: (1) spontaneous fistula closure, or (2) failure of fistula closure but successful nutritional rescue. Prior to being discharged to the rehabilitation center, the PN was adjusted from infusing 24 hours per day to a 12-hour nocturnal schedule to allow for daily activities while untethered from the infusion pump. He was discharged from the rehabilitation center after 3 weeks and went home with continued PN. The fistula spontaneously closed over time, and BT resumed oral intake in consultation with his primary care clinician and an outpatient registered dietitian. Food did not initially taste the same to him, which led him to eat less than desired—a source of major concern to him and his family. His taste gradually returned, oral intake improved, and he was transitioned off PN.

■ INTRODUCTION

Critical illness or injury generates an inflammatory response that increases energy expenditure, leading to a state of catabolism. Catabolism leads to consumption of fat and skeletal muscle that is identified as not only weight loss but also weakness. It is estimated that half of ICU patients are at risk for developing malnutrition. Patients in the ICU and those recovering from critical illness or injury therefore benefit from medical nutrition therapy (MNT) to prevent or treat malnutrition.

MNT typically includes enteral nutrition (EN, nutrition via the GI tract), parenteral nutrition (PN, intravenous nutrition), or oral nutritional supplementation, either alone or in combination. Intensive care patients are usually screened for malnutrition risk and assessed for malnutrition to help select the most appropriate MNT intervention. MNT interventions started in the critical care setting often continue after ICU discharge. For this reason, clinicians caring for ICU survivors need to understand the nutritional needs driven by critical illness as well as the interventions to maintain or improve nutritional status. This chapter describes approaches to screening patients for malnutrition and various interventions that support patients' nutrition during recovery from critical illness.

■ NUTRITION SCREENING AND ASSESSMENT

Nutrition screening tools assist the clinician in identifying patients who may be at risk for developing malnutrition. Malnutrition is graded as mild, moderate, or severe and there are guidelines to help diagnose which one, if any, a patient demonstrates. Medical professional organizations such as the American Society of Parenteral and Enteral Nutrition (ASPEN) and its European Union counterpart (ESPEN) are devoted to nutrition assessment and management. The results generated from the screening process inform the clinician team which patients may benefit most from MNT and potentially predict outcomes. These scores consider age, comorbidities, severity of acute illness, dietary intake following hospital admission, and sometimes additional factors such as laboratory markers of nutritional health or inflammation. Some dietitians take a more nihilistic approach, considering every patient who requires a 48-hour or longer stay in the ICU to be at risk for malnutrition.

Malnutrition is diagnosed using multiple criteria, including weight loss, reduced muscle mass, and a history of reduced intake (Table 11-1). A large proportion, 30-80%, of ICU patients have been found to be malnourished. This diagnosis is associated with longer hospital and ICU length of stay, infectious complications, increased in-hospital mortality, increased

■ TABLE 11-1. AND/ASPEN and GLIM Malnutrition Criteria

Criteria	GLIM[a]	AND/ASPEN[b]
Phenotypic		
Weight loss	X	X
Low BMI[c]	X	
Reduced muscle mass	X	X
Etiologic		
Reduced food/energy intake	X	X
Impaired absorption	X	
Inflammation	X	
Subcutaneous fat loss		X
Fluid accumulation		X
Reduced hand grip strength		X

[a]GLIM recommends at least one phenotypic and one etiologic criteria combination to diagnose malnutrition (Cederholm, T., Jensen, G.L., Correia, M.I.T.D., Gonzalez, M.C., Fukushima, R., Higashiguchi, T., Baptista, G., Barazzoni, R., Blaauw, R., Coats, A.J.S. and Crivelli, A.N., 2019. GLIM criteria for the diagnosis of malnutrition–a consensus report from the global clinical nutrition community. Journal of cachexia, sarcopenia and muscle, 10(1), pp.207-217.) https://onlinelibrary.wiley.com/doi/full/10.1002/jcsm.12383
[b]AND/ASPEN recommends identifying two or more of their six listed criteria to diagnose malnutrition (White, J.V., Guenter, P., Jensen, G., Malone, A., Schofield, M., Force, A.M.T. and Academy Malnutrition Work Group, 2012. Consensus statement of the Academy of Nutrition and Dietetics/American Society for Parenteral and Enteral Nutrition: characteristics recommended for the identification and documentation of adult malnutrition (undernutrition). Journal of the Academy of Nutrition and Dietetics, 112(5), pp.730-738.) https://www.sciencedirect.com/science/article/pii/S2212267212003280
[c]Correlated with age and adaptation for Asian race.
AND, Academy of Nutrition and Dietetics; ASPEN, American Society for Parenteral and Enteral Nutrition; BMI, body mass index; GLIM, Global Leadership Initiative on Malnutrition.

hospital readmissions, as well as long-term postdischarge consequences such as impaired functional capacity and prolonged poor oral intake. For this reason, malnutrition screening, prevention, and treatment measures are common in the ICU and post-ICU phases of care for patients with critical illness.

A patient identified as being nutritionally at risk, or having malnutrition, will prompt a comprehensive nutrition assessment. The nutrition assessment includes communication with ICU team members, engagement with the patient, family, or individuals who provided care prior to admission. Other information obtained may include nutrition intake prior to admission, weight history, physical examination, gastrointestinal function assessment, chewing and swallowing function, laboratory parameters, psychosocial and socioeconomic factors, cultural or religious practices, medication use, comorbidities, and functional capacity. There is growing interest in using imaging tools such as bioelectrical impedance, ultrasound, and computed tomography (CT) imaging to assess muscle and adipose (fat) mass. Imaging guidance may be limited by cost as well as the need for a standardized set of metrics used to report imaging-guided assessments of muscle and adipose as they relate to nutritional health. Presently, such assessments are not standard and may be considered investigational.

■ INVOLVEMENT OF THE REGISTERED DIETITIAN

The registered dietitian (RD) is specifically trained to perform nutrition screenings, assessments, and monitoring. The RD is an expert who has met academic and professional requirements including licensing and certification standards. The RD can assist in deciding the optimal type of MNT by establishing energy and protein calculations, delineating electrolyte and fluid management approaches, nutrition support options to help improve blood sugar management, and EN access device recommendations. Dietitians are positioned to assist in identifying when other members of the care team are needed to optimize the patient's nutrition plan of care. For example, collaboration may be sought from rehabilitation therapists and physiatrists (Chapter 7) to improve or prevent worsening functional status, or to assist with selecting the most appropriate oral diet based on swallowing function. The muscles that are used for chewing and swallowing are skeletal muscles. As such, they too are subject to weakness from catabolism just like the muscles of the legs, arms, and abdominal wall. Dietitians are employed in a variety of units within acute care facilities, as well as within extended care facilities, and the outpatient setting for home care.

■ ESTIMATING ENERGY AND PROTEIN NEEDS

Energy needs are estimated by RDs and other members of the clinical team in multiple ways, including predictive weight-based equations and measurement through indirect calorimetry. Although indirect calorimetry measurement is considered the gold standard for estimating energy needs, it requires specialized equipment and staffing, and is therefore of limited availability. Accordingly, weight-based equations (e.g., 20-30 kcal/kg/day) are often used. These equations work best for patients with BMI 18.5-25 kg/m^2. For patients with BMI <18.5 kg/m^2, "ideal" body weight (IBW) may be used. For patients with BMI >25 kg/m^2, there is considerable variability between approaches used to estimate energy needs.

The amount of energy to provide to a patient classified as overweight (BMI >25 kg/m^2) or obese (BMI >30 kg/m^2) is challenging to determine and remains debated. In the absence of indirect calorimetry measurement, ASPEN guidelines recommend estimating energy requirements using 11-14 kcal per kilogram of *actual* body weight (ABW) for patients with a BMI of 30-50 kg/m^2, and 22-25 kcal per kilogram of *ideal* body weight per day for patients with a BMI

>50 kg/m^2. Recent research suggests that actual caloric needs are higher than this at ~18-21 kcal/kg ABW/day for the patient with a BMI of 30-39.9 kg/m^2 and ~16-17 kcal/kg ABW/day for the patient with a BMI of >40 kg/m^2. These are general guidelines and considerable adjustment typically occurs based upon a patient's degree of illness as well as organ function.

Adjustments to estimated protein needs are common in ICU patients. These may be guided by measurement of urinary nitrogen losses, lean body mass determination (e.g., through CT scanning), or by clinical situations in which increased protein catabolism is expected (e.g., burns, soft tissue losses, polytrauma). Often, a high protein but hypocaloric feeding approach is adopted in the ICU to preserve lean body mass, mobilize adipose stores, and minimize the metabolic complications of overfeeding. In particular, liver failure is a potential consequence of carbohydrate and fat overfeeding that critical care teams strive to avoid. Other clinical conditions such as an open abdomen or a gastrointestinal tract fistula will also increase protein losses out of proportion to the patient's body weight and should be accounted for in the nutritional prescription.

■ NUTRITION IN THE ICU PATIENT

In the early phase of acute illness (the first 48 hours), ICU clinicians often target nutrition below ~70% of energy expenditure to avoid overfeeding in the setting of endogenous energy production by catabolic processes. Patients may also be receiving calories from fluids with dextrose or medications with fat (e.g., propofol) or dextrose. After ICU day 3, goal energy needs are usually increased to 80-100% of total estimated energy needs.

About 40% of ICU patients are able to eat and oral diets are generally initiated as soon as medically appropriate. These oral diets may follow dietary restrictions that take the patient's medical comorbidities into consideration (e.g., carbohydrate-controlled diet for patients with diabetes, low sodium diets for patients with hypertension). Barriers to adequate nutrition intake in the ICU may include poor appetite, early satiety, altered gastrointestinal function (e.g., delayed gastric emptying), taste changes, chewing and swallowing impairment, fatigue, and pain. Texture modifications of liquids and solids may be needed for those with preexisting or acquired chewing and swallowing impairments. These textural modifications (e.g., pureed diet) can be unpleasant to patients, leading to decreased intake. Barriers to optimal nutrition in the ICU may still be present on ICU discharge and may complicate achieving nutritional goals during convalescence.

Often, ICU patients who do eat consume only ~30-50% of their energy needs and ~40% of their protein needs. Therefore, highly restrictive therapeutic diets are usually avoided. If such a diet was in place before ICU admission, it should be reconsidered upon hospital discharge. Oral nutritional supplements (ONS) are often introduced for those patients with suboptimal oral intake, or if suboptimal oral intake is anticipated. ONS consumption has been associated with reduced complications, reduced hospital readmissions, improved hand grip strength, and increased protein and energy intake. ONS are available in a variety of therapeutic options based on disease states, nutrition needs, and even flavoring choices.

When oral intake is not feasible, for example in the mechanically ventilated patient, EN initiation is usually started within 24-48 hours of ICU admission if not contraindicated (e.g., high-dose vasopressor therapy). EN is often started early because it has both nutritive and non-nutritive benefits, including a decreased risk of infection related to preservation of the gut mucosal barrier. EN is also sometimes started for patients who have insufficient (e.g., <70%) caloric intake by mouth. EN is usually administered via a tube placed into a nostril that follows the usual path to reach the stomach (i.e., a nasogastric or nasoenteric feeding tube). There are a number of different nasal tubes that may be utilized for nutrient—and medication—delivery. Some may deliberately have their tip end in the first portion of the small bowel (duodenum) to deliver food past the stomach. Others may have the tip placed even further distally (jejunum) depending on unique patient need. While tubes placed in the stomach may be "blindly" placed but confirmed by an X-ray, some form of either endoscopy or fluoroscopy is commonly required for the more distally placed tubes. Debate remains whether feeding in the stomach compared to a more distal site has a selective outcome advantage or a decreased risk of complication.

A variety of EN formulas are available based on individual needs. Standard, polymeric formulas contain intact protein, fat, and carbohydrate and are appropriate for most ICU patients. Elemental and semi-elemental formulas contain partially or completely hydrolyzed nutrients to maximize absorption without needing processing by gut lumen enzymes. Disease-specific formulas target organ dysfunction or specific metabolic conditions. Patients discharged from the ICU with ongoing EN therapy should have their formula reassessed to determine whether it is still appropriate for the patient once they have survived their ICU stay.

Parenteral nutrition (PN) includes total parenteral nutrition (TPN) and partial parenteral nutrition (PPN). PN can be administered to individuals who have exhausted all strategies to maximize gastrointestinal track luminal nutrition. PN is provided intravenously and requires that the catheter through which it infuses has its tip located in a high-flow centrally located vein (as opposed to a small peripheral vein commonly used to place a standard IV line).

Based on its components, PN formulations may be injurious to small and low-flow peripheral veins. PN contains amino acids, glucose, lipids, electrolytes vitamins, and trace elements. There are a variety of very specific indications for PN that reflect unique clinical conditions, but they may be conveniently grouped into the following two broad categories: (1) the inability to use the GI tract at all, (2) the inability to completely meet nutritional needs using the GI tract. Although PN is most commonly administered in the acute care setting, some patients may need to continue PN after hospital discharge. These patients will need frequent re-evaluation of their formula, review of serum electrolytes, and may need home care nursing support. In-hospital PN is generally delivered using a short-term catheter that is readily placed and removed at the bedside. Long-term catheter approaches exist to support home TPN and are readily cared for by patients, family members, and visiting nursing staff. Maintenance of aseptic technique during PN administration at home is key in preventing catheter-associated bloodstream infections.

■ REFEEDING SYNDROME RISK

Patients may be at risk for refeeding syndrome if they are inadequately nourished for an extended period either prior to, or during, their ICU stay. The reintroduction of carbohydrates or dextrose prompts a metabolic response that may lead to hypokalemia, hypomagnesemia, hypophosphatemia, and thiamine deficiency in an individual who has had a substantial period of undernourishment. Resuming dietary intake of the building blocks to form new cells allows that process to resume throughout the body. The lining of the gastrointestinal tract is continually renewed in health, but that process is severely curtailed during starvation. With feeding and new cell generation, electrolytes such as potassium and magnesium are sequestered inside the cells. Phosphate is consumed to manufacture phospholipids for new cell membranes and to support energy metabolism. The metabolic and physical manifestations of these electrolyte disturbances may lead to mild derangements or contribute to end-organ dysfunction and failure if not treated promptly. If refeeding syndrome is likely to occur, it typically manifests in the ICU. Table 11-2 outlines the ASPEN consensus recommendations for identifying patients at risk for refeeding syndrome.

■ POST-ICU CARE NUTRITION

Upon transitioning out of the ICU, the care team must continue to support patients' nutritional needs. Patients can continue with poor oral intake past their ICU stay, and have been shown to have marked weight loss; weight loss

■ **TABLE 11-2. ASPEN Refeeding Syndrome Consensus Criteria**

	Moderate Risk: 2 Risk Criteria Needed	Significant Risk: 1 Risk Criteria Needed
BMI	16-18.5 kg/m^2	<16 kg/m^2
Weight loss	5% in 1 month	7.5% in 3 months or >10% in 6 months
Caloric intake	None or negligible oral intake for 5-6 days **OR** <75% of estimated energy requirement for >7 days during an acute illness or injury **OR** <75% of estimated energy requirement for >1 month	None or negligible oral intake for >7 days **OR** <50% of estimated energy requirement for >5 days during an acute illness or injury **OR** <50% of estimated energy requirement for > 1 month
Abnormal prefeeding potassium, phosphorus, or magnesium serum concentrations[a]	Minimally low levels or normal current levels with recent low levels necessitating minimal or single-dose supplementation	Moderately/significantly low levels or minimally low/normal levels with recent low levels necessitating significant or multiple-dose supplementation
Loss of subcutaneous fat	Evidence of moderate loss	Evidence of severe loss
Loss of muscle mass	Evidence of mild or moderate loss	Evidence of severe loss
Higher-risk comorbidities	Moderate disease	Severe disease

ASPEN, American Society for Parenteral and Enteral Nutrition: BMI, body mass index.
[a]Please note electrolytes may be normal despite total-body deficiency, which is believed to increase risk of refeeding syndrome.
Reprinted with permission from Wiley (da Silva, J.S., Seres, D.S., Sabino, K., Adams, S.C., Berdahl, G.J., Citty, S.W., Cober, M.P., Evans, D.C., Greaves, J.R., Gura, K.M. and Michalski, A., 2020. ASPEN consensus recommendations for refeeding syndrome. Nutrition in Clinical Practice, 35(2), pp.178-195.) https://aspenjournals.onlinelibrary.wiley.com/doi/epdf/10.1002/ncp.10474

up to 1 kg/day has been reported. Barriers to adequate nutrition intake are remarkably similar in and outside of the ICU. As with patients in the ICU, minimally restricted diets are suggested, when possible, to maximize menu options. Providing ONS to enhance protein and energy intake is also advised.

For patients who are nourished using PN, a plan must be elaborated to help reduce PN intake while increasing oral intake, or EN via a feeding tube. A similar process should occur for those who have been supported using EN and are appropriate to transition to an oral intake regimen. These processes are both termed *transitional feeding* and there are multiple approaches to this process that are successful. However, transitional feeding ultimately relies on the ability to safely swallow.

Dysphagia may persist after transitioning out of the ICU. Rates of dysphagia following breathing tube removal (extubation) have been reported at nearly 40%. Collaboration with a speech and language pathologist (SLP; Chapter 7) may be beneficial to determine the safest option for swallowing liquids and solids.

SLP follow-up is essential for reassessment and diet advancement, as appropriate. If oral intake is unsafe or remains inadequate, an evaluation for semipermanent or permanent (e.g., surgical) EN feeding access is recommended. Because inflammation may persist for weeks—and in some cases months—nutrition support is often indicated after acute care facility discharge. Coordination with RDs at secondary care facilities to ensure that the nutrition support plan is continued is an important part of the care transition plan toward rehabilitation and recovery. Patients with open wounds, and those who need secondary procedures, often benefit from continued nutrition support even after home repatriation to enable wound healing or preparation for additional interventions.

■ CONSIDERATIONS FOR RECOVERY

Patients with malnutrition are more likely to be discharged to long-term care or rehabilitation facilities. They may also have increased postdischarge mortality and hospital readmission rates.

Patients may need to continue modified textured diets and liquids postdischarge as the muscles of chewing and swallowing regain mass and strength and coordination. Patients on modified-texture diets should be followed to move toward a less restrictive diet to optimize intake, as tolerated, and should be administered ONS—sometimes also modified for texture—given their risk of malnutrition. Patients receiving ONS during hospitalization should continue to consume them upon discharge, potentially for as long as 6 months, though more studies in this area are needed. Consumption of ONS posthospitalization has been associated with decreased hospital readmissions and improved functional status leading to improved quality of life.

Patients who are receiving EN or PN in the hospital may need to continue post-hospitalization. EN should be continued for patients at risk for nutritional deterioration or those with malnutrition who cannot meet their needs orally. Some patients, such as those who have suffered a major stroke or those with a high-output fistula, may need to continue EN or PN temporarily or as a permanent form of nutrition. Patients can continue EN or PN in their home, or in other care settings including group homes, long-term care facilities, and rehabilitation centers. Insurance companies have specific criteria that need to be followed post-hospitalization for EN and PN to be a covered expense. Familiarity with these guidelines is important as patients may incur a significant financial burden if payor requirements are not met.

For patients with critical illness related to SARS-CoV-2 (COVID-19), data regarding nutrition are limited. For this reason, established guidelines should still be followed, including screening for malnutrition, limiting therapeutic (i.e., restrictive) diets, and placing enteric feeding tubes, as appropriate. Patients recovering from COVID-19 (Chapter 25) may have a unique symptom burden such as prolonged partial or total loss of smell or taste. There are no treatments specifically aimed at COVID-19 patients with altered taste and smell. However, general postinfectious treatments that target altered taste and smell, such as repeated sampling of a variety of odors like lemon, rose, cloves, and eucalyptus, may be helpful. Vitamin A drops have also shown some promise.

The response to MNT should be monitored using a variety of markers. There are currently no standardized serum biomarkers that can determine the response to MNT, but inpatient acute care monitoring should include weight, adipose and muscle store assessment, abdominal examination including a gastrointestinal function assessment, presence and healing of wounds, drain output(s), respiratory status, hemodynamics, and some laboratory values of inflammation. If a patient is receiving EN, it is recommended *not* to check gastric residual volume, as this measure of tolerance has not been shown to correlate with regurgitation, aspiration, or pneumonia. Assessing actual intake relative to the prescribed oral, enteral, or parenteral nutrition is essential and helps assessing nutritional prescription adequacy, as well as with transition planning. Regardless of whether a patient is in an acute care or in an outpatient setting, a multiprofessional team should follow the patient to optimize nutrition and quality of life.

Tips for Clinicians

1. Patients surviving critical illness have been through major changes in energy expenditure and intake. **Assess the adequacy of the patient's nutritional regimen** (e.g., oral intake, EN or PN regimen) and adjust as needed.
2. **Screen for malnutrition** by assessing weight, lean body mass, muscle mass and tone, and a history that includes dietary intake.
3. **Ensure that the current nutritional regimen is appropriate** given the patient's allergies, intolerances (e.g., lactose intolerance), and cultural or religious preferences and restrictions (e.g., Kosher diet).
4. **Maintain a low threshold for obtaining a consultation from a Registered Dietitian** familiar with the needs of critical illness survivors. Patients who require ongoing EN or PN and those with wound-healing concerns may especially benefit from RD consultation. Some acute care institutions have routine RD consultation for all ICU patients, as well as for all patients receiving EN or PN.

5. **Engage family caregivers in discussions about dietary needs** for critical illness survivors. Family members often help with obtaining food, preparing meals, and ensuring that patient's nutritional needs are met.
6. For patients in institutional settings (e.g., acute rehabilitation, skilled nursing), **ensure that the patient's nutritional needs are known** to the appropriate institution staff.

KEY REFERENCES

Bischoff S, Austin P, Boeykens K, et al. ESPEN guideline on home enteral nutrition. *Clin Nutr.* 2020;39(1):5-22.

Cederholm, T., Jensen, G.L., Correia, M.I.T.D., Gonzalez, M.C., Fukushima, R., Higashiguchi, T., Baptista, G., Barazzoni, R., Blaauw, R., Coats, A.J.S. and Crivelli, A.N., 2019. GLIM criteria for the diagnosis of malnutrition -a consensus report from the global clinical nutrition community. Journal of cachexia, sarcopenia and muscle, 10(1), pp.207-217. https://onlinelibrary.wiley.com/doi/full/10.1002/jcsm.12383

da Silva, J.S., Seres, D.S., Sabino, K., Adams, S.C., Berdahl, G.J., Citty, S.W., Cober, M.P., Evans, D.C., Greaves, J.R., Gura, K.M. and Michalski, A., 2020. ASPEN consensus recommendations for refeeding syndrome. Nutrition in Clinical Practice, 35(2), pp.178-195. https://aspenjournals.onlinelibrary.wiley.com/doi/epdf/10.1002/ncp.10474

Fadeur M, Preiser J, Verbrugge A, Misset B, Rousseau A. Oral nutrition during and after critical illness: SPICES for quality of care!. *Nutrients.* 2020;12(11):3509.

Kondrup J, Allison SP, Elia M, Vellas B, Plauth M; Educational and Clinical Practice Committee, European Society of Parenteral and Enteral Nutrition (ESPEN). ESPEN guidelines for nutrition screening 2002. *Clin Nutr.* 2003;22(4):415-421.

Pironi L, Boeykens K, Bozzetti F, et al. ESPEN guideline on home parenteral nutrition. *Clin Nutr.* 2020;39(6):1645-1666.

van Zanten A, De Waele E, Wischmeyer P. Nutrition therapy and critical illness: practical guidance for the ICU, post-ICU, and long-term convalescence phases. *Crit Care.* 2019;23(1):368.

White, J.V., Guenter, P., Jensen, G., Malone, A., Schofield, M., Force, A.M.T. and Academy Malnutrition Work Group, 2012. Consensus statement of the Academy of Nutrition and Dietetics/American Society for Parenteral and Enteral Nutrition: characteristics recommended for the identification and documentation of adult malnutrition (undernutrition). Journal of the Academy of Nutrition and Dietetics, 112(5), pp.730-738. https://www.sciencedirect.com/science/article/pii/S2212267212003280

Social Worker/ Case Manager's Perspective

Allison Gonzalez

Patient Care Vignette

TG, who goes by the name "Tom," is a 43-year-old man with metastatic rectal cancer. He was brought to the hospital by Fire Rescue due to difficulty breathing (respiratory distress). He was receiving second-line chemotherapy for his rectal cancer due to cancer recurrence after completing first-line therapy. He was admitted through the emergency department and had an endotracheal (ET) tube placed to connect him to a mechanical ventilator as he needed substantial help managing his breathing. Because he was placed on a ventilator, he was transferred to the ICU.

Tom had involuntarily lost 30 pounds in the last 3 months, reducing his weight to 125 pounds. This weight indicated severe malnutrition for this 5 foot, 9 inch man. Social work was consulted upon admission to assist with future planning and family support. Tom has been married to Nikhila for about 15 years. They are first-generation children of Indian immigrants and practice the Hindu religion. Tom has a PhD in economics and Nikhila is a PhD-trained pharmaceutical scientist. Their socioeconomic status is middle class and they are in their early 40s. They own their own house but have spent their savings cushion after Tom was no longer able to work. During that time, Nikhila had to take additional time off from work to get Tom to his multiple doctor's appointments.

They have an 8-year-old daughter who does not come to the hospital due to Nikhila's fears of traumatizing the child. This continues to be a strain for Nikhila because she has struggled with guilt between being wanting to be with her husband and needing to care for their daughter. She tells the social worker that balancing her daughter's needs in school and at home while trying to be present in the hospital has been difficult. She feels as if she is torn between two competing worlds.

Before this unplanned admission, Tom and Nikhila's life was marked by concerns for each other. Tom was not eating and losing weight, and Nikhila increasingly became responsible for everything at home. Nikhila's fears about Tom's future featured prominently in her discussions with the social worker. Throughout surgery, chemotherapy, and radiation they had focused on recovery as they hoped combination therapy would take care of the cancer. Accordingly, they had neither completed Advance Directives nor a living will. The social worker also noted that Tom and Nikhila never had a clear discussion about what would be important, or what goals of care they would value. Relatedly, Tom had not been evaluated by Palliative Care Medicine at any point in time—a consultation that the social worker suggested would be ideal during this ICU admission.

The social worker was initially consulted upon ICU admission to provide multiple services. The first step was to a provide support and develop a rapport with Tom and Nikhila, assess Tom's medical and social situation, and clarify who would serve as Tom's medical decision-maker. In the ICU, Tom did not have the capacity for decision-making. Therefore, care decisions in conjunction with the ICU team and Tom's oncologist were made by Nikhila who served as his surrogate. The scope of actions for which a surrogate is empowered varies by state. Most states, however, define the individuals who may serve as proxies using a tiered hierarchy approach with highest priority provided to spouses, children, and then parents. The social worker must be acutely aware of each state's laws, especially if the patient is being treated in a state different from the one in which they live. As there was no advance care planning, the social worker helped Nikhila make decisions based on what she believed Tom would want if he could share his desires. In addition, the social worker helped the ICU team by gathering information about Tom's anticipated needs including supportive counseling for the wife, psychoeducation and support for their daughter, and education and coordination for post-acute care needs.

■ INTRODUCTION

Social work has been practiced in the United States in some form since the late 1800s and has been steadily evolving. Medical, as opposed to general, social work blossomed in the early 1900s at the Massachusetts General Hospital in Boston. It developed during a time when treatment for the sick was moving into acute care settings instead of being provided within the home. A variety of medical conditions including tuberculosis, syphilis, and polio, coupled with poor urban living conditions, impacted how clinicians were able to care for patients outside of a dedicated facility. With diverse patients being cared for within hospitals, the need for post-acute care management and the coordination of that management drove the need for social workers in and outside of the hospital.

In 1906, Ida Cannon played a key role as a social worker and shifted the profession, centering the work on "bridging the gap between the hospital environment and the patients' usual social environment in order to remove barriers to effective medical treatment." Throughout the 20th century, the profession globally visible when Jane Addams, known for establishing settlement houses in Chicago for immigrants in the early 1900s, was awarded the Nobel Peace Prize. Frances Perkins, also a social worker, was the first woman to be appointed to a Presidential cabinet as Franklin D. Roosevelt's Secretary of Labor. More recently Tamara Grigsby, a former university professor and social worker, served as the Democratic Party member of the Wisconsin State Assembly from 2005 to 2013.

■ ROLE OF THE SOCIAL WORKER IN THE ICU

Not surprisingly, a social worker's role in medical settings, including acute care units, intensive care units (ICU), rehabilitation facilities, and other specialized treatment areas, may not be well understood. The lack of clarity stems, at least in part, from the broad range of services and interventions that social workers provide. It is easier to clearly define the role of the doctor, the nurse, and the respiratory therapist, for example, while it is more problematic to define a precise scope for the social worker (Figure 12-1). The medical

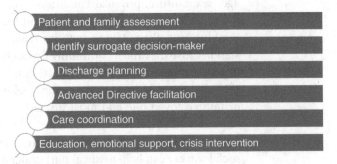

FIGURE 12-1. Key Social Workers Roles in the ICU. This graphic depicts key (but not all) roles for the social worker in an ICU.

social worker assists "behind the scenes" of medical care and engages with patients and families to ensure they have the resources they need to heal, while addressing their emotional and psychosocial needs. Many social worker roles overlap with other disciplines, such as physical or occupational therapy and nursing, which can make it difficult for staff, patients, and family members to distinguish the role of the social worker, and sometimes to identify the individual who is serving as their designated social worker.

In the hospital setting, social workers typically hold a Master's degree in Social Work (MSW) and are able to work in both inpatient and outpatient settings. There are some institutions that employ social workers with Bachelor's degree, but that is not the norm. Relatedly, some schools of social work are offering medical specialization within social work degree granting programs. The National Association of Social Workers (NASW) further defines that social workers' abilities are guided by principles including respect and advocacy for a client's right to self-determination, cultural competency, affirming the dignity and worth of all people bounded by a person-in-environment framework (also known as an "ecological perspective"). The ecological perspective links individuals to their environment on the grounds that "human behavior is to be understood within the social environment in which the behavior takes place." Additional principles of social work focus on individual's strengths instead of weaknesses (strengths perspective), the importance of the client–social worker relationship, social justice, and the value of social work research.

In the current setting of cost containment, social workers must address increasingly complex and varied needs, including the pressure to discharge patients to the next level of care in a timely fashion while maintaining often escalating caseload. Within the ICU, social workers recognize that each person brings their own perspective and experience, which shapes how they respond to stress as well as success during the ICU and recovery phases. A person's age, sex, culture, physical condition, emotional state, and prior experience influence their perceptions of care and the healthcare clinicians with whom they interact. Patients and families react differently than medically trained staff because they most commonly do not have the experience and knowledge of medical terminology and clinical conditions that are common to healthcare clinicians. Moreover, they often feel powerless to help their critically ill or injured loved one and must instead rely on the healthcare team to do so. Experienced social workers are aware of those differences and can help guide patients and families as they make critical medical decisions. Importantly, the social worker can help medical staff understand the goals, values, preferences, and perceptions of the patient and family, including those related to religious and cultural imperatives.

Social workers specialize in psychosocial care and therefore play a key role in helping patients and families navigate complex medical environments, including when there is conflict regarding goals of care, uncertain outcomes, or end-of-life issues. In many ways, ICU social work has become its own subspecialty of medical social work. This hierarchy parallels the subspecialty nature of the different disciplines of critical care (trauma, surgical, cardiac, medical, neurologic, pediatric, etc.). As critical care teams have expanded, the ICU social worker has become an integral member of that multiprofessional team.

Social workers typically support everyone involved in the care of the patient including the patient, the family members or loved ones, and the healthcare team. The ICU social worker also engages in discharge planning—right from the time of admission. Equipment, supplies, or perhaps a different care facility such as a rehabilitation hospital or a skilled nursing facility (SNF) all require time to arrange, and they bear specific costs. Insurance arrangements may be complex and social workers help navigate that process to ensure that when patients are ready to transition out of the acute care facility, everything they need for continued recovery is readily available. Social workers do this by having a broad understanding of services covered by insurance, qualifications for various inpatient stays, as well as a comprehensive knowledge base of available community resources. Other facilities also employ social workers in order to facilitate dialogue and care coordination. Part of ensuring that patients receive care that they wish for is to make certain that they have established boundaries for desired care. Advanced care planning can help with that process.

Advanced care planning is the process where patients either clearly explain, write, or type their wishes for end-of-life care should they become incapacitated and unable to directly guide care. Although advance care planning has not been proven to impact outcomes in the ICU, it does help the healthcare clinicians and families to create goal-concordant treatment plans. Social workers play a central role in advanced care planning primarily through person-to-person education and within team advocacy. Social workers are trained to educate the patients regarding advanced care planning documents, their meaning, and how to complete them. Patients can be intimidated by the content of advance care documents especially because they address scenarios such as advanced life support, cardiopulmonary resuscitation, and withdrawal of life-sustaining treatments. Social workers acknowledge those anxieties and work through them with patients to help them complete what are often complex documents. Social workers also recognize that the Advanced Directive (AD) is a guide rather than an all-inclusive document and must be revisited as a patient's condition evolves. Therefore, the AD serves as a fluid guide for the patient's desires rather than a concrete determination that is final.

This discussion is often facilitated using a series of questions that the social worker poses for the patient and family. Some questions may be emotionally charged and others may be uncomfortable. Examples may be found within public resources offered by the Centers for Disease Control derived from the National Hospice and Palliative Care Organization focused on starting difficult conversations (https://www.cdc.gov/aging/pdf/acp-resources-public.pdf). Nonetheless, supporting patients and families through such difficult determinations is part of the social worker's role. Support can also be sought from the healthcare team, and particularly Palliative Care Medicine clinicians. In Nikhila and Tom's case, their goals are recovery based and are strongly tied to Tom's age. Their spiritual identity and faith-based existence is a major source of strength for them as they desire to pursue continued aggressive care.

Social workers also help coordinate team meetings between family members and healthcare clinicians. Many centers involve families on daily ICU rounds, but some family members cannot be present during the typical time frame for rounds. In those circumstances, the social worker often helps arrange a suitable time for family updates addressing information that supports shared decision-making regarding care. Other team meetings may be more focused and address goals of care—a discussion that is ideally done early during the ICU stay. Other discussions address unique procedures such as a tracheostomy (a breathing tube that is placed through the front of the neck that allows the tube to be removed from the mouth) or a feeding tube. Coordinating to have every relevant team member in a single location for however long it is required is a challenging task, and ICU teams commonly rely on social workers to facilitate those arrangements, and then participate in the meeting.

■ CONSIDERATIONS FOR RECOVERY

As patients improve, they are faced with a variety of transitions in their care. Such transitions include but are not limited to location within the hospital, transfer to another hospital, a change in the healthcare team (different teams often provide care in the ICU compared to the acute care unit), and a change in the intensity of care. In a variety of settings, the social worker does not change and continues to work with the patient and the family and the new healthcare team. In this way, the social worker provides continuity that is quite helpful for all. Transitional care with effective continuity of care (COC) are both goals in primary care systems and a high-priority area for performance improvement and assessment. Safe transitions require multilevel coordination and care as well as knowledge of the patient, the family, and available resources (Fig. 12-2). Social workers are essential in providing quality transitions as they are skilled in assessing and addressing many of the social determinants of health that are addressed during the transition evaluation.

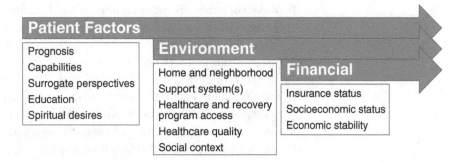

FIGURE 12-2. Transition Considerations. This figure demonstrates three broad group-ings of elements that impact transitions with which the social worker interfaces to support excellent outcomes. Adapted from Social Determinants of Health. https://health.gov/healthypeople/objectives-and-data/social-determinants-health. Accessed on November 26, 2022.

An important element of transition planning is the handoff of the patient and family to a social worker outside of the acute care facility. Just because the patient has survived the ICU and the rest of their acute care episode does not mean that they no longer have care coordination or support needs. An outpa-tient social worker helps fill these needs and is a vital link between the patient and family and resources that span everything from financial assistance pro-grams to Visiting Nurse programs to travel support for ongoing outpatient medical care including rehabilitation. These aspects of care are generally not coordinated by the patient's primary care clinician and rely nearly exclusively on the social worker for success.

Tips for Clinicians

1. **Include social workers and case managers as essential members of the healthcare professional team** in the recovery period for critical illness.
2. Although time is a precious commodity in healthcare encounters, it is often precisely what patients and families need to develop rapport, trust, and to express hopes, desires, concerns, and fears during critical illness recovery.
3. **Use lay language instead of medical terms when explaining condi-tions or procedures.** Try to explain what different procedures mean, and not just what they are. Clarity around daily goals and expectations is particularly helpful in developing trust, and in charting an under-standable course. This also helps patients and families understand prognostication.

4. **Make sure that all the members of the healthcare team understand the plan of care** to ensure that a consistent message is shared.
5. Often the social worker's time with the patient and family garners insights into patient and family goals, values and preferences that will inform how care is offered or deployed. This information is essential and should be specifically sought while crafting a care plan that is to be evaluated using shared decision-making.
6. **Leverage social workers and case managers as early as possible** to help with care planning, family linkage, and care coordination.

KEY REFERENCES

Bernard C, Tan A, Slaven M, et al. Exploring patient-reported barriers to advance care planning in family practice. *BMC Fam Pract*. 2020;21:94.

Bodley T, Rassos J, Mansoor W, Bell CM, Detsky ME. Improving transitions of care between the intensive care unit and general internal medicine ward. A demonstration study. *ATS Scholar*. 2020;1(3):288-300.

Browning ED, Cruz JS. Reflective debriefing: a social work intervention addressing moral distress among ICU nurses. *J Soc Work End-of-Life Palliat Care*. 2018;14(1):44-72.

Bryson SA, Bosma H. Health social work in Canada: five trends worth noting. *Soc Work Health Care*. 2018;57(8):1-26.

Donovan AL, Aldrich JM, Gross AK, et al. Interprofessional care and teamwork in the ICU. *Crit Care Med*. 2018;46(6):980-990.

Gay EB, Pronovost PJ, Bassett RD, Nelson JE. The intensive care unit family meeting: making it happen. *J Crit Care*. 2009;24(4):629.e1-629.e12.

Goh KJ, Wong J, Tien JC, et al. Preparing your intensive care unit for the COVID-19 pandemic: practical considerations and strategies. *Crit Care*. 2020;24(1):1-2.

Hartman-Shea K, Hahn AP, Fritz Kraus J, et al. The role of the social worker in the adult critical care unit: a systematic review of the literature. *Soc Work Health Care*. 2011;50(2):143-157.

Herbst LA, Desai S, Benscoter D, et al. Going back to the ward—transitioning care back to the ward team. *Transl Pediatr*. 2018;7(4):314.

Mason TM, Tofthagen CS, Buck HG. Complicated grief: risk factors, protective factors, and interventions. *J Soc Work End-of-Life Palliat Care*. 2020;16(2):151-174.

McPeake J, Boehm LM, Hibbert E, et al. Key components of ICU recovery programs: what did patients report provided benefit? *Crit Care Explor*. 2020;2(4):e0088.

McPeake JM, Henderson P, Darroch G, et al. Social and economic problems of ICU survivors identified by a structured social welfare consultation. *Crit Care*. 2019;23(1):1-2.

Nelson JE, Mulkerin CM, Adams LL, et al. Improving comfort and communication in the ICU: a practical new tool for palliative care performance measurement and feedback. *Qual Saf Health Care*. 2006;115:264-271.

Raftery C, Lewis E, Cardona M. The crucial role of nurses and social workers in initiating end-of-life communication to reduce overtreatment in the midst of the COVID-19 pandemic. *Gerontology*. 2020;66(5):427-430.

Rivera-Romero N, Ospina Garzón HP, Henao-Castaño AM. The experience of the nurse caring for families of patients at the end of life in the intensive care unit. *Scand J Caring Sci*. 2019;33(3):706-711.

Rose SL, Shelton W. The role of social work in the ICU: reducing family distress and facilitating end-of-life decision-making. *J Soc Work End-of-Life Palliat Care*. 2006;2(2):3-23.

Udelsman BV, Lee KC, Traeger LN, et al. Clinician-to-clinician communication of patient goals of care within a surgical intensive care unit. *J Surg Res*. 2019;240:80-88.

Innovations in ICU Recovery

Music Interventions in ICU and Post-ICU Care

CHAPTER 13

Zhan Liang, Kimberly Sena Moore, and Hilary Yip

> ### Patient Care Vignette
>
> Sylvia was a 63-year-old woman diagnosed with pneumonia complicated by renal failure. When the music therapy research team met her, she had been transferred to a clinical unit after being in the ICU for 11 days. She was resting quietly in bed, with a fall alert bracelet on her left wrist, wearing no-slip yellow hospital socks, with a blanket covering her petite body frame. The television was on, and she was staring at the screen.
>
> Upon seeing the research team, Sylvia turned her head and smiled softly. She shared that she was doing okay and was just waiting to see the doctors; she also mentioned that she missed being home. Her speech was soft and her gestures were minimal. Everything about her movement was slow. The research team asked Sylvia if she would be interested in participating in a research study testing a music and exercise program. She said yes, as she felt that she was not strong and wanted to improve muscle strength.
>
> On the first day of the intervention, Sylvia was provided with instructions: The intervention involved listening to a music playlist that guides patients in completing five exercises: two lower extremity exercises (feet and legs) and three upper extremity exercises (hands, arms, and shoulders), each completed 10 times. In consultation with music therapists, each exercise was facilitated by musical melodies and verbal cues to direct how and when to move the body (e.g., "and down and up"). The intervention was personalized by asking patients to indicate their instrumental sound preferences. (Sylvia preferred the wood and piano sounds.) The intervention took about 10 minutes. Patients were advised to perform the music-guided

exercises at least twice daily for 5 days, with more repetitions allowed if desired. Patients were given an MP3 player preloaded with their playlist and a speaker to use while in the hospital and to take home for further exercise.

It was evident from the first day and throughout the study period that Sylvia was motivated and engaged in the music and exercise program. When the research team entered her room, her face would light up, and she would say she was "ready to exercise." During the first couple of days, she occasionally checked with the team to confirm that she was doing the exercises correctly, especially the bicep curls. After coaching to only move her forearm and not her whole upper arm, Sylvia would occasionally look at her arms while doing the exercise.

In the final days of the study period, Sylvia often listened to the playlist and completed the exercises with her eyes closed. Sometimes she did not want to stop after the tenth time, and would continue to do one or two more repetitions. After each exercise, she smiled and was so proud of herself for doing the movements. At the end of the entire 10-minute set, Sylvia would say, "I feel good," and state how much she looked forward to the next exercise session.

■ INTRODUCTION

Complications of critical illness are varied and include delirium, hospital-acquired weakness, and post-intensive care syndrome, a triad of physical, cognitive, and psychological impairments following an ICU admission. The 2013 Society of Critical Care Medicine Guidelines for the Management of Pain, Agitation, and Delirium in the ICU recommend nonpharmacological interventions, such as music interventions, to foster recovery in ICU survivors experiencing some or all of these complications.

Appropriately designed and implemented music interventions have shown a remarkable ability to improve patient and family function and well-being, ameliorate symptoms, and improve quality of life in patients with chronic disease and disabilities. In this chapter, we will first describe the different intersections of music in healthcare settings, including music therapy, music medicine, and music interventions. Next, we will summarize literature on music interventions in ICU and post-ICU settings, with a primary focus on the adult ICU environment and a short introduction to music therapy in pediatric ICU care. We will then provide considerations and tips for using music to help critically ill patients recover and families cope.

■ THE CONTINUUM OF MUSIC IN HEALTHCARE

There are several ways that music might be used for beneficial purposes in a healthcare setting. Many of these can be considered "music interventions," which involve the application of a music-based experience (e.g., music listening or music-guided movement) for a specific therapeutic aim (e.g., to manage pain or increase endurance). Examples of these are *Arts in Health*, *Music Medicine*, and *Music Therapy.*

Arts in Health

The most recent field to emerge is Arts in Health, which describes the use of arts, including music, to promote health in diverse contexts. Arts in Health professionals bring their creative expertise into the healthcare setting, and may engage in practices that range from enhancing the environment (e.g., performing in the hospital lobby) to interacting with patients and their families (e.g., playing a song for them). Arts in Health programs are typically managed by a coordinator, who organizes visiting artists, artist-in-residence programs, and community partnerships. The National Organization for Arts in Health (NOAH) has published a core curriculum for Arts in Health professionals, as well as practice standards and a code of ethics. In general, the goal for musicians who work as Arts in Health professionals is to enhance the health and reduce stress for patients, families, and professional caregivers by creating a more positive environment through music.

Music Medicine

Music medicine describes the use of music interventions administered in a medical setting, typically by a healthcare professional. The general purpose of a music medicine intervention is to reduce the patient's perception of pain and anxiety. The interventions commonly involve the patient passively listening to prerecorded music, which they may or may not have selected themselves. In most situations, the music is prescribed based on an expectation for how that selection will impact the patient. Although the medical professional administers the intervention, the implementation does not necessarily include a systematic therapeutic process.

Music Therapy

The American Music Therapy Association (AMTA) defines music therapy as "the clinical and evidence-based use of music interventions to accomplish individualized goals within a therapeutic relationship." In the United States, music therapy is considered an allied health profession. Qualified music therapists earn a bachelor's degree or higher in music therapy, complete 1,200 clinical training hours, and hold the Music Therapist-Board Certified (MT-BC) credential issued by the Certification Board for Music Therapists. Following assessment, music therapists develop and implement personally tailored music interventions to address the patient's clinical needs across health domains, including cognition, communication, sensorimotor, and socioemotional. These experiences can include music listening, as well as instrument playing, singing, composing, improvising, and moving to music designed to address individualized treatment goals.

■ MUSIC INTERVENTIONS

Music medicine and music therapy both involve the design and implementation of music interventions, which describe the purposeful application of music to bring about functional change in an individual. Music can either be delivered live or recorded and, depending on the training and skills of the interventionist, can be adapted in-the-moment based on patient preference or needs. Musical elements such as lyrics, tempo, melody, and harmony are specifically chosen, designed, or (if presented live) manipulated to induce a response. Patient-preferred music is typically recommended and can be gleaned by asking patients and/or family members if patients are unable to communicate their interests.

Music interventions can be receptive (listening or moving to music), recreative (making music by playing instruments or singing), compositional (writing music), and/or improvisational (improvising instrumental or vocal music). These may be structured within a session or across multiple sessions to bring about short- or long-term behavioral, physiological, psychological change. The complexity of the music intervention will differ based on the interventionist, specifically their scope of practice, the training required to practice safely and effectively, and expected patient outcomes. In general, music interventions are implemented by medical professionals (e.g., professional music therapists, clinicians, or professionals) or self-administered by an individual. If the intervention delivery involves an interventionist and the patients, the relationship between the two can impact therapeutic outcomes of how the patients understand, process, and manage their emotions, thoughts, and behaviors. The benefit of the intervention can be tested in a variety of ways that include psychological measures, tests of physical performance, or physiologic response.

■ MUSIC IN THE ICU

Music therapy has been shown to decrease patient anxiety and stress levels in many ICU settings, including patients who are and are not mechanically ventilated. These reductions, in turn, may lead to a decrease in the need for sedative and analgesic medications. Smaller studies suggest that music interventions can promote deeper, more restorative sleep and overall sleep quality.

Investigations into the effect that music interventions have on delirium and pain are ongoing.

Music interventions may also be used in pediatric intensive care units (PICU). Music therapists in PICU settings address coping and engagement, pain management, palliative care, bereavement, and motor and speech rehabilitation goals. Music interventions go beyond music listening to include improvisation, songwriting, music-assisted relaxation, and supporting parent/caregiver interactions. Music therapy can be especially beneficial for children with longer lengths of stays and extensive rehabilitation needs.

Music therapy also has benefits for the families and caregivers of ICU patients. Music therapists commonly invite family members to participate in sessions with the patient, which can benefit both the patient and their family members during and after the ICU stay. Through music-based experiences family members can be afforded space to process the situation, discuss medical knowledge, and express their feelings about their loved one's prognosis and related uncertainties. Therapeutic songwriting can allow patients and families to creatively verbalize feelings, support affirmations, and reflect life. Patients and families may choose music with themes that elicit shared memories, soothe feelings, affirm faith, and communicate with each other.

While music interventions are often delivered in person, they can be delivered remotely. In response to the COVID-19 pandemic, hospitals implemented safety protocols that restricted family visitation. In some hospitals, music therapists were allowed on site to continue service delivery, whereas in others music therapists were restricted, leading to profound changes in practice. Telehealth was used to provide virtual services through online platforms. Patients used a hospital tablet or their own tablet/phone to join an individual or group music therapy session while in the hospital.

An alternative virtual method involves the use of recorded video and audio given to patients to use at their leisure. These generally involve either curating online content or creating original content. Music therapists have created, performed, and recorded different music meditations and popular songs for patient use. The music exercise playlist described in the vignette demonstrates how a playlist can be used to motivate patients to self-manage exercises. An alternative involves music therapists compiling songs or meditations on digital playlists, music streaming platforms, or websites with music activities that patients can use during their hospital stay and after discharge.

■ MUSIC IN THE POST-ICU PHASE

As the health-related and clinical needs of patients recovering from critical illness continue after ICU discharge, so too do the potential beneficial effects of music. Music therapists often provide services in settings where ICU patients are discharged, including step-down or transitional care units in medical facilities, rehabilitation centers, long-term care facilities, outpatient rehabilitation clinics, and in private practice. Based on the setting and clinical needs of the post-ICU patient, music interventions can be implemented to address various needs:

- Psychological support, such as facilitating weaning from long-term mechanical ventilation by providing pre-recorded music as a distraction with the goal of reducing anxiety.
- Physical rehabilitation, such as using rhythmic-based music listening to guide movements to improve gait and increase upper and lower extremity strength, endurance, and range-of-motion (the *Move to Music Intervention (M2M)* is one example described in the vignette).
- Psychosocial support, which can range from group instrument playing experiences to increase interpersonal interactions, to music listening for improving mood.
- Cognitive rehabilitation, such as learning to play the ukulele as a way to practice attention regulation, working memory, and learning and memory.
- Speech and language rehabilitation, which often includes singing-based experiences to improve articulation, increase respiratory strength, and practice expressive language.
- Palliative care, which may include engaging the patient in listening to or singing their preferred music as a way to manage anxiety and pain, and increase comfort.

Research continues on the impact that music interventions and music therapy have on post-ICU outcomes. Published studies suggest that these interventions hold promise in decreasing dyspnea and anxiety for patients discharged from the ICU to long-term acute care hospitals for prolonged ventilator weaning. As described in the vignette, these interventions are also used to promote recovery through increasing physical activity and building muscle strength.

Music interventions started in the ICU can and probably should be continued upon ICU discharge. Such continuity can be promoted through sharing music playlists with patients and families. Music therapists may work with patients and families to create playlists of favorite songs for use while in the hospital or at home. This type of activity can extend to a musical life review in which the music therapist helps the patient curate a playlist of songs that represent significant moments, events, or periods in the patient's life. This playlist may also include recordings of the patient and/or family members sharing reflections to accompany select songs. Life review recordings can be used to hold space for reminiscence and acknowledgment of accomplishments, challenges, and the patient's legacy.

Virtual music therapy can also facilitate continuity in music interventions after ICU discharge. Through virtual platforms, music therapists can implement music meditations, music and movement, song discussions, or songwriting to target goals such as reducing anxiety, developing coping skills, promoting self-expression, exercising cognition, and exercising gross or fine motor skills.

■ CONSIDERATIONS FOR RECOVERY

Music interventions provide a holistic, nonpharmacological approach for supporting recovery from critical illness. In this section, we will provide some suggestions on what to consider when designing and implementing a music intervention for patients who are recovering from critical illness.

Type of music interventions should be considered to promote the specific therapeutic purpose. For example, if increasing activity is the goal, moving to rhythmic music can be utilized to motivate or promote adherence to an exercise regimen. If patients experience psychological stress or pain, providing the opportunity to listen to preferred music may be beneficial. Slower music played at 60 to 80 beats per minute might be most beneficial as that pace mimics the average heart rate rhythm. Finally, encouraging patients to sing (and singing with them) may ameliorate stress, promote social support, and improve pain.

When considering the timing, frequency, and dosage for a music listening intervention, there is no consensus in the literature about optimal timing. Many interventions are 30 minutes in duration, but other described music interventions range from 15 to 60 minutes. Because there are is no "gold standard," we recommend that clinicians should start with a 20- to 30-minute session and make adjustments to the length and number of daily listening sessions based on the patient's response to the music.

To achieve the optimal outcomes, it is important to incorporate patients' preferred music. A music preference assessment tool can be used to ask patients or family members to identify their favorite style of music (e.g., classical, country, and jazz), favorite musician, and preferred instruments, as well as music and/or instruments they do not like.

The type of interventionist is another important factor to consider. Music interventions can be delivered by a credentialed music therapist, a nonmusic therapy healthcare provider, such as a nurse or rehab therapist, or via a recorded playlist. We encourage clinicians to consult with a professional music therapist when initially designing music interventions. In collaboration, music therapists can help design a treatment-focused music experience that can be delivered by clinicians with little to no musical expertise.

A vital, yet often overlooked, consideration is the recognition that music has the potential to induce behavioral, affective, and psychosocial harm. This can occur despite the best intentions of the patient, the family, and the health-care clinician. Thus, care should be taken in the selection and delivery of the music, patients should be monitored through the duration of the intervention to ensure beneficial outcomes, and changes made should the patient experience an adverse reaction to the music.

Tips for Clinicians

1. **Observe music therapy sessions**. Observing music therapy will help clinicians identify and refer patients who may be appropriate for music therapy services. For instance, staff can refer patients who need to decrease anxiety, increase relaxation, exercise cognition, express emotion, develop coping skills, and practice gross or fine motor skills. Staff members can give patients reminders of sessions, possibly through the electronic health record system, and communicate the needs of patients, caregivers, and family with music therapists. This information will help music therapists create plans, interventions, and materials specific to those needs.

2. **Remember that music therapy can help with emotion and mood**. Music therapists are uniquely situated to address a patient's psychosocial needs, leveraging the ways that music can regulate mood and emotions.

3. **Keep in mind that music therapy extends beyond playlist curation**. Music therapists can prepare recorded music interventions for the patient to self-implement as part of their daily therapy exercises. These recorded music playlists or songs provide opportunities for patients to continue care and follow their therapeutic needs. These may be accompanied by "homework" the music therapist creates to help motivate regular practice of the therapeutic exercises. This may include listening to the music at specific times of day (e.g., night) or for a specific number of times (e.g., two times a day). A homework program can be completed at the facility when the music therapist is not available, or at home upon discharge. Staff members and family can support patients who are continuing to use music to address their therapeutic needs.

4. **Interdisciplinary collaboration may augment outcomes related to music interventions**. Music therapists can both learn from and contribute to the care and treatment plans created by other members of the patient care team. For example, the music therapist can show the

physical therapist how to use a metronome set at a certain tempo to facilitate gait practice or can design targeted singing interventions for a speech-language pathologist to use for articulation and respiratory exercise.

5. **Music therapy can continue after hospital discharge.** If a patient has initiated music therapy in the hospital, the hospital music therapist can refer the patient for continued music therapy services postdischarge. If there is not a music therapist at the postdischarge facility, there may be a way to work with the care coordinator (e.g., case manager or social worker) to connect the patient and their family to a music therapist in the community to explore contractual services. Finally, a patient and family may visit the website of the Certification Board for Music Therapists (www.cbmt.org) and use the "Find A Therapist" feature to locate and connect with a music therapist in their local area.

KEY REFERENCES

Barr J, Fraser GL, Puntillo K, et al. Clinical practice guidelines for the management of pain, agitation, and delirium in adult patients in the intensive care unit. *Crit Care Med.* 2013;41(1):263-306.

Bradt J, Dileo C. Music interventions for mechanically ventilated patients. *Cochrane Database Syst Rev.* 2014;2014(12):Cd006902.

CBMT. Find a therapist. Available at https://my.cbmt.org/cbmtssa/f?p=CRTSSA:17800: 6480047112754:::17800.

Knott D, Block S. Virtual music therapy: developing new approaches to service delivery. *Music Ther Perspect.* 2020:miaa017. doi:10.1093/mtp/miaa017.

Liang Z, Munro CL, Ferreira TBD, et al. Feasibility and acceptability of a self-managed exercise to rhythmic music intervention for ICU survivors. *Appl Nurs Res.* 2020;54:151315.

Liang Z, Ren D, Choi J, Happ MB, Hravnak M, Hoffman LA. Music intervention during daily weaning trials: a 6-day prospective randomized crossover trial. *Complement Ther Med.* 2016;29:72-77.

MacDonald RA. Music, health, and well-being: a review. *Int J Qual Stud Health Well-being.* 2013;8:20635.

Promoting ICU Recovery: ICU Diaries

Megan K. Zielke, John McGill, and Mark E. Mikkelsen

Patient Care Vignette

A 53-year-old male with past medical history of hypertension, diabetes mellitus, and anxiety was admitted to the medical intensive care unit (MICU) with acute hypoxemic (low oxygen saturation) respiratory failure due to Legionella pneumonia that resulted in the acute respiratory distress syndrome (ARDS; see the chapter on the Respiratory Therapist). On hospital day 2, the patient's oxygenation worsened despite corticosteroids and high-flow nasal cannula O_2, and he required a breathing tube (i.e., intubation) and was supported with invasive mechanical ventilation. On hospital day 3, the patient was sedated, received a neuromuscular blocking medication, and underwent prone position therapy while on the ventilator.

The patient's wife was able to join and participate in multiprofessional rounds in the MICU. By the end of rounds, she had developed a reasonable understanding of her husband's diagnosis and prognosis. When asked how she was doing, she acknowledged being scared and having a difficult time sleeping. She asked whether the patient's preexisting anxiety would worsen and what could be done to mitigate psychological distress after critical illness.

The clinical team introduced her to the ICU's diary program, known as a Healing Journal. The patient's wife agreed to participate, and the MICU pharmacist wrote an initial entry. After 12 days in the MICU, the patient was transferred to the acute care unit to continue his recovery. The clinical team placed 18 entries during his time in the MICU, and the patient's family and friends provided many more separate entries. The patient and his wife visited the MICU 2 months later to express their gratitude for the care and support they received. They were also grateful for the Healing Journal which he read several times since he did not remember most of his MICU stay. He found that the entries helped him to better understand what he experienced. His physical strength has recovered to where he is independent. He acknowledges that he had difficulty sleeping for several weeks, and at times felt anxious that he would fall ill again. Fortunately, these symptoms have decreased in frequency and intensity in recent weeks which he takes as a sign of continued recovery.

■ INTRODUCTION

Millions of patients each year are admitted to an intensive care unit (ICU), many of whom require invasive mechanical ventilation. While ventilated, intravenous sedation is frequently administered to patients to facilitate synchrony with the ventilator and to manage agitation, anxiety, or delirium. Sedatives are often combined with intravenous analgesics, especially when pain is anticipated to be present (i.e., after procedures including surgery). As patients recover, these medications are reduced in dose and then either stopped or replaced with an oral agent depending on the patient's need.

Upon awakening, many patients struggle to recall what occurred to them and to make sense of their lived or perceived experience. In the weeks and months after critical illness, many survivors experience difficulties with cognition, mental health, and physical functioning. These difficulties are known as the post-intensive care syndrome, or PICS. In terms of mental health, depression, anxiety, and symptoms of posttraumatic stress disorder (PTSD) are common after surviving critical illness.

Family members of patients who are critically ill often also experience mental health difficulties including sleep deprivation and a sense of helplessness. These challenges evolve over time. For example, 67% of family members who had a loved one requiring prolonged mechanical ventilation experienced symptoms of depression 7 days into critical illness. At 3 and 12 months, symptoms of depression persisted in 49% and 43% of family members, respectively. Therefore, it is important to recognize that symptoms abate for some, but not all, family members and that interventions are urgently needed to ease their psychological distress. In this chapter, we use the broader definition of family, meaning individuals who have a relationship with, and provide support to, the patient.

To restore a patient's fragmented memories, to preserve patient and family psychological health, and to improve their comprehension of the experience, clinicians began to maintain diaries of a patient's ICU stay. In this chapter, we describe the history and evidence to support the practice of building an

ICU diary program. We then provide practical advice for clinicians interested in starting, and maintaining, an ICU diary program. Finally, we end by discussing complementary strategies to more effectively meet the needs of ICU survivors—a process that begins in the ICU and continues postdischarge.

■ THE HISTORY OF ICU DIARIES

The practice of maintaining ICU diaries began in Scandinavia in the 1980s. The practice spread to Europe and gained greater visibility after a series of publications suggested psychological benefit to both patients and caregivers. In 2016, the practice gained greater traction when the international guidelines for family-centered care for neonatal, pediatric, and adult ICU patients recommended that "ICU diaries be implemented in the ICU to reduce family member anxiety, depression, and post-traumatic stress."

An ICU diary is a log of a patient's clinical course in the ICU. The diary is written in nonmedical language in order to be accessible and understood by patients. Diary entries are placed by clinicians to memorialize the day's events, and family members are encouraged to write entries from their perspective. The initial entry is usually the longest, being written on hospital day 2 or 3, and summarizes the patient's initial presentation to the hospital. Subsequent clinical events may include the following: milestones (e.g., beginning spontaneous breathing trials, ICU discharge), procedures (e.g., central venous catheterization, Foley catheterization, endotracheal tube suctioning), diagnostic tests, transport to and from other locations within the hospital (e.g., radiology, operating room), and functional progress. All clinical team members are encouraged to contribute, as the breadth of unique perspectives can provide the patient with a more comprehensive understanding of their experience. The diary, or journal, is generally left at the patient's bedside.

Family members can document the day's events, and detail who visited. Family member entries can also offer words of encouragement, love, and support, or make entries of community or world events. Clinicians and family may also choose to include pictures of the ICU environment as a means to orient the patient once they are able to review the diary. Of note, taking photographs of the ICU and the patient in the ICU may be subject to hospital policy and should be specifically assessed prior to proceeding.

■ WHAT IS THE EVIDENCE TO SUPPORT THE PRACTICE?

A key study in 2010 assessed the impact of creating an ICU diary and then giving the patient and the family the diary at 1 month after ICU discharge. Patients who received their diary were compared to patients who did not. This study included patients who had an ICU stay of 3 or more days, and all underwent invasive mechanical ventilation just like the patient in the vignette. At 3 months, the incidence of PTSD was significantly less in those who received the diary (5%), compared to 13% in patients who did not. This data is important because it documents that an intervention started in the ICU can improve outcome outside of the hospital, and without ongoing healthcare clinician intervention.

A related study in 2012 introduced ICU diaries into a combined medical–surgical ICU for patients with an ICU length of stay of 4 or more days. In the pre-diary phase of the study, symptoms of severe PTSD were found in 65% of patients and 80% of families. In the diary phase, rates of severe PTSD declined to 50% in patients and 32% in families. When the study ended and ICU diaries were no longer part of clinical care, PTSD rates climbed back to 74% in patients and 68% in families. This data underscores that interventions to shield patients and families from PTSD is a key part of routine care. A more recent trial did not find such robust benefits, suggesting that the benefits of an ICU diary may also rely on how the program is presented and managed.

While further studies are needed to understand the mechanism by which anxiety and depression are less common among patients, and PTSD symptoms less common among family members, experts have suggested several potential mechanisms. First, ICU diaries may facilitate improved communication between clinicians and family members, resulting in a greater understanding of the patient's clinical condition, care and prognosis, greater therapeutic alliance between the clinical team and the family, and less psychological distress as a result. Incorporating a "get to know me" section into the ICU diary is a useful strategy to include in diary design. Second, ICU diaries allow family members to maintain a sense of communication with their loved one during critical illness, and provides a role for family members during this difficult time. For patients, the diary may help to make sense of fractured memories. For example, without proper context, a procedure such as Foley catheterization or endotracheal tube suctioning may be recalled by a patient as an assault, resulting in anxiety, depression, and PTSD. Garrouste-Orgeas described this well: "By providing objective information to patients which could help fill in memory gaps, ICU diaries have allowed them [patients] to abandon unrealistic experiences, reconstruct their experience, gain a sense of reality, and resolve differences in experience with their family."

Studies evaluating the efficacy of this therapy generally include patients who have been mechanically ventilated for greater than or equal to 48 hours. There are several reasons why investigators would use these inclusion criteria. First, it directs the intervention—which requires staff time and dedication— to a vulnerable group of ICU patients who will have an extended ICU length of stay. Further, by targeting patients who require mechanical ventilation, the intervention is being directed to patients who often receive sedation that alters their level of consciousness, and places them at risk to experience fragmented and often intrusive memories that may not accurately reflect reality. However, given the low risk of harm in implementing an ICU diary, we encourage providing ICU diaries for patients with severe critical illness or prolonged ICU stays even if they do not require mechanical ventilation.

■ PRACTICAL TIPS FOR STARTING AND SUSTAINING AN ICU DIARY PROGRAM

To optimize the likelihood of success and sustainability, it is key to have leadership and staff buy-in when developing an ICU diary program. Our institution began by creating an interdisciplinary working group that included the following representatives, who later served as ICU diary champions: physicians, nurses, clinical pharmacists, respiratory therapists, and social workers. We partnered with risk management, whose expertise informed our protocols and procedures (i.e., participation agreement rather than informed consent).

Through this working group, the team was able to set the foundation regarding the immediate and long-term goals for the diary program. This included the short-term goal of increasing communication with the patient's family as well as increasing the humanization of care for their loved ones. Long-term goals included a reduction in the detrimental psychological effects that patients and their family members experience following critical illness. Simultaneously, the team evaluated who we suspected would most benefit from an ICU diary. Ultimately, we agreed that patients would be eligible if they had been intubated for greater than 48 hours, which was approximately 40% of our patients.

Once the team established goals and inclusion criteria, the journal was designed and printed. Further details regarding the creation and organization of the diary, or Healing Journal, is further described by a variety of authors; no single approach is best. Prior to implementing the ICU diary program, members of the working group met with members of the healthcare team for person-to-person education regarding this novel initiative. Key components of this education included who can offer and how to offer a journal, how to write an entry within the journal, and who can write entries since ICU diary use may not be intuitive.

■ WHO CAN OFFER A DIARY?

Any member of the healthcare team can offer a diary to an eligible patient or their family member. In addition to the benefit to the patient and the family of having clinicians contribute different perspectives, there is also the potential that participating can be of benefit to the staff. Specifically, as a form of post-ICU activity, ICU diaries are a means by which clinicians can feel more connected to their profession and their patients. For example, nurses in our ICU reported feeling a "special connection" to their patients through journal writing. This connection has helped some of the healthcare team overcome symptoms of BurnOut syndrome that arise from caring for high acuity patients—an event that seemed to be even more pronounced as a result of the recent pandemic.

■ HOW IS A DIARY OFFERED?

A diary is generally offered to the patient or their family member at the point of meeting inclusion eligibility. The offering is viewed as an invitation to participate, rather than a formal procedure that requires informed consent. The offering member introduces themselves to the patient or family and describes the diary, and diary program's goals, after confirming that the family has time to discuss the program. It is important to use clearly understood language (i.e., avoid medical jargon) when introducing an ICU diary program, and to be mindful of the patient and family's emotional state and level of stress. Anecdotal experience supports describing what the diary is and how the patient and family may benefit from it. Here is an example of an initial communication:

Hi Mrs. Smith, my name is Sally and I am the clinician taking care of your husband today. I wanted to talk to you about a special program that we have in this ICU. Do you have a few moments to talk about it? The initiative is an ICU diary for the patient and their families. Often when patients are critically ill, they may have trouble remembering events during their time in the ICU. This can cause them to be confused or anxious after they recover from being critically ill. The diary is used to journal summaries of daily events using non-medical terms to help them put together the pieces they may have missed while being so sick. Family members may benefit too by using the diary to record visitors, important events, how they felt and what they want their loved one to know about their time in the ICU. Anyone may write in the diary, including family members and healthcare team members that are caring for your husband. Is this something in which you would be interested in participating?"

■ WHAT IS APPROPRIATE ENTRY CONTENT AND STYLE?

Since the goal for the ICU diary is to document the patient's experience in a manner that will be understood by the patient as they recover, each entry should be written in a conversational fashion rather than reporting of objective healthcare information. This is often more difficult for healthcare clinicians than expected. Therefore, prior to rolling out the ICU diaries, our working group spent time writing practice entries with all members of the healthcare team. This allowed for direct and immediate feedback on the content of the entry. The step was well received and appreciated by the multiprofessional team.

■ WHO CAN WRITE ENTRIES?

Any member involved with the care of the patient may write an entry. This includes any member of the patient's family, the bedside nurse, physician, pharmacist, respiratory therapists, physical and occupational therapists, among others. At our institution, members of our consult teams have also taken the time to write entries for the patients. At ICU discharge, the diary is offered to the patient and their family to take with them as they continue onto the next phase of care. If the family chooses not to take the diary with them, the diary is stored in a secure location for a period of time. If the patient or family still does not desire the diary, the diary is disposed of in a secure fashion. If resources are available, patients may benefit from a postdischarge debrief of their ICU diary entries. The ideal time after discharge to pursue a diary debrief has not been established, but a 1-month postdischarge time frame has been used with great success. The debrief can occur by phone, by digital platform, or within the context of a post-ICU clinic.

The above information provides an overview of key information when implementing an ICU diary program from the perspective of one institution. Well-described strategies that aid in the planning, implementation, and sustainment of an ICU diary program include but are not limited to (1) obtaining support of unit members for implementation, (2) addressing patient privacy and professional liability for ICU diary use and content, (3) defining how to resolve potential complaints written within a diary, (4) establishing clear guidelines regarding photographs, and (5) managing diaries following a patient's transition out of the ICU. Distinct from designing and implementing an ICU diary program, an important consideration to explicitly prepare for is the challenge of sustaining an ICU diary program.

To optimize the program's workflow, and to avoid interruptions in the program as a result of leadership transitions and staff turnover, we have found it important to implement the following steps. *First*, at least annually, review the program's process of introducing, completing, and offering an ICU diary. To accomplish this, we kept the ICU diary program as a standing agenda on our weekly ICU leadership meetings, where we would identify and address issues that were identified. We also identified issues through interviews with new and existing staff, accomplished via ICU Healing Journal champion(s) who lead the program and are embedded in our ICU's leadership team. The most common barriers identified included: lack of comfort with introducing and initiating a diary, supply issues (i.e., diary supply not replete), and clinical care and documentation requirements leaving little time for journal entries during a shift. To address these issues, the champion's tasks included: identifying patients for whom the journal is appropriate and facilitating getting the journal started, assessing the unit's journal supply, partnering with the unit educator to meet the educational needs of the unit as it relates to the diary. *Second*, make it visible that the ICU diary program is, and remains, a high priority for the ICU. This is especially important through leadership transitions. *Third*, depending on the ICU's annual case volume and inclusion criteria, calculate the expected number of diaries needed annually and frequently assess and replete supply. *Fourth*, we educate new physicians, advanced practice providers, nurses, pharmacists, and therapists about survivorship in general, and the ICU diary program, in particular. The orientation includes an overview of our ICU website, which includes a section of survivorship. We also review the project's history, our procedure manual, and frequently asked questions' document to acclimate new team members to the process and to be prepared to introduce the diary, obtain agreement to participate, and to make entries. We also provide examples of cases in which the journal was beneficial to patients and their family as a motivational tool.

We have found that implementing and sustaining a successful ICU diary program requires embracing family presence in the ICU and other recommended patient- and family-centered care practices. Specifically, an ICU diary program is best layered into an ICU that afford the family open and flexible visiting hours, where family members are invited to join multiprofessional team rounds, and offered the option of being present during care—including procedures—as well as resuscitation efforts. Further, an ICU diary program should be viewed as a part of a family education program, since providing families with information about the ICU setting reduces anxiety, depression, and PTSD symptoms. Other complementary strategies such as those that reduce ventilator duration, decrease sedation, and mobilize patients out of bed are just as important as those that occur after discharge including ICU survivor support groups and post-ICU clinics. These topics are addressed in other chapters within this book.

Tips for Clinicians

1. Patients and families sustain significant stress during an episode of critical illness. There are multiple strategies that can help reduce the impact of those stressors during an episode of critical care as well as after acute care facility discharge. **Understanding which approaches are used in your facility, or the facilities that care for your patients is essential** in helping them understand those resources and how to use them during recovery.

2. An ICU diary program is one approach that is relatively straightforward to implement and delivers benefits during convalescence for patients and family members. Even if the patient expires, family members may derive benefit from having a journal that captures significant events during the end of the patient's life.

3. If the facility that cared for the patient and their family has an ICU diary program, **it is useful to explore whether they have the diary** and are reading it during outpatient office visit during recovery.

4. **Clinicians benefit from specific training regarding how to author entries within an ICU diary** to avoid medical jargon and instead adopt a conversational tone that is easily understood—and legible!

5. **ICU diaries are suitable for every team member to use,** just as they are ideal for family members and other loved ones. Recall that with critical illness or injury, ICU events may be difficult to recall, and some may be inaccurately remembered in an intrusive fashion that triggers anxiety of fear. PTSD is common in both ICU survivors and their family members. An ICU diary is one way to help reduce PTSD by providing a useful chronicle of events that can be examined at one remove from when those events occurred.

6. **PTSD after critical illness or injury should be specifically queried** and addressed to support mental health and wellness following acute care facility discharge.

KEY REFERENCES

Berning JN, Poor A, Buckley SM, et al. A novel picture guide to improve spiritual care and reduce anxiety in mechanically ventilated adults in the intensive care unit. *Ann Am Thorac Soc.* 2016;13(8):1333-1342.

Cameron JI, Chu LM, Matte A, et al. One-year outcomes in caregivers of critically ill patients. *N Engl J Med.* 2016;374:1831-1841.

Davidson JE, Aslakson RA, Long AC, et al. Guidelines for family-centered care in the neonatal, pediatric, and adult ICU. *Crit Care Med.* 2017;45(1):103-128.

Davidson JE, Jones C, Bienvenu OJ. Family response to critical illness: postintensive care syndrome-family. *Crit Care Med*. 2012;40(2):618-624.

Garrouste-Orgeas M, Coquet I, Périer A, et al. Impact of an intensive care unit diary on psychological distress in patients and relatives. *Crit Care Med*. 2012;40(7):2033-2040.

Garrouste-Orgeas M, Flahault C, Vinatier I, et al. Effect of an ICU diary on posttraumatic stress disorder symptoms among patients receiving mechanical ventilation: a randomized controlled trial. *JAMA*. 2019;322(3):229-239.

Geense WW, Zegers M, Peters MAA, et al. New physical, mental, and cognitive problems 1-year post-ICU: a prospective multicenter study. *Am J Respir Crit Care Med*. 2021;203: 1512-1521.

Govindan S, Iwashyna TJ, Watson SR, et al. Issues of survivorship are rarely addressed during intensive care unit stays. Baseline results from a statewide quality improvement collaborative. *Ann Am Thorac Soc*. 2014;11(4):587-591.

Haines KJ, Sevin CM, Hibbert E, et al. Key mechanisms by which post-ICU activities can improve in-ICU care: results of the international THRIVE collaboratives. *Intensive Care Med*. 2019;45(7):939-947.

Jones C, Backman C, Capuzzo M, et al. RACHEL group. Intensive care diaries reduce new onset post-traumatic stress disorder following critical illness: a randomized, controlled trial. *Crit Care*. 2010;14(5):R168.

Jones C, Backman C, Griffiths RD. Intensive care diaries and relatives' symptoms of posttraumatic stress disorder after critical illness: a pilot study. *Am J Crit Care*. 2021;21(3):172-176.

Marra A, Pandharipande PP, Girard TD, et al. Co-occurrence of post-intensive care syndrome problems among 406 survivors of critical illness. *Crit Care Med*. 2018;46(9):1393-1401.

McIlroy PA, King RS, Garrouste-Orgeas M, et al. The effect of ICU diaries on psychological outcomes and quality of life of survivors of critical illness and their relatives: a systematic review and meta-analysis. *Crit Care Med*. 2019;47(2):273-279.

Mikkelsen ME, Jackson JC, Hopkins RO, et al. Peer support as a novel strategy to mitigate post-intensive care syndrome. *Advanced Crit Care*. 2016;27(2):221-229.

Mikkelsen ME, Still M, Anderson BJ, et al. Society of Critical Care Medicine's international consensus conference on prediction and identification of long-term impairments after critical illness. *Crit Care Med*. 2020;48(11):1670-1679.

Needham DM, Davidson J, Cohen H, et al. Improving long-term outcomes after discharge from intensive care unit: report from a stakeholders' conference. *Crit Care Med*. 2012;40(2):502-509.

Nydahl P, Knück D, Egerod I. The extent and application of patient diaries in German intensive care units. *Connect—World Crit Care Nurs*. 2010;7(2):122-126.

Pun BT, Balas MC, Barnes-Daly MA, et al. Caring for critically ill patients with the ABCDEF bundle: results of the ICU liberation collaborative in over 15,000 adults. *Crit Care Med*. 2019;47(1):3.

Rogan J, Zielke M, Drumright K, Boehm LM. Institutional challenges and solutions to evidence-based, patient-centered practice: implementing ICU diaries at 2 U.S. sites. *Crit Care Nurse*. 2020;40(5):47-56.

Sullivan DR, Liu X, Corwin DS, et al. Learned helplessness among families and surrogate decision-makers of patients admitted to medical, surgical and trauma ICUs. *Chest*. 2012;142(6):1440-1446.

CHAPTER 15

Post-ICU Clinics

Patrick Holman, Kristin E. Schwab, and Jason H. Maley

Patient Care Vignette

A 52-year-old woman who works as a software engineer is admitted to the intensive care unit (ICU) with acute respiratory distress syndrome due to Streptococcal pneumonia. She requires 10 days of mechanical ventilation, including the use of deep sedation, neuromuscular blockade (temporary chemical paralysis), and prone-positioning therapy. She experiences delirium upon extubation (removal of the breathing tube), which continues for several days in the ICU. She is discharged to an acute rehabilitation facility and ultimately returns home after 6 weeks in the rehabilitation facility.

At home, she continues to experience ongoing vivid dreams related to her ICU stay and feels intrusive thoughts about her illness, anxiety over getting sick again, and persistent shortness of breath that limits her activity. She is assisted at home by her husband and she is able to perform activities of daily living independently. She finds that focusing on tasks, such as cooking or reading, is still challenging and she often loses her train-of-thought. She is not sure if she will be able to return to work. She visits her primary care doctor who recently learned about a post-ICU clinic with multidisciplinary expertise to help with her recovery.

■ INTRODUCTION TO POST-ICU CLINICS

As the population of ICU survivors grows, there is an increasing need for healthcare clinicians to understand the sequelae that these patients experience and how to best care for them after their ICU stay. Over the past two decades, some healthcare institutions have established multidisciplinary "post-ICU" clinics to address this goal. Previously, these clinics primarily existed in Europe, and to only a limited extent elsewhere. Interest in post-ICU care has globally increased as a result of both the COVID-19 pandemic and the increasing recognition of long-term sequelae of critical illness.

Limited data exist to inform the structure and implementation of post-ICU clinics. However, substantial evidence now describes the sequelae of critical illness. Further, experts within the critical care and rehabilitation communities advocate for novel follow-up care for ICU survivors re-entering the community. For example, the National Institute for Health and Care Excellence (NICE) guidelines for post-acute care recommend that "adults in critical care for more than 4 days should have a review by a healthcare professional 2 to 3 months after leaving critical care to talk about their recovery and any problems they might have." This review is specifically designed to identify those who have problems that they might not recognize (e.g., post-intensive care syndrome; see Introduction and Chapter 4), issues that they have not been able to address with locally available resources (e.g., certain kinds of specialty rehabilitation), or new conditions that have developed as a result of prior care (e.g., ventral hernia; see Chapter 23).

This chapter will explore the current landscape of post-ICU clinics including current evidence, best practices for clinic structure, ongoing challenges, and future directions.

■ HOW AND WHY THIS PROGRAM WORKS

Post-ICU clinics are ideally informed by the epidemiology of critical illness survivorship, and are ideal for those who no longer need inpatient management whether in a long-term acute care hospital, a rehabilitation facility, or a skilled nursing facility. Post-ICU clinic participants have ideally returned home after surviving their critical illness. A multitude of studies have evaluated patient outcomes after the ICU, including neurocognitive, psychiatric, physical, financial, social, and quality-of-life outcomes. The data support that the post-ICU clinics work for patients suffering from difficulties in each of these areas, the reasons for which are set forth below.

Neurocognitive (Higher Level Brain Function) Outcomes

There is robust evidence that following life-threatening critical illness patients commonly suffer some degree of cognitive impairment. The landmark Brain-ICU study enrolled 821 survivors of respiratory failure or shock for longitudinal cognitive assessment. At 12 months, roughly 25% of these patients had cognitive impairment similar to patients with mild Alzheimer's disease and 33% had impairment similar to patients with moderate traumatic brain injury.

This cognitive decline was present for patients regardless of age, surprisingly including those less than 50 years old. Therefore, family members should be aware that when their loved one's brain does not seem to have returned to its previous level of function, a healthcare professional should evaluate them. A post-ICU clinic can do just that as a matter of routine.

Psychiatric Outcomes

After life-threatening critical illness, ICU survivors often experience anxiety, depression, and/or posttraumatic stress disorder (PTSD) months to years after their critical illness. In the first year, 50-75% of ICU survivors may experience at least one psychiatric condition (e.g., depression, anxiety, and mood disorder), with high rates of having more than one at the same time. Studies evaluating outcomes beyond 1 year suggest that these impairments remain present in up to half of the patients. Many have less intense symptoms over time, but some continue to benefit from professional guidance and medication therapy. In addition, a large cohort study reviewing nearly 500,000 ICU survivors found an increased risk of suicide and self-harm among ICU survivors compared to non-ICU hospitalized patients.

Strength and Endurance Outcomes

Similar to other domains, physical impairments (e.g., weakness and reduced endurance) are commonly persistent following ICU discharge and substantially impact ICU survivors' health-related quality of life. Studies examining survivors of sepsis and mechanical ventilation suggest that up to 75% of patients have impairments in physical function in the months following discharge, including difficulty with activities of daily living. Such limitations may persist for 5 years after discharge, establishing a clear need to assess patients for physical limitations when they present for postdischarge care. If it is not part of the routine assessment, persistent weakness or limited endurance may be missed. Such sequelae may be addressed using directed physical therapy as well as occupational therapy. Post-ICU clinics routinely explore how well patients are returning to their pre-illness level of function.

Financial and Social Outcomes

ICU survivors often bear substantial financial costs that persist after discharge. When the cost of ongoing care—including new medications or therapies—create financial difficulty for patients and their family, it is known as financial toxicity. Other terms have been applied including financial stress, financial hardship, economic burden, and more. Originally described for cancer patients, this condition also occurs after serious injury or critical illness.

Drivers of financial toxicity include medical bills not covered by insurance (i.e., balance billing as well as services such as home care that are not authorized by the insurance carrier), changes in insurance coverage, and lost employment, which may substantially impair recovery and access to follow-up care. A systematic review of over 50 studies and 10,000 patients found that 64%, 40%, and 32% of previously employed ICU survivors were jobless 3, 12, and 60 months after an ICU stay, respectively. Furthermore, patients commonly have difficulty driving (when they own a vehicle) in the immediate postdischarge period with a little over half of the patients in one study not yet driving at the time of follow-up (median 1 month). This creates a barrier to accessing care that would otherwise be available, potentially including a post-ICU clinic. Therefore, costs for driving services add to financial toxicity, or family members serve as drivers, often limiting their ability to continue to work. Understanding and overcoming these barriers is essential for post-ICU clinics to provide accessible and equitable care.

■ POST-ICU CLINIC BARRIERS AND FACILITATORS

A number of studies have explored the potential benefits of post-ICU clinics, as well as the barriers to implementation; randomized controlled trials are summarized in Table 15-1. In one such study, Haines and colleagues explore the perceived barrier to and facilitators of post-ICU clinics among members of the Society of Critical Care Medicine THRIVE post-ICU clinic initiative (https://sccm.org/MyICUCare/THRIVE). They identified nine major barriers: lack of staff in clinics, inability to identify appropriate patients, lack of collective identity of ICU survivorship, patient and family limitations to accessing clinics, lack of funding, lack of space, practice variation between clinicians, limitations of clinicians as volunteers, and hospital billing infrastructure (Fig. 15-1). Major enablers of clinic success included interprofessional teamwork, defined operational processes, the human connection, motivated clinicians, creative problem solving, and the support of the SCCM THRIVE collaborative (Fig. 15-2).

In a single-center descriptive study of the ICU clinic at Vanderbilt, Sevin and colleagues described additional challenges. They noted that many patients were discharged to rehab facilities or the homes of friends or family that resulted in inaccurate home contact information. There was substantial lag time in follow-up, and many care transitions took place between the ICU and home, which led to fragmented care in the absence of planned longitudinal follow up. In addition, many patients did not understand the importance or potential benefit of ICU specific follow-up. This is an aspect of care that can be readily reinforced upon discharge home as well as during primary care outpatient office follow-up.

▦ TABLE 15-1. Randomized Controlled Trials of Post-ICU Clinics and Their Interventions

Study	Year	Authors	Study Design	Outcomes/Discussion
PRaCTICaL	2009	Cuthbertson et al	• **Intervention: RN led physical rehabilitation program** • Pragmatic, nonblinded, multicenter RCT • 286 patients from three UK hospitals	• No difference in primary or secondary outcomes evaluating HRQoL • Noted one-third of patients required specialty referral indicating gaps of care in leaving the hospital
RECOVER	2015	Walsh et al	• **Intervention: Post-hospital rehabilitation & dietary program** • 240 patients in two Scottish hospitals	• No difference in primary outcome—Rivermead Mobility Index • Improved patient satisfaction regarding their recovery
RAPIT	2016	Jensen et al	• **Intervention: RN led post-ICU recovery program (mixed in-person & telephone)** • Two-arm, nonblinded, parallel group, multicenter, pragmatic RCT • 386 patients in Denmark	• No differences in HRQoL and prevalence of mental health impairments
SMOOTH	2016	Schmidt et al	• **Intervention: Post-ICU support program with RN trained case managers to support PCPs vs. PCP alone** • Multicenter RCT • 291 patients in Germany	• No difference in primary or secondary outcomes looking at mental HRQoL • Patients with more severe cognitive dysfunction were excluded
REVIVE	2017	McDowell et al	• **Intervention: Supervised outpatient exercise program** • Prospective, multicenter, Phase II RCT, with blinded outcome assessment • 60 patients	• No difference in primary outcome of SF-36 scores • Early improvement in secondary outcomes including: incremental shuttle walk test, functional limitations profile, self-efficacy to exercise, readiness to exercise. However, findings were not sustained at 6-month follow-up
Vanderbilt ICU Recovery Program	2019	Bloom et al	• **Intervention: Pilot inter-disciplinary post-ICU clinic** • Single institution, nonblinded, RCT • 232 patients	• Demonstrated feasibility (primary outcome) by study group having more support interventions done • No significant difference in secondary outcome of 30-day readmission rate • Longer time to readmission for intervention group

RCT, randomized controlled trial; RN, registered nurse.

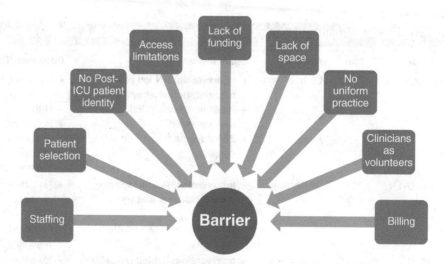

FIGURE 15-1. Post-ICU Clinic Barriers. This figure presents commonly identified barriers to establishing a post-ICU clinic.

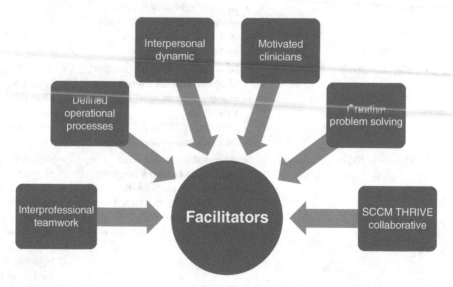

FIGURE 15-2. Post-ICU Clinic Facilitators. These six elements each help facilitate the smooth and effective functioning of a post-ICU clinic.

In 2019, Haines and colleagues also explored the mechanisms by which post-ICU activities resulted in perceived improvements in the ICU care. Their findings revealed important potential benefits of post-ICU clinics, including:

- Identifying otherwise unseen targets for ICU quality improvement or education programs

- Creating a new role for survivors in the ICU
- Educating ICU colleagues by having them visit the post-ICU clinic
- Understanding the patient experience
- Improving staff morale

To provide further insight into the potential benefits of post-ICU care, McPeake and colleagues interviewed patients to explore the need for post-ICU clinics, describing five key components associated with patient-perceived success of post-ICU programs:

- Providing continuity of ICU recovery care
- Improving post-ICU syndrome (PICS) symptoms
- Managing expectation and normalizing the postdischarge course
- Validating internal and external patient progress
- Reducing feelings of guilt and helplessness

■ POST-ICU CLINIC STRUCTURE

Patient Identification

Identifying patients who are most likely to benefit from a post-ICU clinic is an essential step—and one that is quite challenging. Since no healthcare systems is equipped to follow every ICU survivor in a dedicated clinic, patients at particularly high risk for PICS should be identified. Moreover, patients get admitted to an ICU for a variety of reasons other than life-threatening critical illness or injury, including: (1) monitoring that must occur at a frequency that cannot occur on the general floor, (2) management with a device that cannot be managed on the general floor, (3) transient use of a medication that cannot be administered on the general floor, (4) overflow when there are no general floor beds, and (5) monitoring for events that are time sensitive. Most of those patients have an ICU length of stay (LOS) that is 24 hours or less. Therefore, stratifying patient risk for PICS would help select the ideal post-ICU population.

This risk-stratification can be performed by considering baseline patient characteristics—such as baseline cognitive, mental health, or physical impairments—as well as ICU-specific risk factors, including delirium, prolonged sedation, invasive mechanical ventilation, sepsis, shock, the acute respiratory distress syndrome, or the need for a tracheostomy or transabdominal wall feeding catheter. Others such as new organ failure, recurrent infections, and conditions that affect cognition, mental health, strength, or endurance are additional factors to guide patient selection. We recommend considering both ICU LOS (e.g., greater than 72 hours) and a high severity of acute illness to identify as many patients as possible who may benefit from post-ICU follow-up. Since there is no "one-size fits all" approach to identify all at-risk patients, clinical judgment including the factors identified above should inform referral to a post-ICU clinic.

Timing of Referral

The ideal timing for post-ICU clinic follow-up remains largely unstudied. Consensus guidelines recommend an assessment 2-4 weeks after hospital discharge; this may be a convenient and comfortable time frame rather than one driven by evidence. Furthermore, many individuals may receive care in a facility that does not have a post-ICU clinic. Their initial postdischarge medical care may be with their primary care clinician. Therefore, those clinicians will benefit from developing a familiarity with PICS and PICS-F so that they can screen for either condition and make the appropriate referral to a post-ICU clinic as well as a PICS support group.

For facilities that do have a post-ICU clinic, facilitating clinic evaluation timing can be challenging, particularly as many patients are first discharged to transitional care facilities such as skilled nursing facilities, acute rehab units, or long-term acute care hospitals. A discharge navigator/coordinator may be useful to connect with patients while they're still in the hospital, introduce the post-ICU program, provide anticipatory guidance, and schedule the post-ICU clinic follow-up appointment. The discharge navigator role may be filled by a nurse, social worker, respiratory therapist, or case manager, among others; patients value the continuity of care that a navigator and a focused clinic provides. Employing a discharge coordinator is associated with decreased readmission rates and decreased loss-to-follow-up in the vulnerable post-ICU population.

Team Members

Post-ICU clinics typically engage a multiprofessional team to best address the many domains of PICS. Clinicians and survivors have advocated for clinics led by ICU physicians, as this both facilitates longitudinal care delivery for the patients and provides a portal for feedback to improve processes for future patients in the ICU. In addition to the intensivist, these clinics may include a physiatrist (rehabilitation medicine physician), physical therapist, respiratory therapist, psychologist, psychiatrist, social worker (to assess for psychological sequelae), occupational therapist, speech/language pathologist, or neurocognitive specialist. Additional team members may include a pharmacist, registered dietitian, chaplain, geriatrician, and palliative care medicine specialist. In this way, the post-ICU clinic recapitulates the typical multiprofessional team that works together to care for patients during their episode of acute critical illness or injury.

■ POST-ICU CLINIC VISIT PATIENT ASSESSMENT

While each survivor's recovery journey is unique, standardized tools to evaluate for PICS should be employed during the clinic visit (Fig. 15-3). This allows clinicians to track progression over time as well as better map what patients or their family members report to objective criteria. Expert consensus recommends using the Hospital Anxiety and Depression Scale (HADS) to assess for anxiety and depression and either the Impact of Events Scale-Revised (IES-R) or the shorter IES-6 to evaluate for posttraumatic stress disorder. The Montreal Cognitive Assessment (MOCA) or MOCA-Blind can be used to screen for cognitive impairment, and the Six-Minute Walk Test (6MWT) can be used to evaluate physical function. Manual muscle testing and hand-grip dynamometry may be incorporated to evaluate for ICU-acquired weakness, including critical illness myopathy and critical illness neuropathy. To assess health-related quality of life, experts recommend starting with the EuroQol-5D (EQ-5D) questionnaire, which can also be used to evaluate pain. While the specifics of each tool are not explored in this chapter, there is an important aspect to be emphasized—there are precise methods to assess patients for complications of critical illness. Therefore, when patients and

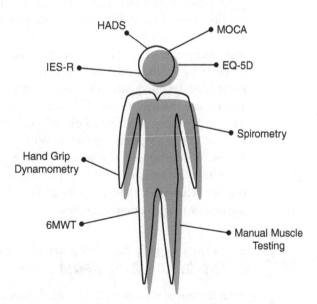

FIGURE 15-3. Post-ICU Clinic Patient Assessment Tools. This figure presents a variety of tools that can be used to help assess post-ICU clinic patients and help decide on the need for specific kinds of rehabilitative therapy. EQ-5D, EuroQol-5D; HADS, Hospital Anxiety and Depression Scale; IES-R, Impact of Event Scale-Revised; MOCA, Montreal Cognitive Assessment; 6MWT, Six-Minute Walk Test.

family members are asked what seems to be a lot of questions, there is a solid underpinning reason for those questions, and the answers help to guide referrals for medical or physical therapy, or other unique interventions.

In addition to these screening tools, we recommend considering the following: medication reconciliation (this helps eliminate unnecessary medications and reduces "polypharmacy"), screening for new or persistent symptoms, summarizing the patient's ICU course to help fill in any gaps and answer any questions (this is also supported by an ICU journal, see Chapter 4), counseling on expected ICU recovery, and performing relevant healthcare maintenance tasks such as vaccinations. Moreover, the post-ICU clinic's multiprofessional approach may also address and inform postcritical illness sexual health—an aspect of well-being that is multidimensional and should be aligned with each patient's individual needs and recovery trajectory. We regularly ask for feedback from patients and families on their ICU experience to contribute to process improvement within the ICU. As has become increasingly recognized under the term "PICS-Family," an ICU stay can lead to adverse psychological effects on family members (see Chapter 4). For this reason, and because of their important role as caregivers and facilitators of recovery, it is important to include family/caregivers in the clinic visit as well.

Due to the multidisciplinary nature of the clinic, these visits may be longer than typical specialist visits and may span 1-2 hours. These appointments have traditionally been performed in-person, although that presents an access and equity barrier for patients with limited mobility, large geographical distances between the center and the patient's home, and reduced access to transportation. Telemedicine provides an attractive solution to increase access and reduce barriers to care—a tool well leveraged during the SARS-CoV-2 pandemic across a variety of digital platforms including Microsoft TEAMS, ZOOM, Bluejeans, and Doximity. While the recommended screening tools for psychological and cognitive function can be performed over a digital video link, assessment of physical function is more challenging. For this reason, we believe that there remains an important role for in-person visits when feasible from the patient's standpoint.

■ INTERFACING WITH PRIMARY CARE CLINICIANS, AND GRADUATION FROM CLINIC

After the initial visit, post-ICU clinics may consider performing follow-up visits at regular intervals until the patient is able to "graduate" back to their primary care provider. Those with established plans of care for PICS may be able to graduate after one or two visits, while those with ongoing symptoms of PICS often need ongoing follow-up for years. For those with significant impairments, we typically perform more frequent initial interval follow-up (e.g., every 1-2 months) and later space this out (e.g., every 3-6 months) over subsequent visits. Regular visits and relationships with longitudinal providers remain essential, as survivors often voice desires to better understand their long-term recovery trajectory and better reintegrate into daily life during this extended clinic follow-up period. Therefore, post-ICU clinics benefit from having regular staffing rather than rotating staff who change on a weekly or monthly basis.

■ CONCLUSIONS

Critical illness ICU survivors commonly suffer impairments in mental health, cognition, and physical function that substantially impact quality of life. These health impairments may be compounded by the financial toxicity of critical illness, including medical expenses and unemployment. It is therefore essential that healthcare systems meet the needs of these survivors. One way to do so is through structured longitudinal follow-up care that enhances recovery and helps restore quality of life. These clinics ideally should enroll patients with a high-risk of PICS, such as those who have experienced prolonged critical illness, sepsis, shock, and respiratory failure. Planned clinic follow-up may flow from the ICU team's recognition that a patient has a high risk for PICS, but may also result from an initial postdischarge visit with a primary care clinician. Patients will benefit from standardized screening for impairments in mental health, cognition, and physical function at an initial post-ICU clinic visit, or during primary care postdischarge evaluation. These impairments are then best addressed by a multiprofessional team using in-person visits, digital telemedicine platforms, or a combination of both. Lessons from post-ICU clinic patients and family members should be brought back to the ICU to facilitate continuous quality of improvement of ICU care and optimize the ICU experience. Post-ICU clinics are a key step in improving the long-term quality of life for survivors of critical illness or injury.

Tips for Clinicians

Post-ICU Care Prior to Hospital Discharge

1. Prior to hospital discharge, **educate patients and families about post-intensive care syndrome (PICS) and post-intensive care syndrome-family (PICS-F)** and the importance of post-ICU rehabilitative care—empowering them to advocate for post-ICU care as needs arise.
2. **Provide educational materials regarding PICS and PICS-F**, such as those which are available through professional societies.

3. **Ensure outpatient follow-up is scheduled** for patients in a post-ICU clinic or with a primary care clinician within 2-4 weeks after hospital discharge to specifically address post-ICU recovery.
4. Schedule telemedicine follow-up as an alternative for patients who may not be able to follow-up in-person during the early post-acute recovery period.

Establishing a Post-ICU Clinic and Conducting a Post-ICU Clinic Visit

1. **Establish patient selection criteria** to focus on those at high risk for PICS.
2. **Consider engaging a multiprofessional group** to serve as core members of a post-ICU clinical program, or key consultants if a formal clinic is not feasible. These members should have expertise to address cognitive (e.g., neurology, occupational therapy, speech therapy), mental health (e.g., psychiatry, psychology, social work), and physical (e.g., physical therapy, physiatry, pulmonary medicine, respiratory therapy) impairments.
3. Validated screening measures may be used during post-ICU visits to measure impairments in mental health, physical function, and cognition.
4. Based on screening, patients may be referred to other members of a multiprofessional post-ICU clinic or scheduled with consultants who can address their key needs.
5. **Include family members in the post-ICU evaluation** and recovery process, given their essential role as caregivers and their risk for PICS-F.
6. **Provide social work support** to address the social and financial needs that many patients and family members experience as barriers to recovery.
7. When there is a PICS Support group, **encourage clinic attendees to participate**.
8. Bring lessons learned from the post-ICU clinic back to the ICU on a regular basis.

KEY REFERENCES

Bloom SL, Stollings JL, Kirkpatrick O, et al. Randomized clinical trial of an ICU recovery pilot program for survivors of critical illness. *Crit Care Med*. 2019;47(10):1337-1345.

Cuthbertson BH, Elders A, Hall S, et al. Mortality and quality of life in the five years after severe sepsis. *Crit Care*. 2013;17(2):R70.

Cuthbertson BH, Rattray J, Campbell MK, et al. The PRaCTICaL study of nurse led, intensive care follow-up programmes for improving long term outcomes from critical illness: a pragmatic randomised controlled trial. *BMJ*. 2009;339:b3723.

Fernando SM, Qureshi D, Sood MM, et al. Suicide and self-harm in adult survivors of critical illness: population based cohort study. *BMJ.* 2021;373:n973.

Griffiths JA, Barber VS, Cuthbertson BH, Young JD. A national survey of intensive care follow-up clinics. *Anaesthesia.* 2006;61(10):950-955.

Haines KJ, McPeake J, Hibbert E, et al. Enablers and barriers to implementing ICU follow-up clinics and peer support groups following critical illness: the thrive collaboratives. *Crit Care Med.* 2019;47(9):1194-1200.

Haines KJ, McPeake J, Hibbert E, et al. Enablers and barriers to implementing ICU follow up clinics and peer support groups following critical illness: the thrive collaboratives. *Crit Care Med.* 2019;47(9):1194-1200.

Haines KJ, Sevin CM, Hibbert E, et al. Key mechanisms by which post-ICU activities can improve in-ICU care: results of the international THRIVE collaboratives. *Intensive Care Med.* 2019;45(7):939-947.

Herridge MS, Tansey CM, Matté A, et al. Functional disability 5 years after acute respiratory distress syndrome. *N Engl J Med.* 2011;364(14):1293-1304.

Hopkins RO, Suchyta MR, Farrer TJ, Needham D. Improving post-intensive care unit neuropsychiatric outcomes: understanding cognitive effects of physical activity. *Am J Respir Crit Care Med.* 2012;186(12):1220-1228.

Huang M, Parker AM, Bienvenu OJ, et al. Psychiatric symptoms in acute respiratory distress syndrome survivors: a 1-year national multicenter study. *Crit Care Med.* 2016;44(5):954-965.

Iwashyna TJ, Ely EW, Smith DM, Langa KM. Long-term cognitive impairment and functional disability among survivors of severe sepsis. *JAMA.* 2010;304(16):1787-1794.

Jackson JC, Pandharipande PP, Girard TD, et al. Depression, post-traumatic stress disorder, and functional disability in survivors of critical illness in the BRAIN-ICU study: a longitudinal cohort study. *Lancet Respir Med.* 2014;2(5):369-379.

Jalilian L, Cannesson M, Kamdar N. Post-ICU recovery clinics in the era of digital health and telehealth. *Crit Care Med.* 2019;47(9):e796-e797.

Jensen JF, Egerod I, Bestle MH, et al. A recovery program to improve quality of life, sense of coherence and psychological health in ICU survivors: a multicenter randomized controlled trial, the RAPIT study. *Intensive Care Med.* 2016;42(11):1733-1743.

Kamdar BB, Suri R, Suchyta MR, et al. Return to work after critical illness: a systematic review and meta-analysis. *Thorax.* 2020;75(1):17-27.

Kosinski S, Mohammad RA, Pitcher M, et al. What is post-intensive care syndrome (PICS)? *Am J Respir Crit Care Med.* 2020;201(8):P15-P16.

Lainscak M, Kadivec S, Kosnik M, et al. Discharge coordinator intervention prevents hospitalizations in patients with COPD: a randomized controlled trial. *J Am Med Dir Assoc.* 2013;14(6):450.e1-6.

Lee CM, Herridge MS, Matte A, Cameron JI. Education and support needs during recovery in acute respiratory distress syndrome survivors. *Crit Care.* 2009;13(5):R153.

Maley JH, Brewster I, Mayoral I, et al. Resilience in survivors of critical illness in the context of the survivors' experience and recovery. *Ann Am Thorac Soc.* 2016;13(8):1351-1360.

Marra A, Pandharipande PP, Girard TD, et al. Co-occurrence of post-intensive care syndrome problems among 406 survivors of critical illness. *Crit Care Med.* 2018;46(9):1393-1401.

McDowell K, O'Neill B, Blackwood B, et al. Effectiveness of an exercise programme on physical function in patients discharged from hospital following critical illness: a randomised controlled trial (the REVIVE trial). *Thorax*. 2017;72(7):594-595.

McPeake J, Boehm LM, Hibbert E, et al. Key components of ICU recovery programs: what did patients report provided benefit? *Crit Care Explor*. 2020;2(4):e0088.

Mehlhorn J, Freytag A, Schmidt K, et al. Rehabilitation interventions for postintensive care syndrome: a systematic review. *Crit Care Med*. 2014;42(5):1263-1271.

Mikkelsen ME, Still M, Anderson BJ, et al. Society of Critical Care Medicine's International Consensus Conference on prediction and identification of long-term impairments after critical illness. *Crit Care Med*. 2020;48(11):1670-1679.

Needham DM, Davidson J, Cohen H, et al. Improving long-term outcomes after discharge from intensive care unit: report from a stakeholders' conference. *Crit Care Med*. 2012;40(2):502-509.

Needham DM, Sepulveda KA, Dinglas VD, et al. Core outcome measures for clinical research in acute respiratory failure survivors. An International Modified Delphi Consensus Study. *Am J Respir Crit Care Med*. 2017;196(9):1122-1130.

NICE. 2018 surveillance of rehabilitation after critical illness in adults. NICE guideline CG83. 2018.

Pandharipande PP, Girard TD, Jackson JC, et al. Long-term cognitive impairment after critical illness. *N Engl J Med*. 2013;369(14):1306-1316.

Pratt CM, Hirshberg EL, Jones JP, et al. Long-term outcomes after severe shock. *Shock*. 2015;43(2):128-132.

Schmidt K, Worrack S, Von Korff M, et al. Effect of a primary care management intervention on mental health related quality of life among survivors of sepsis: a randomized clinical trial. *JAMA*. 2016;315(24):2703-2711.

Sevin CM, Bloom SL, Jackson JC, Wang L, Ely EW, Stollings JL. Comprehensive care of ICU survivors: Development and implementation of an ICU recovery center. *J Crit Care*. 2018;46:141-148.

Sevin CM, Jackson JC. Post-ICU clinics should be staffed by ICU clinicians. *Crit Care Med*. 2019;47(2):268-272.

Walsh TS, Salisbury LG, Merriweather JL, et al. Increased hospital-based physical rehabilitation and information provision after intensive care unit discharge: the RECOVER randomized clinical trial. *JAMA Intern Med*. 2015;175(6):901-910.

Family Presence on Critical Care Rounds

Caitlin C. ten Lohuis, Heather Meissen, Katherine R. Casey, and
Craig M. Coopersmith

Patient Care Reflection

It is human nature to yearn for safety, protection, support, and love when one is scared or sick—a familiar face, the touch of a loved one, a family member's soothing voice. The SARS-CoV-2 pandemic with its associated limitations on hospital visitation has stripped patients of these vital human needs. There are new innovative avenues by way of FaceTime or Zoom calls to connect patients and loved ones from a distance; nonetheless, there is no substitution for in-person human presence.

During this time when visitors are extremely limited and oftentimes not permitted within hospital walls, the bedside staff are the sole bridge connecting patients and loved ones. Prepandemic, it was a common sight to walk by a critically ill patient's room and see a loved one perched in a chair with their hand blanketed overtop the patient's fingers. Albeit sometimes in silence, hearing the hum of the ventilator, their presence provided a sentiment of comfort and familiarity. The pandemic created a starkly contrasting reality. Once a SARS-CoV-2 patient becomes ill enough to require ICU care, their fear is borderline insurmountable. They are in a closed room, isolated and alone, and their only human compassion and support is the frontline providers at the bedside. Suddenly strangers become family, and the importance of human care surpasses that of medical care. Taking the time to sit in a patient's room and quietly keep them company so they feel safe to close their eyes is the most valuable intervention you can provide.

Once a patient deteriorates enough to require ventilator support, many do not survive. One occurrence that has been pivotally impactful has been the number of times that I as a frontline provider am the last person to speak with a patient. Generally, SARS-CoV-2 patients are completely lucid, just extremely hypoxemic. Once the hypoxemia progresses beyond the limits of noninvasive oxygen support, intubation is the next step. There is chaos and buzzing activity around the patient's bed including gathering supplies and setting up machines in preparation for placing the patient on the ventilator. Meanwhile the patient sits in the hospital bed, terrified of the uncertainty and staring down the barrel of mortality. Once SARS-CoV-2 patients get intubated, it is typically a tumultuous and long recovery, including prolonged periods of time on the ventilator, significant muscular atrophy, and almost always severe encephalopathy. Many of the patients suffer complications leading to death or never wake up to full neurologic functioning. It dawned on me that there is a "golden window"—this period of time just before intubation may be the patient's final moments awake in life. Secondarily, it dawned on me how significant it is during this "golden window" to put forth great effort in connecting the patient with the family via telephone or video call, as it may be the final time they speak. Honoring the "golden window" is now incorporated into my intubation checklist.

In a time where it is extremely busy, hectic, and easy to get frazzled in completing innumerable tasks, the SARS-CoV-2 pandemic has reminded me to slow down. It has reminded me to be human, to hold the patient's hand, and to provide them as safe and caring of a space as possible amid the terror and unpredictability. During a time when families are not physically present at the bedside due to SARS-CoV-2 transmission risk, a provider is no longer solely focused on practicing the best medicine. There is a new role to be that human presence, to be that bridge connecting patients and loved ones as effectively as possible. The SARS-CoV-2 pandemic has magnified how inexplicably valuable it is to have the presence of loved ones at the bedside to advocate for, support, and provide a space of calm familiarity.
—Katherine Casey

■ HOW AND WHY FAMILY MEMBERS ON ICU ROUNDS WORK TO SUPPORT POST-ICU RECOVERY

Beyond the physical stressors of critical illness that a patient experiences during their stay in an ICU, patients are in a foreign environment and completely isolated from the outside world. Well before the COVID-19 pandemic, there was a clear understanding that an ICU stay could result in patients having major psychological disorders including depression, anxiety, and posttraumatic stress disorder (PTSD) both during their ICU and hospital stay and after discharge. In fact, 30-50% of ICU patients experience post-intensive care syndrome (PICS) which is characterized by physical, cognitive, and emotional impairments. PICS continues to affect the quality of life of patients as well as families after discharge and its effects can persist for months to years. During the COVID-19 pandemic, hospital visitation ceased or was severely curtailed, and frontline ICU professionals became the bridge between patients and families in the ICU. Hospitals relied on virtual forms of communication with family members. While methods varied, telephones were used for clinician–family communication and videoconference was predominately used for patient–family communication. During this time, patient- and family-centered care was derailed and the regular communication between the ICU team and the family became increasingly difficult. The COVID-19 pandemic highlighted the integral role family members play in a patient's ICU stay, and the loss that occurs when they are absent.

In addition to the mental and emotional stress on patients and families caused by ICU admission, the severity of illness of critically ill patients can limit their ability to be involved in decision making. Patients depend on family members for emotional support, to help navigate healthcare decisions, and to serve as surrogate decision-makers if the patient cannot participate due to illness or ongoing therapy. Therefore, family members should be recognized not only as "visitors," but also as "partners in care" who should be encouraged to actively participate in their loved one's care. Importantly, family members understand the patient's goals, values, and preferences in ways that the ICU team cannot. This knowledge renders family members key team members in ensuring the delivery of goal-concordant care.

With the shift from physician-directed care to patient autonomy, patients and their family members were provided information about care and then needed to select the path they desired. This approach recognized the value of individual decision-making but provided less than desired support during the process of arriving at a care decision. The early 2000s brought a new model—shared decision-making. With shared decision-making, there is a mutual understanding between clinician and patient of the diagnosis, treatment options, prognosis, within the context of the patient's goals, values, and preferences. Shared decision-making is ideal when the patient can participate in the process. With acute critical illness or injury, and the need for complex critical care, patients are often unable to share their thoughts and values. Accordingly, family members or other legally authorized representatives must serve in the patient's stead as a surrogate to share what the patient would likely have thought about their condition and care if they were able.

Surrogate decision-makers clearly benefit from seeing, hearing, and sometimes smelling the ICU room and the patient attached to life-sustaining devices to garner an accurate picture of their loved one. Therefore, effective communication between family and the healthcare team is essential in providing patient-centered care.

Shared decision-making helps relieve families of the tremendous anxiety and stress that accompanies their loved one's illness and helps facilitate difficult decision-making for patients in the ICU. Families of patients facing terminal illness do not want to make end-of-life decisions alone. Instead, through shared decision-making, a genuine partnership between the ICU team, patients, and families is preferred. This importance of families in patient care has created a family-centered care model in addition to the patient-centered care model. The goals of patient- and family-centered care are to (1) enable patients and families to actively engage in medical decision-making and self-management, (2) coordinate and integrate patient care across groups of clinicians, (3) provide physical comfort and emotional support, (4) understand patients' concepts of illness as they relate to cultural and spiritual beliefs, and (5) understand and apply principles of disease prevention and behavioral change appropriate for diverse populations. While the latter goal is more appropriate for outpatient care, the first four readily apply to the ICU.

Patient- and family-centered care is also one of the six elements of the Society of Critical Care Medicine's (SCCM) ICU Liberation Bundle. SCCM's ICU Liberation Bundle provides evidence-based care to liberate ICU patients from pain, oversedation, delirium, mechanical ventilation, immobility, and isolation through easy-to-implement daily interventions. Implementation of SCCM's ICU Liberation Bundle has been shown in more than 20,000 patients to decrease the likelihood of hospital death within 7 days by 68%, reduce delirium and coma days by 25-50%, reduce physical restraint use by more than 60%, decrease ICU readmission by 50%, and reduce discharges to nursing home and rehabilitation by 40%. Social isolation is a major risk factor for morbidity and mortality and negatively impacts health. While critical illness or injury separates patients from families as they receive care in a hospital, family engagement and empowerment to participate in the patient's care is to encourage family participation in ICU rounds.

Family presence on rounds is an encouraged element of the SCCM's ICU Liberation bundle. Having a family member or members participate in rounds has been studied in the adult, pediatric, and neonatal ICU. A wide variety of studies demonstrated that family members who attend rounds are more involved with decision making and have greater satisfaction with the care team than those who do not attend rounds. Rounds that are performed without family or patient inclusion can hinder the patient, family, and ICU team relationship, especially if there is no other communication that flows to the family. Complications, untoward events, and unfavorable and unanticipated outcomes are likely to be viewed with suspicion and distrust when there is an absence of a collaborative relationship between the patient's family and care teams, particularly during the course of ICU care.

■ IMPLEMENTATION OF FAMILY MEMBERS ON ROUNDS IN THE ICU

Family presence is the attendance of family members on daily bedside rounds during a discussion of the patient's condition and the daily plan for care. Family members that should be included on rounds are those that the patient has selected as decision makers. Additional family members can join once consent is given by the patient (or their legally authorized representative) for the non–decision makers to be present. The healthcare team should invite family members to rounds everyday while highlighting the family member's role as a valuable member of the care team (see Figure 16-1 for benefits of including family members on ICU rounds). As an attempt to welcome and ease any fear or anxiety a family member may feel about attending rounds for the first time, some hospitals give families a written and verbal explanation of rounds (Fig. 16-2). This helps prepare the family member for the usual conduct of rounds, and often includes a description of team members that are regularly present. Some ask the family to designate one of the patient's decision makers who participates in rounds as the family spokesperson. This individual fields phone calls from the rest of the interested family members to share information as appropriate. Importantly, this also decreases the number of phone calls that the critical care nurse fields during the day as family members try to secure information about their loved one.

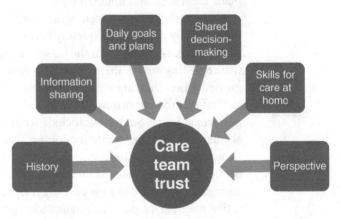

FIGURE 16-1. Benefits of Family Members on ICU Rounds.

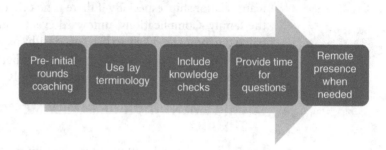

FIGURE 16-2. **Process Aspects of Family Members on Rounds.**

In addition to being present on rounds, families and patients should have the opportunity to participate in the discussion of the patient's care. There are often pieces of history, life quality, plans, and related elements that help the ICU team. Healthcare teams can encourage participation by suggesting family members make a list of questions that they would like to have answered during rounds. Throughout the rounds, the patient and family should remain the focal point to further promote engagement. After the plan is discussed, a healthcare provider should provide a summary for the family using understandable language without confusing medical jargon. At the conclusion of rounds, the family and the patient (when able) should have an opportunity to voice any final concerns that need clarification or may have not been covered in sufficient detail. When well done, family members who participate in critical and shared decision-making feel less like visitors and more like family members. If family members are unable to attend, a virtual option is ideal to support continuity and engagement and to ensure that daily events and care plans are shared and understood.

Since complex care often results in care that needs to be continued at home, family members frequently become uncompensated caregivers. Seeing the complexity of care from the outset, family members gain a useful perspective regarding where their loved one started and how much they have progressed when they are ready to return home. Furthermore, family presence also affords the opportunity to help train them in tasks that they will need to perform at home. Such tasks include wound packing, ostomy appliance management, and tracheostomy suctioning. Family members who are used to participating in ICU rounds may also be comfortable doing so if post-ICU care is required at long-term acute care hospital or a rehabilitation facility. Their additional exposure to how care evolves lends a certain comfort in being an active member of post-hospitalization care. Having a complete perspective on what worked well, or how their loved one appeared when they develop intercurrent illness, helps family members advocate for their loved one after leaving the acute care setting as well. Ongoing physical therapy or occupational therapy exercises can be taught to family members so that between visits therapy continues in a consistent fashion. Clearly essential, family members that are present during ICU rounds impact bedside workflow in anticipatable—and manageable—ways.

■ THE IMPACT OF FAMILY MEMBER DURING ICU ROUNDS ON CLINICIANS

Despite the benefits discussed above, family members on rounds has the potential to adversely impact clinician workflow. Common concerns healthcare clinicians express when involving family members in rounds primarily focus on how having nonclinicians will impact discussion content, the time required to complete rounds, trainee education, and when there are complex issues with unfavorable trajectories, family stress. Furthermore, some clinicians may be concerned about how family presence will impact their workflow related to other time-consuming tasks such as note writing and care coordination activities—much of which often occurs during rounds.

Total Rounding Time

With heavy caseloads and the many obligations that being an ICU clinician brings, an increased time spent on rounds can be an undesired byproduct of having families on rounds. While this is a true observation, there is a benefit that generally offsets any additional time spent during rounds. Without families on rounds, update and difficult discussion conferences typically occurred during the afternoon within the confines of the ICU conference room. That room is aptly named the "fishbowl" since several sides often housed large windows or were principally glass walls. Instead, when families are engaged on rounds, those family conferences are far less frequent, and when they do occur, are crisply focused. This change evolves from families understanding the care plan and daily goals, but is closely driven by increased satisfaction with the healthcare team. The daily exploration of the prior 24 hours' events, the patient's condition using an organ system approach, education of trainees, and the opportunity to ask questions and receive answers helps build trust, avoid conflict, and enhance satisfaction. Moreover, family members feel as if they are an integral team member, establishing family presence as a way of providing patient- and family-centered care.

Teaching on Rounds

Daily ICU patient rounds are optimally multiprofessional and generally involve nurses, advanced practice providers (nurse practitioners, physician assistants [APPs]), physicians, respiratory therapists, pharmacists, physical therapists, registered dietitians, social workers, speech pathologist, case managers, and pastoral care; other team members such as specialty consultants are engaged as needed. In teaching institutions, learners from multiple specialties are often present during bedside rounds with active teaching happening throughout rounds. Some clinicians may be concerned that rounds-based teaching will decrease if families are present on rounds—especially since a lot of teaching occurs by asking questions that define the learner's knowledge boundaries. Incorrect answers have the potential to be perceived by family members as the inability to provide quality care to the patient. It is helpful to share the expectation that family members will hear trainees provide answers that trigger more education. When this process is studied, neither the amount of teaching nor the quality of teaching changes if family is present on rounds.

Relatedly, despite concerns that rounds may increase family stress, families choose to be present during teaching rounds when offered the choice to have teaching occur without them. Families ultimately report feeling more equipped to serve as surrogates to make healthcare decisions when included on teaching rounds. In addition to engaging families in the treatment plan, family presence on rounds creates more opportunities for bidirectional communication. Healthcare clinicians can hone their communication skills with family members present on rounds and receive immediate feedback if communication is not clear. The ability to translate medical jargon into readily understandable language is a key skill that also translates into establishing informed consent. Rounds with family members present is an ideal way to repeatedly practice, refine, and perfect communication and presentation skills that span all of the specialties that provide care in the ICU.

Team Dynamics

Another concern is that team members cannot be honest—especially in disclosing medical errors, care delays, or related events—in front of families during rounds, or that family presence will preclude common intrateam communication methods that leverages humor. Part of the benefit of having families on rounds is that they do learn about care processes including what went well and what went awry. Honesty in identifying errors—and their correction—builds trust. Furthermore, when family members attend rounds there is often less side conversation between team members. Instead, communication principally focuses on patient care issues. Having family members as part of the rounding team encourages professional behavior by decreasing cynicism and judgmental assessments of other clinicians, administration, or the healthcare system. While these are changes in the usual workflow, they are also positive ones to be embraced in the pursuit of patient- and family-centered care.

■ REMOTE FAMILY PARTICIPATION DURING ROUNDS

Most ICU rounds happen in the morning so that patients are evaluated early in the day and if required changes to care plans can be initiated. While this time frame is ideal for patient care, it is less ideal for many families. Rounds frequently occur during working hours or when childcare duties may be paramount. Commonly identified barriers for family members to attend rounds include work and family responsibilities, distance to the hospital, and the rounding time frame. In addition, restrictive visitation policies—common during COVID-19 care—often precluded families from joining rounds. Thus, logistical concerns that prevent family presence on rounds are frequent and disconnect the care team from the patient's family.

Digital communication platform flourished in large part in response to the COVID-19 pandemic. ZOOM (Zoom Video Communications, San Jose, CA), Skype (Skype Technologies, Redmond, WA), Microsoft TEAMS (Microsoft, Redmond, WA), FaceTime (Apple, Cupertino, CA), or commercial systems available for hospital purchase (Angel Eye [AngelEye Health, Little Rock, AR] and NICView [Natus, San Carlos, CA]) linked people around the world and permeated all levels of education during periods of lockdown. This global connectivity was particularly leveraged by the medical community to share insights, new practices, and fresh discoveries in a rapid fashion. Those same platforms also brought families back to the bedside and into the office space in a virtual fashion. While many families still have a strong preference for physical presence on rounds when they are able, virtual presence is a practical alternative when families are unable to attend rounds in person. Videoconferencing advantages include (1) generating care plans that are family- and patient-centered, (2) improving family member understanding of daily goals and care plans, (3) presenting and sharing nonverbal communication cues, and (4) enabling family members to feel part of the team. In particular, having a family–clinician conference that occurs outside of rounds in a private space such as the clinician's office allows the clinician to remove personal protective equipment (PPE) that would otherwise hide facial expressions. These cues are essential parts of communication that videoconferencing within rounds fails to provide as PPE is required for safety. Therefore, more than one digital connection may be required for difficult discussions, especially when addressing goals of care or end-of-life issues.

Improving communication between the healthcare team and family has been consistently shown to improve shared decision-making, relieve caregiver stress, and increase family satisfaction level of patient care. Therefore, implementation of family virtual presence on rounds when physical presence cannot occur should enhance patient-centered care. Care should be taken to maintain digital communication security and privacy when such platforms are utilized. Emerging technologies that specifically enable remote participation in rounds by families should inform new ICU design and existing ICU renovation.

Tips for Clinicians

1. Family members are key team members in providing patient- and family-centered care.
2. Family member coaching prior to participating in rounds helps prepare them for team members, discussion content, and their role within rounds.
3. Workflow changes while incorporating families on rounds are anticipatable, manageable, and, on balance, positive regarding information exchange and shared decision-making.
4. Participation in rounds helps ready family members for post-ICU care, especially procedural tasks that are required after home repatriation.
5. Remote participation in rounds by families with distance, time, or responsibility constraints is intensely valuable and should leverage a digital platform with which the family is comfortable, or on which they can be readily trained.
6. Privacy and security during digital communication is essential and it is worthwhile to engage your facility's Information Technology team to help with both aspects.
7. Some discussions are emotionally charged and benefit from facial cueing that is derailed by PPE, especially when undertaken using telepresence. Consider a separate discussion where the clinician and the family can both share key nonverbal facial cues.

KEY REFERENCES

Allen SR, Pascual J, Martin N, et al. A novel method of optimizing patient-and-family-centered care in the ICU. *J Trauma Acute Care Surg.* 2017;82(3):582-586.

Au SS, des Ordons AR, Soo A, et al. Family participation in intensive care unit rounds: comparing family and provider perspectives. *J Crit Care.* 2017;38:132-136.

Brown SM, Azoulay E, Benoit D, et al. The practice of respect in the ICU. *Am J Respir Crit Care Med.* 2018;197(11):1389-1395.

Cacioppo JT, Hawkley LC. Social isolation and health, with an emphasis on underlying mechanisms. *Perspect Biol Med*. 2003;46(3 Suppl):S39-S52.

Curtis JR, Sprung CL, Azoulay E. The importance of word choice in the care of critically ill patients and their families. *Intensive Care Med*. 2014;40(4):606-608.

Cypress BS. Family presence on rounds: a systematic review of literature. *Dimens Crit Care Nurs*. 2012;31(1):53-64.

Davidson JE, Powers K, Hedayat KM, et al. Clinical practice guidelines for support of the family in the patient-centered intensive care unit: American College of Critical Care Medicine Task Force 2004-2005. *Crit Care Med*. 2007;35(2):605-622.

Epstein EG, Arechiga J, Dancy M, et al. Integrative review of technology to support communication with parents of infants in the NICU. *J Obstet Gynecol Neonatal Nurs*. 2017;46(3):357-366.

Epstein EG, Sherman J, Blakcman A, Sinking RA. Testing the feasibility of skype and facetime updates with parents in the neonatal intensive care unit. *Am J Crit Care*. 2015;24(4):290-296.

Halpern NA, Anderson DC, Kesecioglu J. ICU design in 2050: looking into the crystal ball! *Intensive Care Med*. 2017;43(5):690-692.

Heyland DK, Cook DJ, Rocker GM, et al. Decision-making in the ICU: perspectives of the substitute decision-maker. *Intensive Care Med*. 2003;29(1):75-82.

Jacobowski NL, Girard TD, Mulder JA, Ely EW. Communication in critical care: family rounds in the intensive care unit. *Am J Crit Care*. 2010;19(5):421-430.

Johnson CC, Suchyta MR, Darowski ES, et al. Psychological sequelae in family caregivers of critically III intensive care unit patients. A systematic review. *Ann Am Thorac Soc*. 2019;16(7):894-909.

Levy MM. Shared decision-making in the ICU: entering a new era. *Crit Care Med*. 2004;32(9):1966-1968.

Meert KL, Clark J, Eggly S. Family-centered care in the pediatric intensive care unit. *Pediatr Clin North Am*. 2013;60(3):761-772.

Murray PD, Swanson JR. Visitation restrictions: is it right and how do we support families in the NICU during COVID-19? *J Perinatol*. 2020;40(10):1576-1581.

Nin Vaeza N, Martin Delgado MC, Heras La Calle G. Humanizing intensive care: toward a human-centered care ICU model. *Crit Care Med*. 2020;48(3):385-390.

Secunda KE, Kruser JM. Patient-centered and family-centered care in the intensive care unit. *Clin Chest Med*. 2022;43(3):539-550.

Stelson EA, Carr BG, Golden KE, et al. Perceptions of family participation in intensive care unit rounds and telemedicine: a qualitative assessment. *Am J Crit Care*. 2016;25(5):440-447.

Valley TS, Schutz A, Nagle MT, et al. Changes to visitation policies and communication practices in michigan ICUs during the COVID-19 pandemic. *Am J Respir Crit Care Med*. 2020;202(6):883-885.

Wong P, Redley B, Digby R, et al. Families' perspectives of participation in patient care in an adult intensive care unit: a qualitative study. *Australian Crit Care*. 2020;33(4):317-325.

Pet Therapy

Sara Holland and Juliane Jablonski

Patient Care Vignette

JK was a 65-year-old man initially admitted to the hospital with acute cholecystitis for which he would need a cholecystectomy. His course was complicated by delirium, sepsis, and the inability to breathe well on his own, requiring a long-term breathing tube. After 2 weeks of hospitalization, JK remained in the intensive care unit. He had undergone tracheostomy placement to support ventilator weaning and feeding tube placement for nutritional support. JK's mental clarity slowly improved but he became increasingly depressed, communicated feelings of hopelessness, had limited eye contact with his family or healthcare team, and did not want to participate in physical therapy. Psychiatry was consulted and JK's family was present at the bedside every day trying their best to support him.

On day 21 of JK's hospitalization, the nurses lifted him out of bed to a bedside lounge chair. His wife and daughter were sitting next to him. They were surprised to see JK opening his eyes to look outside of his ICU room. There stood a hospital therapy dog, a brown Labrador retriever named Tugger. JK lifted his arm to wave at Tugger. Glenn, Tugger's handler, asked the bedside nurse if it was okay to visit JK and his family. The clinical team and JK's family were encouraged by JK's engagement since little else had captured his attention. Tugger and Glenn entered the room. Glenn placed a towel on a chair for Tugger to jump up and sit face-to-face next to JK. Within seconds, the first smile anyone had seen on JK's face since his admission appeared; his wife and daughter began to cry. Tugger and Glenn spent an hour with JK. Two days later, Tugger and Glenn came by for a second visit. During this second visit, the physical therapist was doing routine patient care rounds and session scheduling. Previously, JK would not engage in sessions beyond getting out of bed to the chair. Today was different. With Tugger at his side, JK wrote to the physical therapist, "Can I try to stand and take a few steps with Tugger?" That moment was a turning point in JK's care. He found the strength and the drive to participate in his recovery. JK later described his experience by saying, "Tugger ignited in me a good feeling for the simple joys of life that I truly missed and want to experience once again."

Hospital environments are complex, fast-paced, and at times, chaotic that are very different from other spaces. Moreover, much of a patient's time in an acute care facility is spent in their room, and often in bed or in a bedside chair. For most, it is a very different environment than what they were used to before becoming ill. The intensive care unit (ICU) environment may be even more overwhelming, given its continuous flow of personnel, the loss of privacy, frequent alarms, and bright lighting at all hours of the day and night. With critical illness or injury, ICU care also leads to restricted movement that results from care devices. An unfamiliar environment and unfamiliar voices may be complicated by sleeplessness that can lead to anxiety, fear, and delirium. Often during the initial phase of care, medications that address pain and sedation—especially when a breathing tube and mechanical ventilation is required—are used for management. Sometimes, those medications may trigger or worsen delirium. Therefore, nonpharmacologic approaches have been intensively explored as alternatives to more medication. Animal-assisted therapy (AAT; also called "pet therapy") is one nonpharmacological approach to supporting recovery by reducing stress in the ICU as well as other areas of the hospital.

■ BENEFITS OF THE HUMAN–ANIMAL BOND

Human and animal companionship has existed for thousands of years. As far back as 1869, Florence Nightingale wrote nursing notes about using animals in a therapeutic setting. In the 1970s, researchers concluded that dogs provided a critical "social lubricant," making it easier for hospitalized psychiatric patients to communicate with each other as well as with staff. Since then, research into the benefits of pet ownership and human–animal interaction has demonstrated improved mobility, decreased blood pressure, decreased anxiety, decreased perceived pain, and even mortality benefits in some patient groups. Animals may also help people discover a sense of purpose, provide company, and decrease feelings of loneliness. Increasing recognition of the positive effects of human–animal interaction and companionship helps explain the growing presence of animals in previously people-only spaces, such as airplanes, public transportation, as well as acute and chronic health-care settings.

■ ANIMAL ROLES IN HEALTHCARE

Animals may participate in healthcare in a variety of specified roles including as a service animal, or one that participates in AAT. Other newly designated non-healthcare unique roles include that of an emotional support or comfort animal. Each role has explicit definitions and unique criteria. Under updates to the US Americans with Disabilities Act (ADA), *service animals* are dogs or miniature horses that have been specifically trained to do work or perform tasks that mitigate a person's disability; the disabled person and their service animal form a dyadic partnership that is recognized by law. An example of a service animal is a guide dog trained to complete tasks that a human can no longer perform due to blindness. Under the ADA, state and local governments, businesses, and nonprofit organizations that serve the public must allow service animals to accompany people with disabilities in all areas of the facility where the public is allowed to convene, including hospitals. Only sterile areas or isolation areas may exclude service animals. Moreover, while the facility must allow the service animal to enter, the facility is not required to provide care for the service animal. The owner's family, friends, or on occasion, a service animal agency will do so. Service animals must meet specific requirements for behavioral training as well as veterinary care, and are required to be badged as a service animal (commonly presented on their harness).

A subset of service animals includes *psychiatric service animals.* Such uniquely trained animals are quite different from animals that provide emotional support. Rather, the psychiatric service animal performs tasks to mitigate a person's legally recognized disability from a psychiatric illness as opposed to a physical disability. Such tasks could include protecting a person experiencing a dissociative episode from wandering into danger or preventing or interrupting impulsive or disruptive behavior such as self-mutilation. There are many more service animals than psychiatric service animals. Often, psychiatric service animals have their task assumed by the healthcare facility during episodes of illness.

Emotional support animals (ESA) are simply pets that are not required to meet any behavioral training or veterinary certification requirements. People with an ESA require documentation from a psychiatrist or psychologist that they have a condition whose management is supported by the animal's presence. Indeed, unlike service animals, ESAs may be any kind of animal ranging from a dog to a cat to a chinchilla to a miniature goat; others including a peacock and a tarantula have been featured in the lay press. ESAs do not qualify as service animals under the ADA. For this reason, access to public spaces is not guaranteed for ESAs as it is for service animals. Moreover, because the ESA is not required to meet behavior training standards, they may represent a danger to staff especially in unfamiliar and often loud spaces (ICU alarms). Therefore, they are commonly excluded from the ICU and the acute care unit. Outpatient spaces are often more welcoming of ESAs, but this is institution—and healthcare clinician—specific. Of note, the not infrequent staff allergy to animals may inform decisions regarding the presence of ESAs as well. Visitation by a patient's home pet is generally not supported due to all of the concerns noted for ESAs. On occasion, and principally around the end-of-life some acute care facilities allow quite limited visitation by a home pet, but this is not a standard practice.

There are key differences between service animals, ESAs, and *therapy animals*. A therapy animal is any animal that is handled by a human trainer (also called a *handler*) and that provides therapeutic benefit to people experiencing illness or suffering. Therapy animals provide comfort through their presence—and commonly their response to being touched—but are not trained to perform a specific job or tasks. Animals with fur such as miniature horses, rabbits, llamas, guinea pigs, miniature pigs, as well as birds and certain snakes often serve in this capacity. Therapy animals are trained to be capable and competent in navigating specific circumstances they are likely to encounter during a hospital visitation or therapy session, such as smells, sounds, and the presence of a variety of unfamiliar people. The companionship offered by therapy animals is especially useful in hospitals, where patients are often alone despite increasingly liberal hospital visitation policies. Therapy animals always enter and exit the ICU with their handler. Quite often, the handler and the therapy animal live together, but some therapy animals live at a zoo and work with a variety of handlers who can bring them to the hospital.

According to the International Association of Human-Animal Interaction Organization, therapy animals provide *animal-assisted therapy* (AAT), a goal-oriented intervention that intentionally includes or incorporates animals in health, education, and human service for the purpose of therapeutic gain in humans. Multiple terms are used to describe AAT programs within healthcare facilities, including pet therapy, animal-assisted activities, AAT, pet volunteer programs, animal visitation programs, among others. Hospital-based pet therapy programs are rapidly increasing in the United States.

■ IMPLEMENTING AN ANIMAL-ASSISTED THERAPY PROGRAM

Allowing an animal to come into a hospital would have been unheard of at the beginning of the 21st century. Over time, however, AAT has been successfully implemented in numerous healthcare settings including nursing homes and children's and adult hospitals. While the growth in AAT is notable, there is a lack of consistent practice standards, measures of program efficacy, and regulatory oversight. AAT programs can be safely implemented, but structured program planning and oversight is necessary to avoid potential risks to patients, staff, visitors, therapy animals, and animal handlers.

Expert practice guidelines are available to help facilities implement an AAT program. These include guidelines published by the US Centers for Disease Control and Prevention (CDC), the American Veterinary Medical Association (AVMA), and the Society for Healthcare Epidemiology in America (SHEA). The SHEA guidelines are comprehensive and directed at overall implementation practices for healthcare AAT programs. AVMA guidelines target the welfare of animals involved in AAT programs and how to maximize the therapeutic benefit of the human–animal bond. CDC guidelines specifically address optimizing infection control and focuses on preventing animal to human transmission; little guidance exists on preventing human to animal transmission of pathogens such as methicillin-resistant *Staphylococcus aureus* (MRSA)—a common hospital encountered and drug-resistant bacteria. Where evidence is limited, the AAT guidelines provide practical, expert opinion–based recommendations to reduce risks. Additional guidelines are available through Tufts University and the Cummings School of Veterinarian Medicine, where an AAT program, Paws for People, has been in place since 1998.

US hospital-based animal-assisted program names often have creative and endearing titles. Examples of active hospital-based programs include *Paws for People* (Tufts University), *Dogs on Call* (Virginia Commonwealth University School of Medicine), *Caring Canines* (Mayo Clinic), *SOUL—Source of Unconditional Love* (Mercy Hospice in Sacramento), and *HUPs Pups* (Hospital of the University of Pennsylvania), among others. The critical first step in building a sustainable AAT program is to form a planning, development, and implementation committee that includes key stakeholders. These stakeholders include, but may not be limited to, hospital administrators, infection control practitioners, bedside nurses, clinicians, clinical and nonclinical staff, facility security (or Police as appropriate), volunteer services, guest services, veterinary consultants, marketing and media professionals, and patient advisory consultants. This committee should lead the development of organizational AAT policies and submit them for review by facility committees and the legal department. Broad organizational expertise is needed to standardize safety protocols to protect both humans and animals. The potential path that an AAT animal and handler will take should be walked by members of the committee to identify strategies for success and potential pitfalls alike.

AAT policies should include clearly stated program goals, allowable animal species and their role within the program, screening procedures for therapy animals and their handlers, and standard protocols that address facility entry, patient contact, and facility exit. Once agreement is reached on policy standards, department oversight of the AAT program should be determined. Animal handlers participating in the AAT program are typically volunteers; therefore, hospital volunteer offices or departments typically assume organizational oversight. Other important partnerships include community therapy animal organizations, and veterinary services. Box 17-1 summarizes the key components for organizations to consider when writing policies and creating a hospital-based AAT program.

According to the 2015 SHEA guidelines, "facilities should consider use of certification by organizations that provide relevant formal training programs." Organizations that use certified animals and handlers can potentially decrease organizational liability risk around the animal and handler's ability to provide competent and safe interactions within a healthcare facility.

Box 17-1—Key Components in Building and Regulating a Hospital-Based AAT Program

1. Clearly written program goals
2. Primary organizational oversight (i.e., Volunteer Office or Department)
3. Animal species included in the AAT program
4. Designated hospital entrance for animals to enter the facility
5. Organizational champions to work with handlers and animals to navigate the environment and move between units
6. Screening procedures for animals and handlers before joining the AAT program
7. Training requirements and/or certification of animals and handlers
8. Evidence of previsitation veterinary evaluation (vaccination status, pathogen screening)
9. Immunization status of handlers
10. Orientation program for animals and handlers
11. Patient populations that are included and excluded from receiving AAT
12. Criteria to determine who receives a visit, and how to request a visit
13. Organizational staff education requirements
14. Evaluation of handlers' compliance with standard occupational health practices
15. Mechanism for safety concern reporting
16. Program outcome measures

Nationally recognized programs exist for handlers to register and certify a therapy animal. Most of these programs are restricted to canines (i.e., Alliance of Therapy Dogs, Delta Dogs International). Although variation exists between these programs, foundational requirements for age and veterinary care, education, and training must be met by the animal and the handler. Some programs include observation testing by a trained handler to evaluate the animal's skill and aptitude. General features of all programs include educational components for infection control practices, rigorous health and grooming, and human–animal interaction.

■ INFECTION CONTROL MEASURES

Infection control is one of the most important issues to address in AAT organizational policies. Standardized processes must be designed to decrease risks associated with potential zoonotic pathogen transmission (animal to human), cross-transmission of human pathogens, patient injury, and exacerbation of patient symptoms; animal injury or infection is less robustly addressed. *Zoonosis* is a disease that can be transmitted from animals to humans. *Zoonotic pathogens* are viruses, bacteria, fungi, or parasites transmitted to a human by an animal. Zoonosis outside of healthcare is well-understood, with examples of *Staphylococcus aureus*, *Campylobacter*, and *Salmonella* transmission documented between animals and humans. In healthcare settings, there is a theoretical risk of zoonotic pathogen transmission from an animal to a human, including transmission of pathogens by an animal between patients. There are unfortunately few scientific studies that address this risk, though we recommend several commonsense measures to ensure effective infection control measures during an animal visit (Box 17-2).

Box 17-2—Key Components of a Successful Animal Visit

1. Animals bathed and groomed before each facility visit
2. Prohibited raw meat diet for therapy animals
3. Use of clean linen or bath towel on patient's bed or chair for animal to sit; discard to dirty linen after visit
4. Patient, staff, and handler hand hygiene before and after all animal visits
5. Cleaning and disinfection of surfaces soiled by animal waste
6. Discouragement of animal from licking
7. Discouragement of petting of animal's paws
8. Animal wellness assessment and procedures including limitations on visiting time and provision of a designated space for animal toileting

ANIMALS IN CRITICAL CARE

AAT penetrance into critical care spaces is consistent with a growing trend toward humanizing the intensive care environment, providing patient-centered nonpharmacological interventions, and providing more frequent and intensive rehabilitative care. Since AAT in the ICU is relatively new, data regarding outcomes as well as risks are scant. It should be noted that critical care environments and isolation rooms are considered restricted areas by the SHEA guidelines, and special care should be taken when considering AAT for patients deemed by facility guidelines to be immunocompromised. Critical care environments present the additional challenges of crowding, noise, urgency, and care devices compared to other areas of the hospital. These environmental elements can create additional stressors for not only the animal and handler, but also the patient and staff. Perhaps for these reasons, AAT is more commonly encountered in noncritical care units. Furthermore, since patients are often much less mobile in the ICU, the ability to directly engage with a therapy animal may be restricted and might also be frustrating for the patient. Patients who have delirium are inappropriate for animal visitation as there is a real risk of animal injury, but a related risk of patient misinterpretation of the animal or its intentions. When there is an AAT program within an ICU, it is essential to screen patients—and their visitors—for specific animal aversion or fear. Some people are afraid of dogs but are delighted by cats, and this knowledge should inform the kind of animal that might visit that patient for therapy. A similar screen should occur for animal allergy because pet dander, even after grooming, may trigger an allergic response in susceptible individuals. The same kinds of screening should occur for staff as well. Despite limitations, AAT can be very helpful for a variety of patients in the ICU.

CONSIDERATIONS FOR RECOVERY

Hospitalized patients recovering from critical illness may experience emotional distress and loneliness that could be addressed by interactions with animals, including AAT. This same kind of therapy can be continued at a rehabilitation or longer-term care facility prior to returning home. Adopting a new pet upon returning home may be a decision that is informed by a patient's ability to care for that animal as well as aspects of recovery that include the presence of open wounds, the need for temporary assistance devices, and the ability of family members or other caregivers to help with pet care. Most commonly as a result of injury, some patients acquire a disability that may be addressed with a service animal. Specific referral for such services should be made when the need—and the patient's desire to be helped in that way—is recognized.

Tips for Clinicians

1. Interactions with animals have multiple potential benefits for patients during an episode of critical illness or injury. However, a specific program is required to support those interactions in a safe and effective fashion.
2. It is ideal to understand your facility's rules and regulations regarding service animals, therapy animals, and emotional support animals; only service animals are addressed by federal law.
3. Service animals (dogs and miniature horses) are excluded from sterile areas and isolation areas but are allowed by law in all other spaces. The facility is not required to provide care for the animal; family members, friends, and sometimes service animal agencies will do so. The facility's requirement is to provide care for patients.
4. Developing an animal therapy program is a multiprofessional venture for which multiple guidelines exist to inform implementation and safety practices.
5. Therapy animals must meet specific criteria in order to serve in this manner while emotional support animals or home pets do not.
6. Animal therapy programs can be deployed in critical care spaces but are more common on acute care units.
7. Pet therapy is not limited to the acute care facility and at-home programs also exist to meet the needs of individuals who are recovering from critical illness or injury who cannot care for a pet on their own.
8. Service animals can help critical illness survivors who have developed new disabilities navigate the world and accomplish daily tasks. Timely referral once the disability is recognized, and the patient being interested in service animal aid, is key.

KEY REFERENCES

Barker SB, Gee NR. Canine-assisted interventions in hospitals: best practices for maximizing human and canine safety. *Front Vet Sci*. 2021;8:615730.

Centers for Disease Control and Prevention https://www.cdc.gov/infectioncontrol/guidelines/environmental/background/animals.htmlimals.html. Guidelines for Environmental Infection Control in Healthcare Facilities (2003). Last Reviewed November 5, 2015. Content source: Centers for Disease Control and Prevention, National Center for Emerging and Zoonotic Infectious Diseases (NCEZID), Division of Healthcare Quality Promotion (DHQP).

Cherniack E, Cherniack A. The benefit of pets and animal-assisted therapy to the health of older individuals. *Curr Gerontol Geriatr Res*. 2014; Article ID 623203. https://doi.org/10.1155/2014/623203.

DiSalvo H, Haiduven D, Johnson N, et al. Who let the dogs out? Infection control did: utility of dogs in health care settings and infection control aspects. *Am J Infect Control.* 2006;34(5):301-307.

Freeman L, Linder D, Mueller M, Gibbs D. Animal assisted interventions: how to guide for facilities. Available at https://hai.tufts.edu/animal-assisted-intervention-manual-for-facilities-now-available-to-download. Accessed November 1, 2021.

Hetland B, Bailey T, Prince-Paul M. Animal assisted interactions to alleviate psychological symptoms in patients on mechanical ventilation. *J Hosp Palliat Nurs.* 2017;19(6):516-523.

Hosey MM, Jaskulski J, Wegener ST, Chlan LL, Needham DM. Animal-assisted intervention in the ICU: a tool for humanization. *Crit Care.* 2018;22(1):22. https://www.avma.org/resources-tools/avma-policies/animal-assisted-interventions-guidelines.

Jegatheesan B, Beetz D, Ormerod E, et al. *The IAHAIO Definitions for Animal Assisted Intervention and Guidelines for Wellness of Animals Involved.* 2018. Available at http://www.iahaio.org/new/fileuploads/9313IAHAIO%20WHITE%20PAPER%20TASK%20FORCE%20-%20FINAL%20REPORT.pdf.

Martin N, Pascual JL, Crowe DT Jr, et al. Comfort at the crossroads: Service, therapy and emotional support animals in the intensive care unit and at the end-of-life. *J Trauma Acute Care Surg.* 2018;84(6):978-984.

Murthy R, Bearman G, Brown S, et al. Animals in healthcare facilities: recommendations to minimize potential risks. *Infect Control Hosp Epidemiol.* 2015;36(5):495-516.

US Department of Justice, Civil Rights Division, Disability Rights Section ADA Requirements, Service Animals. Originally issued July 12, 2011. Last updated on site February 24, 2020. Available at https://www.ada.gov/service_animals_2010.htm. Accessed October 1, 2021.

Writing Panel of Working Group, Lefebvre SL, Golab GC, et al. Guidelines for animal assisted interventions in health care facilities. *Am J Infect Control.* 2008;36(2):78-85.

Special Populations

Pediatrics

Neethi P. Pinto and Vinay Nadkarni

Patient Care Vignette

Twelve-year-old Maya wasn't quite herself at her Saturday soccer game, complaining of headache. The next morning she couldn't walk to the bathroom. Her parents took her to the emergency department where her symptoms worsened. By early Monday, Maya had difficulty breathing. She was quickly transported to the nearest pediatric intensive care unit (PICU) across the state border. Upon arrival, she was intubated and found to be completely paralyzed with the exception of the ability to open her eyes. Initially, Maya's differential diagnosis included a paralysis recently seen among children in the western United States who had been infected with Enterovirus d68 as well as Guillain-Barre syndrome (GBS). Even after confirmation of a diagnosis of atypical GBS, Maya's family faced uncertainty about her long-term prognosis. The medical team told them that Maya might not regain function of her arms or legs. Maya's family, school, and church communities were instrumental in supporting Maya and her family during their arduous journey, taking turns to stay with Maya's siblings while her parents juggled being at the hospital, work, or home.

The medical team was also tireless; after several courses of plasmapheresis and intravenous immunoglobulin treatment in tandem with ongoing physical, occupational, and speech therapy, Maya slowly regained the ability to move. After a few weeks in the PICU, she underwent tracheostomy tube placement to facilitate chronic mechanical ventilation support, ongoing therapies, and discharge to a rehabilitation facility. After 1 month, she was discharged home, and within 6 months, Maya made a full physical and psychological recovery—walking without assistance, undergoing tracheostomy decannulation, playing soccer again, returning to school, and eventually graduating from high school on time with plans to attend college. Her parents and siblings were also able to resume work and return to leisure routines that had been interrupted and put on hold during Maya's PICU admission and lengthy recovery.

■ INTRODUCTION

Children admitted to the PICU have experienced life-threatening critical illness or injury. Stories like Maya's illustrate the fundamental importance of the multiprofessional team in healthcare. Each team member has a pivotal role in supporting the child and family, contributing to their care, and facilitating recovery. With a shortage of intensivists and the increasing medical complexity of patients, the core PICU team is dependent not only on intensivists and nurses but advanced practice providers (e.g., physician assistants, nurse practitioners, hospitalists, etc.), pharmacists, therapists (respiratory, physical, occupational, and speech-language), dietitians, social workers, case managers, and a host of other hospital-based clinicians. Professionals trained in each of those different disciplines must work collaboratively, using their diverse training and experience to address patient needs and improve care. This collaboration results in improved outcomes related to all aspects of acute care.

Critically ill children are often evaluated by a wide range of specialists during their PICU stay, making it difficult for the child and the parents to keep track of who is involved in care. Importantly, the bedside nurse commonly serves as an anchor for the parents, and interfaces with the multiprofessional ICU team as well as subspecialty consultants to link parents and team members around their child's care. Child life specialists are unique to pediatric care and use a patient- and family-centered approach to identify and meet the life stage needs of a patient and their family. Based on their size and complexity, PICU team use regularly scheduled meetings to review outcomes, tailor care approaches, and identify opportunities for quality improvement.

■ ICU CARE CONSIDERATIONS

While many of the general care processes are similar across adult and pediatric ICUs, there are quite important differences that impact outcomes and the consequences of ICU survivorship.

Key Differences Between PICU Survivorship and Adult Intensive Care Unit (ICU) Survivorship

Effective team communication in centralized PICUs with high-intensity staffing is associated with lower pediatric mortality compared to pediatric care delivered in an adult setting or outside of the PICU. Advances in science and technology have helped reduce the PICU mortality rate to 2-3% which is strikingly lower than the adult ICU mortality rate of 10-29%. However, morbidity among PICU survivors has concomitantly increased over the past several decades. Nearly 40% of PICU survivors remain medically vulnerable years after discharge, with the development of new morbidities, functional impairments, and decreased health-related quality of life (HRQL). These ICU survivorship consequences contribute to the growth of a population of chronically critically ill children who repeatedly require hospital care, as well as a distinct population of children who live with chronic complex conditions. In addition, this rise in PICU-related morbidity may durably impact the child survivor (new technology dependence, medical complexity, inability to reside in the family home), the child's siblings (increased responsibility, decreased time with parent or the affected sibling), parents (ability to return to work, need to advocate for resources or public services for the child, psychological well-being), as well as the family in a collective fashion (stress on relationships, posttraumatic stress, financial toxicity, decreased leisure activities, medicalization of the home, and a family schedule centered on the survivor). Children are much more adaptable than their adult counterparts, a process known as "neuroplasticity" when it applies to brain function. Therefore, despite suffering from severe critical illness, children are more apt to survive and be more functional than adults who survive similar illness. Pediatric outcomes are indeed related to developmental stage and comorbidities prior to PICU admission—a strong parallel to adult care that is influenced by age and chronic diseases as well. Since PICU mortality is quite low, there is substantial investment in a comprehensive and high-intensity approach to care. However, that survivorship comes as the price of engendering some less desirable outcomes such as the post-intensive care syndrome (PICS).

Post-Intensive Care Syndrome-Pediatrics (PICS-p)

PICU survivors may experience new cognitive, physical, social, and emotional difficulties after discharge, recognized as the post-intensive care syndrome-pediatrics (PICS-p) (Fig. 18-1). PICS impacts adults, families (PICS-F), as well as pediatric patients (PICS-p). These long-term outcomes are influenced by pre-existing comorbid conditions, the severity of illness, and for pediatric patients, developmental status. The conceptual framework for PICS-p also recognizes that the child survivor is interdependent upon parents and siblings who may

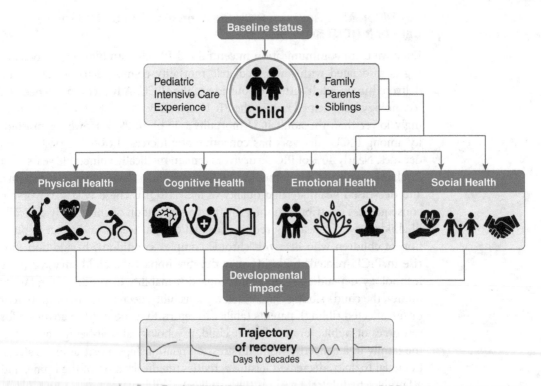

FIGURE 18-1. Post-Intensive Care Syndrome-Pediatrics. This image represents PICS-p and how the syndrome impacts various aspects of the child's development and recovery trajectory over time. Manning JC, Pinto NP, Rennick JE, et al. Conceptualizing post intensive care syndrome in children-the PICS-p framework. *Pediatr Crit Care Med.* 2018;19(4):298-300.

also experience emotional and social difficulties attributable to the child's critical illness. In turn, the family's response may influence the child's outcomes. The trajectory for recovery may span days to decades with periods of improvement, decline, or relative constancy. Some children may be more resilient while others may be medically vulnerable. Recovery across the different domains of PICS-p may occur at very different rates as the process toward health is often asymmetric. PICU survivors face challenges in recovering physical function, cognitive health, emotional and social health, as well as family dynamics. Below we explore these difficulties and strategies to support successful convalescence.

■ PHYSICAL FUNCTION

The recognition of PICS-p, persistent and long-lasting morbidities following critical illness in children, has prompted us to broaden our focus of outcomes assessment beyond in-hospital survival to survivorship that includes patient and family priorities. While diagnosis, acute therapy, prognosis, and survival are key priorities *early* in critical illness, functional status, quality of life, and rehabilitation needs are the focus once *survival* is clear. Therefore, substantial attention has been paid to determine how best to assess and quantify residual and persistent morbidity during critical illness recovery.

What Is Functional Status?

Functional status is an important, patient-centered outcome that is relevant for healthcare clinicians and administrators since the degree of functional decline following critical illness is a significant predictor of hospital length of stay and resource utilization. This metric describes the degree of independence—and not just strength or physical capability—following critical illness. Many consider functional status and its impact on the quality of life to be the most important outcomes for survivors of critical illness. Previous definitions of function focused on one's capability and performance, describing function as "an individual's ability to perform normal daily activities required to meet basic needs, fulfill usual roles and maintain health and well-being." We currently define functional status as a multidimensional construct that integrates biological, psychological, social, and environmental aspects of human functioning (Fig. 18-2). This model resonates with the PICS-p framework's recognition of the interdependence of a child's environment and family on physical, cognitive, emotional, and social health outcomes.

This conceptual framework for functioning has been adopted in several fields, including rehabilitation medicine, mental health, social service, population-based health, policy development, and monitoring, and is now

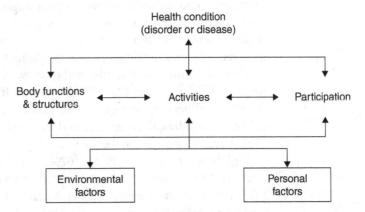

FIGURE 18-2. A Framework for Functional Status. This figure demonstrates the interlinked aspects of the global assessment known as functional status.

increasingly applied in adult and pediatric critical care. Having a multidimensional measure of function is relevant in critical care, as not all domains may be affected to the same degree or recover at the same rate, and domains are influenced by different risk factors. For example, the effect of ICU delirium on cognitive function is quite distinct compared to the effect of prolonged immobility on strength.

Assessing Functional Status in Critically Ill Children

Functional status in critically ill children has been measured using numerous unique and overlapping tools. Many tools are reliable, easy, and quick to administer scales. The clinician can assess these scales and provide a single composite score that may be most useful during an episode of critical illness. Nonetheless, contemporary recommendations stress the importance of using patient-reported outcome measures in critical care, particularly when evaluating survivorship. It is important to note that functioning reflects one's ability to perform a task, whereas HRQL indicates one's perception of their functional ability. Functional status measures are therefore designed to be objective, while HRQL is subjective.

Long-Term Functional Outcomes in Critically Ill Children

Persistent morbidity and less than desired functional outcomes shape the current demographic PICU populations. Between 44 and 50% of critically ill children admitted to a PICU demonstrate some degree of functional disability ahead of the critical illness that has brought them to the hospital. Acquired functional decline from admission baseline to PICU discharge occurs in 10-36% of critically ill children who survive their PICU stay. Relatedly, based on patient-reported outcome measures, a staggering 82% of children experience functional deterioration in one or more domains following critical illness. Currently identified risk factors for acquired functional disability are multifactorial and include: (1) baseline patient characteristics such as older age, baseline functional status, malignancy, chronic complex disease, and immunodeficiency, and (2) critical care and illness-related factors such as severity of illness, neurologic insult, and PICU-acquired morbidities (e.g., delirium, withdrawal syndrome, and prolonged bedrest). While seemingly dismal, recovery occurs in the vast majority.

Slightly more than two-thirds (67%) of patients exhibit some functional recovery by 6 months, but one-third fail to recover their baseline function. Longer-term studies suggest that up to 20% of survivors experience persistent morbidities 1-2 years post-PICU discharge. Postdischarge factors that influence functional recovery include demographics such as preexisting comorbidities and increasing age, as well as the contextual and environmental factors such as family functioning and social or peer support. It is important to note that not all children decline in function following PICU admission, and a small proportion of patients, primarily those electively—as opposed to emergently—admitted for surgical correction, may experience functional improvement at hospital discharge. Those who experience functional disability benefit from rehabilitation.

■ REHABILITATION DURING AND FOLLOWING CRITICAL ILLNESS

Acute Rehabilitation in the PICU

Acute rehabilitation in the PICU encompasses a wide spectrum of activities and therapies aimed to prevent physical, cognitive, and psychological impairment related to critical illness. For infants and children undergoing rapid neurologic and physical development, the importance of early and progressive rehabilitation cannot be overemphasized. Importantly, children under the age of 3 comprise two-thirds of all PICU patients admitted for more than 72 hours. Thus, unlike adults, children are at risk of not only decline in function but also delay in achieving key developmental milestones. Therefore, early intervention to support recovery and minimize disability is key. Early rehabilitation in critically ill adults (within 72 hours of ICU admission) is associated with decreased duration of mechanical ventilation and improved physical function at discharge. While pediatric data are still emerging, there is ample reason to translate these findings to children since rehabilitation during a PCIU stay is both safe and feasible. The major question is how to pursue rehabilitation in the most effective fashion across a broad range of ages and developmental stages.

Optimizing Acute Rehabilitation in the PICU

Critically ill children are at a high risk of functional impairments as a result of concerns of safety and comfort which lead to oversedation and bedrest. This approach is amplified by a seemingly ubiquitous PICU culture of immobility. In fact, recent international studies have shown that one-fifth of all PICU patients admitted for more than 2 days are *completely immobile* on any given day. An intense focus on resuscitation and stabilization in the early phases of critical illness may delay addressing mobility and rehabilitation needs. These needs can be readily met by physical and occupational therapists (PT and OT) as well as speech-language pathologists (SLP). Even if a child is deemed to be "too sick" to participate in a rehabilitation evaluation in the first 48 hours of admission, PTs and OTs can provide crucial information at this early stage of critical illness regarding baseline function, developmentally appropriate positioning, and strategies to prevent ICU-acquired weakness. All of this can occur even when in-bed exercises and out-of-bed mobility are contraindicated by the severity of illness.

While early rehabilitation effort is key to optimizing functional outcomes for PICU patients, nurses are the foundation underlying patient mobilization efforts. Over two-thirds of all mobilization activities in the PICU are initiated by nurses alone or in collaboration with other staff. As such, engaging PTs and OTs early on can facilitate increased nursing comfort, with activity and mobility promotion, and provide a conduit for staff education. Furthermore, family presence and engagement in ICU rounds and direct patient care are independently associated with increased out-of-bed mobility.

Even with robust interprofessional buy-in and family engagement, creating a culture of mobility and promoting early and safe rehabilitation in the PICU are dependent on related strategies. These include many of the ICU Liberation approaches that are used so effectively in adults (see Chapter 4: The Nurse's Perspective Fig. 18-2), including minimal but effective sedation, adequate pain management, delirium prevention, early mobilization, and family empowerment and engagement. Each of these actions helps patients participate in their own care, spend less time on mechanical ventilation, and engage with their family. Thus, each of these elements should be addressed for "every kid, every day" through a streamlined process, often on morning rounds with adaptation throughout the day as needed. It is ideal to set and communicate developmentally appropriate goals. The nurses, PTs, and OTs can work each day toward achieving these goals. Moreover, clear documentation of rehabilitation progress and unmet goals helps outpatient clinicians to continue the work that was started within the PICU or on the acute care unit or within the rehabilitation facility.

■ IMPACT OF CRITICAL ILLNESS ON COGNITIVE FUNCTION

Evaluating the scope of PICS-p-induced cognitive dysfunction helps in identifying when children have lost milestones they previously achieved, changes in the progress of normal development, and challenges in reintegrating into normal activities. Once any of these are identified, focused cognitive rehabilitation may be undertaken to support recovery. The most commonly affected cognitive domains are executive functioning (higher level thinking), attention regulation, processing speed (how rapidly children think), memory, and the ability to utilize adaptive skills in school and at home. Unsurprisingly, cognitive dysfunction impedes learning and keeping up with the developmental stage of children of a similar age.

Risk Factors for Poor Cognitive Outcomes

Besides the obvious risk factor of traumatic brain injury (TBI), critical illness also places a child at risk for poor cognitive outcomes. Similar to TBI, brain inflammation, low oxygen saturation, reduced brain blood flow, certain medications, invasive mechanical ventilation, and a variety of brain-focused surgical procedures all increase the risk for cognitive dysfunction. While those with TBI are often readily referred for cognitive rehabilitation, pediatric critical illness survivors are less commonly referred. The lack of robust PICS-p evaluation programs is likely to reduce the frequency of referrals as well.

■ CONSIDERATIONS FOR RECOVERY

Post-PICU Interventions to Mitigate Cognitive Problems

Given that the pediatric brain is still in the stage of development, understanding the cognitive morbidities related to surviving critical care is of paramount importance to design age-appropriate interventions that improve outcomes and address the consequences of PICU survivorship (Figure 18-3). Return to school presents a substantial challenge for critical illness survivors. Developing patient-specific plans in conjunction with educators and a cognitive specialist helps support success. Cognitive specialists include neuropsychologists, as well as developmental pediatricians; their engagement is not mutually exclusive in designing a recovery or reintegration program. Programs often

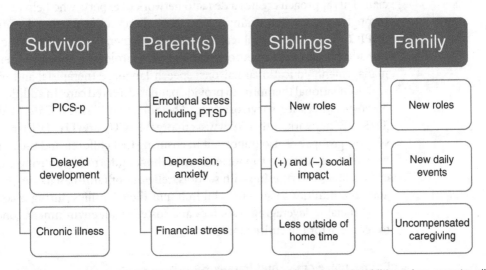

FIGURE 18-3. Consequences of PICU Survivorship. PICU survivorship impacts the child survivor, parents, siblings, and the entire family in readily identifiable ways. Note is made that many children have only one parent, while some are cared for by other family members such as grandparents. Others still are in foster care and as such do not have a traditional family composition.

include those that help re-establish previously learned behaviors or establish new ways to compensate for cognitive difficulties. Some approaches include daily attention training, self-instruction, physical fitness, structured work stations, diary training, behavioral coaching, family-delivered support, and cognitive behavioral therapy as well as psychoeducation. Each of these improves attention, memory, adaptive functioning, mood, and how children with a history of critical illness respond to new stressful events. Medication may help with attention and mood concerns, but those approaches are beyond the scope of this chapter.

Outpatient healthcare clinicians are often tasked with managing a multitude of symptoms related to PICS-p during recovery. They are also tasked with objectively identifying new deficits and morbidities related to an episode of critical illness. This can be a daunting task due to the breadth of PICS-p domains that need to be assessed. Therefore, clinicians are encouraged to develop collaborative relationships with cognition experts and to utilize their skillset as management plans for PICS-p-related issues are being developed and implemented. In the adult space, post-ICU clinics staffed in a multiprofessional fashion, including intensivists, critical care nurses, pharmacists, respiratory therapists, psychologists, social workers and more, often help in identifying patients with PICS and direct them to a variety of resources, including cognitive care specialists (see Chapter 15). The post-ICU clinic assessment and guidance is then shared with the patient's outpatient clinician. This approach creates a de facto network of experts who help the patient through recovery. For example, post-ICU clinics allow for the identification of PICS-p-associated problems as well as partnership between critical care providers, physiatrists, neuropsychologists, neurologists, social workers, case management, educational liaisons, speech-language therapists, and physical and occupational therapists to provide patient-centered care. In addition, web-based resources for survivors (e.g., The Society of Critical Care Medicine's THRIVE network: https://www.sccm.org/MyICUCare/THRIVE) and peer support groups are also important in ensuring that children and their families have routine access to support and educational information during and after critical illness. Partnering with schools, religious or faith-based organizations, and communities to support children and their families during recovery is also crucial to leveraging resources and fostering an environment conducive to recovery for the entire family.

Emotional, Social, and Family Health

The PICS-p framework highlights the impact that surviving critical illness and injury after a PICU stay can have on the experience and health outcomes of children. This conceptual framework also recognizes that when the child is part of a family, PICS-p affects family members as well. Therefore, intensive care survivorship can impact the experience and outcomes of parents and siblings, particularly with regard to emotional and social health. This is separately identified in adults as PICS-F (PICS-Family).

PICU Experience for Families

Having a critically ill or injured child is a hugely stressful and emotionally turbulent experience for most parents and may be magnified when there is only one parent. Stressors are numerous and include the unfamiliar and foreign PICU environment, changes to parental or caregiver role and family functioning, the degree of illness or injury, and uncertainty regarding their child's outcome. Differences in parental roles and stress responses have been noted, with mothers reported to have greater levels of stress than fathers. Complex medical conditions and unfamiliar medical jargon may make it difficult for parents or caregivers to understand what is happening on a daily basis, let alone from an overarching perspective. Even when the child has recurrent critical illness—a growing cohort of PICU patients—a variety of factors make the experience quite stressful for parents or caregivers who are familiar with the PICU environment. Chief among those stressors are medical care failures during outpatient care, less than ideal care coordination, and a perceived lack of individualized care between critical illness episodes. Care outside of the home, such as within a rehabilitation facility, also increased parental or caregiver stress. Siblings also experience stress which is driven by a different but interrelated array of factors.

The impact on siblings spans both emotional and social health domains. Siblings experience changes in parental behavior as well as parent presence and availability as parent(s) spend time with the ill child in the PICU. Even if siblings can visit their ill sibling, the well siblings are typically cared for by a substitute caregiver such as a relative or family friend while the parent(s) are at the PICU. During substitute caregiver time, siblings may be expected to take on age-inappropriate responsibilities such as the care of other siblings or domestic duties. Siblings who do visit the PICU can have repetitive exposure to distressing contact such as the foreign and sometime frightening environment (including other patients, technology, and interventions), uncertain outcomes, and the negative emotions expressed by relatives. Whether in the PICU or in the home setting, siblings experience negative emotions such as fear, sadness, anxiety, and relative neglect of their own needs including emotional support. These effects can be magnified during a prolonged episode of critical illness for an ill sibling.

Clinicians must recognize the unique and emotionally dynamic state of parents and siblings—and minimize modifiable stressors as much as possible. Family engagement and involvement needs to be optimized, including opportunities for parents or caregivers to ask questions, be present, be involved, and have choice. The "SIBS" framework may help both PICU and non-PICU healthcare professionals meet sibling needs. This framework includes: Support—which includes preparing siblings for hospital visitation; Information—ensuring that information is delivered in a developmentally appropriate fashion; Balance—mechanisms to help parents spend quality time with siblings who visit; and Sensitivity to time and resources and sustainable solutions across the duration of a child's critical illness. These are not the only approaches that can be used, but they do provide a starting point if no systems are already in place.

Post-PICU Discharge—Survivor Emotional and Social Health

Emotional and social health challenges are not limited to the PICU hospitalization and persist among children who survive critical illness. More than one-third of PICU survivors experience emotional impairment. Key risk factors for developing negative psychological outcomes such as fear of future medical care, concerns regarding the loss of control over one's health, and posttraumatic stress disorder include the number of invasive procedures, the severity of illness, and younger age. Inaccurate and intrusive memories of actual care events during PICU care are associated with posttraumatic stress—a process that is identical in adults. Since undesirable outcomes occur in a substantial proportion of PICU survivors, there is a driving need to identify and manage modifiable risk factors to improve postdischarge outcomes. Importantly, such interventions may involve school resources, home health, and psychologic counseling as well as out-of-home therapies. Ensuring that the PICU survivor can access required services may need input and management from a social worker to help arrange transportation, finances, and care coordination (see Chapter 12: Social Worker/Case Manager's Perspective).

Post-PICU Discharge—Family Emotional and Social Health

Up to one-third of parents report having an acute stress disorder and 12.3% meet the criteria for posttraumatic stress disorder at 3 months after their child is discharged from the PICU. Furthermore, up to 60% of parents report symptoms of anxiety and up to 50% report depression at 3 months after PICU discharge. Factors associated with impaired parental emotional health relate to the child having an unexpected PICU admission, the number of procedures the child required, parental preexisting psychological or emotional conditions, limited social support, and the child's and sibling's outcomes after critical illness including social and emotional dysfunction.

Social disruptions after PICU discharge are well described, including substantial changes in family roles and functioning. Parenting styles may change to address new and perhaps undesirable behaviors of the child—a critical illness survivor. New time demands can derail parental friendships as they struggle to balance convalescing child care with usual family activities including work. Unsustainable time away from work to facilitate child convalescence may lead to employment loss. Financial toxicity related to complex care and aftercare is also well described. Not all changes are negative. Some parents report a greater degree of expressiveness and openness which enhances family dynamics and minimizes conflict. For siblings, a mixture of positive and negative social health impacts are reported. Family dynamics may change due to parents and caregivers taking on more medicalized roles to meet the physical health needs of the child that has survived. Quite often, parents, family members, and friends serve as uncompensated caregivers, especially in those with limited access to aftercare agencies and resources. Relatedly, siblings may also adopt novel roles to support changes to the family unit which may adversely impact their ability to engage in activities outside of the home including age-appropriate activities with friends, as well as athletic or scholastic activities. However, siblings also report positive effects related to enhanced kinship between family members.

Tips for Clinicians

1. Critically ill children demonstrate a quite high survival rate especially when compared to adults with critical illness.
2. PICU survivors increasingly experience long-term physical, cognitive, emotional, and social health deficits.
3. Because children are dependent on and an integral part of their families, their morbidity also has a profound impact on their siblings, parents, and family unit during the immediate months after hospitalization and through years of recovery.
4. Approaches to mitigate against these undesirable consequences ideally starts in the PICU using prevention strategies such as those identified in the ICU Liberation Bundle.
5. Communication between critical care teams, families, and outpatient healthcare clinicians is essential to improving transitions of care and long-term outcomes.

6. Routine screening for the potential negative sequelae of pediatric critical illness will allow for timely identification of new morbidities, and implementation of targeted interventions to facilitate physical, cognitive, and psychological rehabilitation and improve the quality of life and the well-being of children and their families.
7. Consider referral to a post-ICU clinic, especially in those with long duration PICU care, multiple procedures, or in patients with features of PICS-p, which will engage a multiprofessional team to help guide care during convalescence.

KEY REFERENCES

Abela KM, Wardell D, Rozmus C, LoBiondo-Wood G. Impact of pediatric critical illness and injury on families: an updated systematic review. *J Pediatr Nurs.* 2020;51:21-31.

Als LC, Nadel S, Cooper M, et al. A supported psychoeducational intervention to improve family mental health following discharge from paediatric intensive care: feasibility and pilot randomised controlled trial. *BMJ Open.* 2015;5(12):e009581.

Andrews B, Rahman N, Pinto N. Family support and ICU survivorship: lessons learned from the pediatric critical care experience. In: Netzer G, ed. *Families in the Intensive Care Unit: A Guide to Understanding, Engaging, and Supporting at the Bedside.* Cham: Springer International Publishing; 2018:101-118.

Babikian T, Asarnow R. Neurocognitive outcomes and recovery after pediatric TBI: meta-analytic review of the literature. *Neuropsychology.* 2009;23(3):283-296.

Babikian T, Merkley T, Savage RC, et al. Chronic aspects of pediatric traumatic brain injury: review of the literature. *J Neurotrauma.* 2015;32(23):1849-1860.

Bele S, Chugh A, Mohamed B, et al. Patient-reported outcome measures in routine pediatric clinical care: a systematic review. *Front Pediatr.* 2020;8:364.

Bennett TD, Niedzwecki CM, Korgenski EK, Bratton SL. Initiation of physical, occupational, and speech therapy in children with traumatic brain injury. *Arch Phys Med Rehabil.* 2013;94(7):1268-1276.

Betters KA, Hebbar KB, Farthing D, et al. Development and implementation of an early mobility program for mechanically ventilated pediatric patients. *J Crit Care.* 2017;41:303-308.

Bone MF, Feinglass JM, Goodman DM. Risk factors for acquiring functional and cognitive disabilities during admission to a PICU*. *Pediatr Crit Care Med.* 2014;15(7):640-648.

Bradbury KR, Williams C, Leonard S, et al. Emotional aspects of pediatric post-intensive care syndrome following traumatic brain injury. *J Child Adolesc Trauma.* 2021;14(2):177-187.

Bronner MB, Peek N, Knoester H, et al. Course and predictors of posttraumatic stress disorder in parents after pediatric intensive care treatment of their child. *J Pediatr Psychol.* 2010;35(9):966-974.

Bulic D, Bennett M, Georgousopoulou EN, et al. Cognitive and psychosocial outcomes of mechanically ventilated intensive care patients with and without delirium. *Ann Intensive Care.* 2020;10(1):104.

Choong K, Canci F, Clark H, et al. Practice recommendations for early mobilization in critically ill children. *J Pediatr Intensive Care.* 2018;7(1):14-26.

Choong K, Fraser D, Al-Harbi S, et al. Functional recovery in critically ill children, the "WeeCover" multicenter study. *Pediatr Crit Care Med.* 2018;19(2):145-154.

Choong K, Zorko DJ, Awojoodu R, et al. Prevalence of acute rehabilitation for kids in the PICU: a Canadian multicenter point prevalence study. *Pediatr Crit Care Med.* 2021;22(2):181-193.

Colville G, Kerry S, Pierce C. Children's factual and delusional memories of intensive care. *Am J Respir Crit Care Med.* 2008;177(9):976-982.

Colville G, Pierce C. Patterns of post-traumatic stress symptoms in families after paediatric intensive care. *Intensive Care Med.* 2012;38(9):1523-1531.

Cramer CL, Orlowski JP, DeNicola LK. Pediatric intensivist extenders in the pediatric ICU. *Pediatr Clin North Am.* 2008;55(3):687-708, xi-xii.

Devlin JW, Skrobik Y, Gelinas C, et al. Clinical practice guidelines for the prevention and management of pain, agitation/sedation, delirium, immobility, and sleep disruption in adult patients in the ICU. *Crit Care Med.* 2018;46(9):e825-e873.

Dinglas VD, Faraone LN, Needham DM. Understanding patient-important outcomes after critical illness: a synthesis of recent qualitative, empirical, and consensus-related studies. *Curr Opin Crit Care.* 2018;24(5):401-409.

Dodd JN, Hall TA, Guilliams K, et al. Optimizing neurocritical care follow-up through the integration of neuropsychology. *Pediatr Neurol.* 2018;89:58-62.

Ebrahim S, Singh S, Hutchison JS, et al. Adaptive behavior, functional outcomes, and quality of life outcomes of children requiring urgent ICU admission. *Pediatr Crit Care Med.* 2013;14(1):10-18.

Edwards JD, Lucas AR, Boscardin WJ, Dudley RA. Repeated critical illness and unplanned readmissions within 1 Year to PICUs. *Crit Care Med.* 2017;45(8):1276-1284.

Fayed N, Cameron S, Fraser D, et al. Priority outcomes in critically ill children: a patient and parent perspective. *Am J Crit Care.* 2020;29(5):e94-e103.

Fink EL, Beers SR, Houtrow AJ, et al. Early protocolized versus usual care rehabilitation for pediatric neurocritical care patients: a randomized controlled trial. *Pediatr Crit Care Med.* 2019;20(6):540-550.

Fink EL, Maddux AB, Pinto N, et al. A core outcome set for pediatric critical care. *Crit Care Med.* 2020;48(12):1819-1828.

Hall TA, Leonard S, Bradbury K, et al. Post-intensive care syndrome in a cohort of infants & young children receiving integrated care via a pediatric critical care & neurotrauma recovery program: a pilot investigation. *Clin Neuropsychol.* 2022;36(3):639-663.

Hardy KK, Olson K, Cox SM, et al. Systematic review: a prevention-based model of neuropsychological assessment for children with medical illness. *J Pediatr Psychol.* 2017;42(8):815-822.

Henderson CM, Williams EP, Shapiro MC, et al. "Stuck in the ICU": caring for children with chronic critical illness. *Pediatr Crit Care Med.* 2017;18(11):e561-e568.

Herrup EA, Wieczorek B, Kudchadkar SR. Characteristics of postintensive care syndrome in survivors of pediatric critical illness: a systematic review. *World J Crit Care Med.* 2017;6(2):124-134.

Hopkins RO, Suchyta MR, Farrer TJ, Needham D. Improving post-intensive care unit neuropsychiatric outcomes: understanding cognitive effects of physical activity. *Am J Respir Crit Care Med*. 2012;186(12):1220-1228.

Ista E, Scholefield BR, Manning JC, et al. Mobilization practices in critically ill children: a European point prevalence study (EU PARK-PICU). *Crit Care*. 2020;24(1):368.

Jee RA, Shepherd JR, Boyles CE, et al. Evaluation and comparison of parental needs, stressors, and coping strategies in a pediatric intensive care unit. *Pediatr Crit Care Med*. 2012;13(3):e166-172.

Kachmar AG, Irving SY, Connolly CA, Curley MAQ. A systematic review of risk factors associated with cognitive impairment after pediatric critical illness. *Pediatr Crit Care Med*. 2018;19(3):e164-e171.

Khetani MA, Albrecht EC, Jarvis JM, et al. Determinants of change in home participation among critically ill children. *Dev Med Child Neurol*. 2018;60(8):793-800.

Killien EY, Farris RWD, Watson RS, et al. Health-related quality of life among survivors of pediatric sepsis. *Pediatr Crit Care Med*. 2019;20(6):501-509.

Kostanjsek N. Use of The International Classification of Functioning, Disability and Health (ICF) as a conceptual framework and common language for disability statistics and health information systems. *BMC Public Health*. 2011;11(Suppl 4):S3.

Kudchadkar SR, Nelliot A, Awojoodu R, et al. Physical rehabilitation in critically ill children: a multicenter point prevalence study in the United States. *Crit Care Med*. 2020;48(5):634-644.

Kudchadkar SR, Yaster M, Punjabi NM. Sedation, sleep promotion, and delirium screening practices in the care of mechanically ventilated children: a wake-up call for the pediatric critical care community. *Crit Care Med*. 2014;42(7):1592-1600.

Lenker H, Kim Y, Wieczorek B, Kudchadkar SR. Acute rehabilitation and early mobility in the pediatric intensive care unit. In: Zimmerman J, ed. *Fuhrman and Zimmerman's Pediatric Critical Care*. 6th ed. Philadelphia: Elsevier, Inc.; 2021:845-854.

Manning JC, Pinto NP, Rennick JE, et al. Conceptualizing post intensive care syndrome in children-the PICS-p framework. *Pediatr Crit Care Med*. 2018;19(4):298-300.

Meert KL, Clark J, Eggly S. Family-centered care in the pediatric intensive care unit. *Pediatr Clin North Am*. 2013;60(3):761-772.

Murphy Salem S, Graham RJ. Chronic illness in pediatric critical care. *Front Pediatr*. 2021;9:451.

Needle JS, O'Riordan M, Smith PG. Parental anxiety and medical comprehension within 24 hrs of a child's admission to the pediatric intensive care unit. *Pediatr Crit Care Med*. 2009;10(6):668-674.

Patel RV, Redivo J, Nelliot A, et al. Early mobilization in a PICU: a qualitative sustainability analysis of PICU up! *Pediatr Crit Care Med*. 2021;22(4):e233-e242.

Pinto NP, Rhinesmith EW, Kim TY, et al. Long-term function after pediatric critical illness: results from the survivor outcomes study. *Pediatr Crit Care Med*. 2017;18(3):e122-e130.

Pollack MM, Holubkov R, Funai T, et al. Pediatric intensive care outcomes: development of new morbidities during pediatric critical care. *Pediatr Crit Care Med*. 2014;15(9):821-827.

Pollack MM, Holubkov R, Glass P, et al. Functional status scale: new pediatric outcome measure. *Pediatrics*. 2009;124(1):e18-e28.

Riley AR, Williams CN, Moyer D, et al. Parental posttraumatic stress symptoms in the context of pediatric post-intensive care syndrome: impact on the family and opportunities for intervention. *Clin Pract Pediatr Psychol*. 2021;9(2):156.

Rodriguez-Rubio M, Pinto NP, Manning JC, Kudchadkar SR. Post-intensive care syndrome in paediatrics: setting our sights on survivorship. *Lancet Child Adolesc Health*. 2020;4(7):486-488.

Saliski M, Kudchadkar SR. Optimizing sedation management to promote early mobilization for critically ill children. *J Pediatr Intensive Care*. 2015;4(4):188-193.

Silver G, Doyle H, Hegel E, et al. Association between pediatric delirium and quality of life after discharge. *Crit Care Med*. 2020;48(12):1829-1834.

Stocker M, Pilgrim SB, Burmester M, et al. Interprofessional team management in pediatric critical care: some challenges and possible solutions. *J Multidiscip Healthc*. 2016;9:47-58.

Treble-Barna A, Beers SR, Houtrow AJ, et al. PICU-based rehabilitation and outcomes assessment: a survey of pediatric critical care physicians. *Pediatr Crit Care Med*. 2019;20(6): e274-e282.

Watson RS, Asaro LA, Hutchins L, et al. Risk factors for functional decline and impaired quality of life after pediatric respiratory failure. *Am J Respir Crit Care Med*. 2019;200(7):900-909.

Watson RS, Choong K, Colville G, et al. Life after critical illness in children-toward an understanding of pediatric post-intensive care syndrome. *J Pediatr*. 2018;198:16-24.

Zimmerman JJ, Banks R, Berg RA, et al. Trajectory of mortality and health-related quality of life morbidity following community-acquired pediatric septic shock. *Crit Care Med*. 2020;48(3):329-337.

Obstetrics

Arthur Jason Vaught

Patient Care Vignette

A 33-year-old patient at 28 weeks gestation presents to the emergency department with a fever, and back and flank pain as well as symptoms that suggest a urinary tract infection (UTI). This is her first pregnancy and she and her partner are quite anxious about the developing baby. She has a history of obstructive kidney stones that have required treatment multiple times over the last 5 years. Her current symptoms were similar to symptoms she had experienced about 3 weeks into her current pregnancy when she was also treated for a UTI. Because she was pregnant, she was initially evaluated in Obstetrical Triage where blood and urine cultures were obtained. Based on a high heart rate and a low blood pressure, she had two IV lines placed and she was administered 2 liters of intravenous fluid. She was also started on pregnancy-compatible antibiotics to treat her UTI as well as any urinary bacteria that were in her bloodstream.

Despite fluid resuscitation, her blood pressure remained low and her laboratory profile demonstrated an increasing amount of acid in her bloodstream (lactic acid, a lab marker of poor blood flow and oxygen delivery). To help with blood pressure of both mother and baby, a continuous infusion of a blood pressure–raising medication (vasopressor agent) was started. To assess the developing baby, fetal heart rate monitoring was initiated. It demonstrated indeterminate tracings that required ongoing surveillance as they were neither normal nor completely reassuring. The patient started to have contractions every 2 minutes, which were tracked by the monitor. Given her low blood pressure that needed fluid resuscitation and a vasopressor infusion, frequent uterine contractions, and indeterminate fetal heart rate tracings, she was admitted to the ICU for septic shock management.

■ INTRODUCTION

Approximately 1-10 per 10,000 pregnant patients are admitted to the ICU in the United States each year, with most patients being admitted immediately following delivery. The majority of these patients require critical care due to postpartum hemorrhage or complications of preeclampsia. ICU stay is typically short (~2 days) and patients are more likely to be Black, are older than 35 years of age, and have their child or children delivered by cesarean section. Internationally, epidemiologic risk factors are similar to that of the general intensive care population, but the United States continues to have higher rates of maternal mortality compared to other developed countries. This chapter addresses special considerations of the obstetric population in the ICU, and the importance of a collaborative approach between the intensivist, obstetric care clinicians, other consultants, and bedside staff. It will also help patients and families understand the kinds of medical or surgical conditions that impact pregnancy and how the required care influences post-ICU survivorship.

■ ICU CARE CONSIDERATIONS FOR THE OBSTETRIC POPULATION

Obstetrical and Postpartum Bleeding

The majority of obstetrical patients admitted to an ICU have either obstetrical (still pregnant) or postpartum hemorrhage. Postpartum hemorrhage is defined as a blood loss greater than 1,000 mL, a decrease in hematocrit of 10%, or other acute signs of hypovolemia (low blood volume). The majority of patients with obstetric hemorrhage can be managed on obstetric units, especially if in a tertiary care center. The specific capabilities of the obstetrical care unit influence whether the patient should be moved to the ICU, a more common occurrence in less well-resourced sites. Alternatively, an ICU clinician can help guide critical care in the obstetrical unit, but this is much less frequent than patient admission to the ICU.

A wide variety of techniques are available to the obstetrician to control bleeding, which include medications, devices, procedures in the Interventional Radiology suite, as well as operation that may include emergency hysterectomy if there is life-threatening hemorrhage. When there is large volume bleeding, some centers also engage with the Acute Care Surgery or Trauma Service staff for additional aid, especially if the facility's massive transfusion protocol is activated. This protocol brings red blood cells, plasma, and platelets to the patient's bedside for rapid infusion and is most commonly used to rescue injured patients with life-threatening bleeding. Nonetheless, other places in the hospital including ICUs, the operating room, and procedure suites all may need this rescue protocol.

Major shifts in fluid volumes occur around delivery. These shifts also influence laboratory values and should be expected by the care team. Since patients have access to values posted to their remotely accessible chart, such changes may also need to be explained to the patient and family members. Relatedly, the "hypervolemia of pregnancy" (increased total body salt and water volume) resolves after delivery through frequent and large volume urination. This is normal and should be interpreted in a positive fashion since the loss of excess fluid via the urine does not occur when there is ongoing bleeding.

Cardiac Disease and Hypertensive Disorders of Pregnancy

Cardiac disease and preeclampsia are also among the leading causes of maternal ICU admission as well as morbidity and mortality. Both preeclampsia and cardiac disease are notably more common in patients with advanced maternal age, preexisting comorbid conditions, and survivors of congenital heart disease correction. Risk factors for admission to the ICU include HELLP (hemolysis, elevated liver enzymes, low platelet count) syndrome, eclampsia, pulmonary edema, or hypertension that does not respond to intermittent medications and instead requires continuous infusion therapy. In particular, patients with HELLP syndrome may also have bleeding, and this is one of the conditions that often requires transfusion therapy to correct.

Medication selection for hypertensive disorders of pregnancy is different from how outpatient high blood pressure is managed. The specific agents reflect the need for immediate blood pressure control (i.e., intravenous instead of oral agents) as well as the concomitant pregnancy. While many agents may afford tight control of blood pressure and are reasonably safe during pregnancy, nitroglycerin should only be used with caution as it may cause uterine relaxation and increase the likelihood of postpartum hemorrhage. Patients with eclampsia may also develop seizures that drive ICU admission for monitoring and anticonvulsant medication management. The typical therapies for eclamptic seizures are rapid fetal delivery and magnesium sulfate infusion; magnesium is another ideal antihypertensive agent around delivery. Seizure activity should also prompt CT scan imaging to evaluate for structural causes such as a brain tumor or intracranial bleeding.

Pregnancy may be complicated by myocardial ischemia (just as in nonpregnant patients) but also by cardiomyopathies that are unique to pregnancy. Myocardial ischemia in the setting of pregnancy is typically attributed to the same causes as those in nonpregnant individuals. Urgent therapy (often performed in the cardiac catheterization lab) is needed to correct myocardial ischemia during pregnancy, but certain therapies will increase bleeding risk including aspirin and anticoagulation agents. Obstetric, critical care, and cardiac clinicians should collaboratively weigh the risk and benefits of specific interventions along with their attendant risk of bleeding; many approaches may be successful. Other agents such as β-blockers or other blood pressure–lowering agents are well tolerated by both the mother and the fetus.

It should be noted that immediate delivery is not indicated in the setting of acute myocardial ischemia. In fact, delivery within the first 2 weeks after acute myocardial ischemia or infarction (AMI) is associated with recurrent AMI. If the patient is beyond the acute event, postponing birth for 2-3 weeks to allow for cardiac healing is reasonable. Unfortunately, there is little data on the optimal gestational age of birth that should be targeted after the mother has suffered an AMI. In settings of massive myocardial ischemia causing cardiogenic shock or cardiac arrest, a multiprofessional approach should determine delivery timing, method, and postdelivery disposition as plans should reflect the individual patient circumstance.

Peripartum cardiomyopathy is a distinct entity that may result in cardiogenic shock and the need for ICU care. Pregnant patients with any kind of cardiac history—especially any kind of cardiomyopathy—optimally undergo consultation with both cardiology and critical care clinicians in a complex care center to plan management that supports safe fetal delivery. This kind of consultation is of great benefit as it may lead to changes in medications, and also craft plans for rescue interventions, should the need arise. Rescue may require a mechanical circulatory support device but the need for such rescue is associated with an increased risk of both fetal and maternal death.

Embolic Disease

Embolic events including pulmonary embolism (PE) as well as amniotic fluid embolism (AFE) are rare but significant events in pregnancy. Risk factors include postpartum hemorrhage, preeclampsia, and certain kinds of platelet disorders. Deep vein thrombosis (DVT) is a common precursor to PE; emboli may be quite small or so large as to cause cardiac arrest. Therapy for PE ranges from anticoagulation to thrombolysis therapy (thrombo = clot; lysis = destruction; similar to what is given to some stroke patients). Each of these approaches carries a significant risk of bleeding, especially around delivery.

Another approach is known as catheter-directed thrombolysis that only delivers the clot-lysing drug right at the site of the clot instead of providing it throughout the entire bloodstream. Catheter-directed thrombolysis requires a skilled proceduralist and is not available at all centers. Some centers have a Pulmonary Embolism Response Team (PERT) that provides consultation to other facilities, can help select the most appropriate therapy, and even help arrange transfer when needed to access specialists who may not be present in the outside hospital. Surgical thrombectomy, while feasible during pregnancy, is a last resort that carries a much higher risk of fetal death (up to 20%). After nonmassive PE (no cardiac arrest), maternal and fetal survival is nearly 90%, a success rate that should prompt the care team, the patient, and family to readily pursue therapy.

AFE is a rare phenomenon (2-6 in 100,000 births) that results in cardiogenic shock (neither side of the heart pumps well and leads to low blood pressure), acute respiratory failure (unable to support their own breathing), and disordered clotting (too much or too little and in inappropriate locations). The precise mechanisms that lead to AFE remain unclear, but AFE has some features that are similar to an allergic response. Patients who sustain AFE are critically ill and require care in an ICU. The lungs are particularly injured, and many require a breathing tube to be placed to allow them to receive invasive mechanical ventilation. Since the lungs are so sensitive to the AFE process, the patient may develop acute respiratory distress syndrome (ARDS; see Chapter 5: The Respiratory Therapist's Perspective and below) and therefore may require days to weeks on the ventilator to recover. Because there are no straightforward diagnostic criteria for AFE, it remains a diagnosis of exclusion. This means that other potential causes are examined and excluded, leaving AFE as the remaining plausible explanation. Treatment is largely supportive and typically involves blood pressure–raising agents (vasopressors) given by intravenous infusion, invasive mechanical ventilation, and blood product transfusion as needed.

Acute Respiratory Failure and ARDS

In the setting of acute COVID-19 infection, acute respiratory failure and ARDS occurred much more commonly in pregnant patients. Furthermore, COVID-19-infected pregnant women demonstrated a higher risk of requiring mechanical cardiopulmonary support which is associated with higher fetal and maternal mortality. As with all patients who require invasive mechanical ventilation, lung protective ventilation is also appropriate for the pregnant patient (see Chapter 5: The Respiratory Therapist's Perspective). Some strategies that are commonly used for nonpregnant patients who have ARDS may be dangerous for the unborn child. Allowing higher than normal carbon dioxide concentration or slightly lower than normal oxygen concentration may be poorly tolerated by the fetus and can lead to complications including fetal demise. Therefore, the ICU team may need to treat the pregnant patient with ARDS slightly differently than the nonpregnant patient, and such approaches are ideally shared with the family during ICU rounds (see Chapter 16). Other standard therapies remain useful throughout pregnancy and include prone position therapy, inhaled pulmonary vasodilating agents, and extracorporeal membrane oxygenation (ECMO) and should be employed if indicated. Given the risks of bleeding as well as clotting with ECMO, those risks should be explicitly clear to the patient's decision-maker(s). A variety of online resources may help with shared decision-making (see Appendix C).

Sepsis and Septic Shock

Sepsis is a specific condition that is triggered by infection and is characterized by how the infected person responds to that infection. There are specific criteria for sepsis as well as the related condition of septic shock that are used by clinicians to help guide care. The Surviving Sepsis Campaign (SSC; www.sccm.org/SurvivingSepsis) has developed and published guidelines and care approaches that are designed to improve the timeliness of care as well as survival in adults; a pediatric version has also been developed. Maternal sepsis and septic shock are leading causes of severe maternal morbidity and mortality and benefit from rapid care as identified in the SSC guideline and bundle. Most importantly, sepsis and septic shock (as soon as they are recognized) should be treated as medical emergencies with a variety of aspects of care started within the first hour. These key aspects include obtaining cultures to identify what bacteria (or more rarely fungal of viral pathogens) are present, starting empiric antibiotic therapy, checking specific laboratory measures, and starting fluid resuscitation. During pregnancy the amount of required fluid administered may be less than anticipated due to the hypervolemia of pregnancy. For patients like the one in our vignette, starting an infusion of a vasopressor may be life-saving.

During pregnancy, most infections that lead to sepsis or septic shock are related to either the urinary track or the uterus. Knowing the common sites that lead to infection helps guide assessment and select appropriate antibiotics. The pregnant patient with sepsis or septic shock who requires ICU care benefits from the usual ICU team-based care to which obstetric clinicians and neonatologists are added as key members. Because there are unique monitors and medications that are uncommonly deployed in the ICU—but are common in Labor and Delivery—the obstetric team helps guide relevant aspects of ICU care that address both maternal and fetal support. Two major aspects of care upon which the ICU team relies on the obstetric care team are fetal monitoring and the timing of delivery.

Fetal Monitoring in the ICU

Critical illness or injury care for the pregnant patient is routinely accompanied by fetal monitoring after a certain estimated fetal age. An estimated gestational age of 23 weeks correlates to an estimated fetal weight of 500 grams. Many institutions will include some form of fetal monitoring after 23 weeks, especially in resource-replete institutions. While the needs of the mother take precedence over the needs of the unborn child, the best care for the fetus is excellent maternal care. Only fetal monitoring can identify how well—or how poorly—the fetus is doing while the mother undergoes necessary care (such as resuscitation and antibiotics for the patient in the vignette). Fetal monitoring can also be used if the mother requires surgical care in the operating room. Because there is no consensus on the best way or the optimal timing to use, fetal monitoring decisions are individualized based upon fetal gestational age and local resources.

Fetal surveillance is most commonly performed using ultrasound monitoring in an intermittent or continuous fashion by the obstetric clinician. Intermittent monitoring can be readily performed with a handheld Doppler device that detects and then transmits fetal heart sounds to track the fetal heart rate. A larger ultrasound machine is typically used to obtain ultrasound images as well as detailed fetal evaluation termed the "biophysical profile." The biophysical profile, which includes real-time sonography of the fetus, includes five important components—a nonstress test, fetal breathing, fetal movement, fetal tone, and amniotic fluid volume. A score (maximum of 10) is generated from each component and results are used to predict fetal health. A score of 8 or more is considered normal; 6 is considered equivocal (uncertain); and 4 or less is abnormal. The score is used by the obstetric and ICU teams to help determine the urgency and timing of planned delivery. The ICU clinicians may also use ultrasound to assess a variety of aspects of the mother's care, including blood volume, how well the heart is contracting, as well as some aspects of lung function.

Cardiac Arrest and Perimortem Cesarean Section

Maternal cardiac arrest is a rare complication. Acute management is detailed by the Advanced Cardiac Life Support (ACLS) program and does not differ with pregnancy. When the mother suffers a cardiac arrest, the fetus' blood flow through the placenta also stops. Rescue CPR (cardiopulmonary resuscitation) only restores a small portion of the blood flow that the fetus normally receives. Therefore, maternal cardiac arrest carries a huge risk for fetal death as well. Fetal rescue—when of an age sufficient for survival outside of the uterus—uses a resuscitative hysterotomy (incision of the uterus identical to a cesarean section) to rapidly deliver the fetus. This procedure is optimally performed by an obstetrician or a suitably trained surgeon and should occur where the arrest occurs (as opposed to moving to an OR) to maximize survival. Fetal care by a neonatologist is essential as the fetus is generally preterm and will need specialized neonatal critical care to survive derailing the usual expectation of immediate pairing with mother and other family members—a substantial hardship regardless of maternal survival.

CPR occurs most commonly with the patient flat on their back to take advantage of a hard surface against which compressions can push blood out of the heart. Because the pregnant uterus compresses the main vein that returns blood to the heart from the lower half of the body, rapid fetal delivery using a resuscitative hysterotomy relieves that compression and helps restore maternal heart function. Therefore, this approach benefits both the fetus and the mother. Previously, resuscitative hystererotomy was used only following four minutes of failed ACLS measures, but now this approach is now utilized sooner in the resuscitation. Newer guidance suggests that the use of immediate resuscitative hysterotomy is warranted when the mother's heart rhythm is not one that will respond to a countershock. These specific considerations must be thoroughly shared with the mother (if she survives), as well as other family or loved ones as the decision to pursue fetal delivery in the setting of maternal cardiac arrest is quite uncommon and is likely to be rather unsettling.

Considerations for Recovery

Pregnant patients who require critical care, but who do not deliver their baby (or babies) may be generally considered to be similar to nonpregnant patients with regard to post-ICU recovery, besides the need for ongoing obstetrical care (see Chapter 15). When delivery accompanies hospitalization for critical illness or injury, there are a variety of issues that the multiprofessional team should anticipate and manage to enhance recovery. Even if the mother remains in the ICU for a period of time after delivery, standard postpartum care should proceed, including routine baby visitation to provide mother-baby skin-on-skin contact, lactation consultant care (especially for first-time mothers and to facilitate pumping as needed), and provisions to support parent/partner/family visitation. COVID-19 isolation measures tended to derail visitation; the long-term consequences of which continue to be discovered (see Chapter 25).

When the mother is so critically ill that analgesia and sedation and invasive mechanical ventilation (for example) is required for care, she may have little to no recall of delivery or any bonding episodes following delivery. Therefore, the ICU and obstetric teams in conjunction with family should work together to record key events that can be explored later. An ICU diary (see Chapter 14) may help fill in maternal memory gaps, as can digital photographs or video recordings (if permitted by the institution). Ongoing maternal critical illness will preclude neonatal ICU visitation if the delivered baby also requires critical care. Telemedicine resources that are often present in complex care institutions can link the baby and the mother to support at least visual and auditory linkage. Otherwise, digital videoconferencing platforms that can be accessed via computer, smartphone, or tablet may be used to great effect. Such linkages may be particularly important if the delivered baby requires interfacility transfer based on the need for neonatal critical care resources that are not present in the facility in which the delivery occurred. Consideration of maternal interfacility transfer to render care in the same institution supports recovery as well.

Fetal demise may occur during maternal critical illness or following critical injury. This life-altering event requires great sensitivity to support the surviving mother who continues to require ICU care. That care must also include family or other loved ones important to the mother. Grief is expressed in a variety of ways and may impact critical care in nonbeneficial ways including anger, depression, withdrawal, and a lack of engagement in self-care. Survivor guilt is not uncommon and should be specifically sought perhaps especially following fetal demise as a result of maternal injury.

Tips for Clinicians

1. **Optimal team-based care for pregnant patients is multiprofessional** and leverages typical clinical teams in conjunction with obstetric care clinicians. Other specialists such as Pediatricians, Pediatric Intensivists, or Neonatologists may be essential depending on specific clinical circumstances.
2. Maternal, fetal (before delivery), and infant (after delivery) care needs may outstrip available resources at the initial receiving facility. **Maintain a low threshold for referral or transfer** to a facility with appropriate clinical capabilities.
3. **Post-ICU survival care should include evaluation for typical issues in critical care survivorship** that are detailed elsewhere throughout this book, such as post-intensive care syndrome. A post-ICU clinic may be an ideal location to perform these multiprofessional evaluations.

4. If critical illness coincides with delivery, conventional postdelivery education and supports such as lactation consultation may not have been provided to the patient. **Consider referring the patient for postdelivery services as needed.**

5. **Consider early referral to mental health services** as needed for bereavement, postpartum depression, and/or depression and anxiety related to critical illness.

KEY REFERENCES

American College of Obstetricians and Gynecologists Practice Bulletin No. 202: Gestational hypertension and preeclampsia. *Obstet Gynecol.* 2019;133(1):e1-e25.

American College of Obstetricians and Gynecologists Practice Bulletin No. 211: Critical care in pregnancy. *Obstet Gynecol.* 2019;133(5):e303-e319.

American College of Obstetricians and Gynecologists' Presidential Task Force on Pregnancy and Heart Disease and Committee on Practice Bulletins—Obstetrics. ACOG Practice Bulletin No. 212: pregnancy and heart disease. *Obstet Gynecol.* 2019;133(5):e320-e356.

Antepartum Fetal Surveillance: American College of Obstetricians and Gynecologists Practice Bulletin Summary, Number 229. *Obstet Gynecol.* 2021;137(6):1134-1136.

Balgobin CA, Zhang X, Lima FV, et al. Risk factors and timing of acute myocardial infarction associated with pregnancy: insights from the National Inpatient Sample. *J Am Heart Assoc.* 2020;9(21):e016623.

Beacher L, Mauermann S, Cruz M, et al. ECMO outcomes in pregnant and peripartum women. *J Am Coll Cardiol.* 2020;75(11 Supplement 1):1062.

Bienstock JL, Eke AC, Hueppchen NA. Postpartum hemorrhage. *N Engl J Med.* 2021;384 (17):1635-1645.

Coggins AS, Gomez E, Sheffield JS. Pulmonary embolism and amniotic fluid embolism. *Obstet Gynecol Clin.* 2022;49(3):439-460.

Elkayam U, Goland S, Pieper PG, Silverside CK. High-risk cardiac disease in pregnancy: Part I. *J Am Coll Cardiol.* 2016;68(4):396-410.

Elkayam U, Hall S, Lansky A, et al. The use of Impella heart pump for management of women with peripartum cardiogenic shock. *J Am Coll Cardiol.* 2019;73(9 Supplement 1):1015.

Evans L, Rhodes A, Alhazzani W, et al. Surviving sepsis campaign: international guidelines for management of sepsis and septic shock 2021. *Intensive Care Med.* 2021;47(11):1181-1247.

Hennemeyer C, Khan A, McGregor H, et al. Outcomes of catheter-directed therapy plus anticoagulation versus anticoagulation alone for submassive and massive pulmonary embolism. *Am J Med.* 2019;132(2):240-246.

Jackson AM, Dalzell JR, Walker NL, et al. Peripartum cardiomyopathy: diagnosis and management. *Heart.* 2018;104(9):779-786.

Lisonkova S, Razaz N, Sabr Y, et al. Maternal risk factors and adverse birth outcomes associated with HELLP syndrome: a population-based study. *BJOG.* 2020;127(10):1189-1198.

Manuck TA, Rice MM, Bailit JL, et al. Preterm neonatal morbidity and mortality by gestational age: a contemporary cohort. *Am J Obstet Gynecol.* 2016;215(1):103.e1-103.e14.

Medcalf KE, Park AL, Vermeulen MJ, Ray JG. Maternal origin and risk of neonatal and maternal ICU admission. *Crit Care Med.* 2016; 44(7):1314-1326.

Rose CH, Faksh A, Traynor KD, et al. Challenging the 4-to 5-minute rule: from perimortem cesarean to resuscitative hysterotomy. *Am J Obstet Gynecol.* 2015;213(5):653.

Rose CH, Wyatt MA, Narang K, et al. Timing of delivery with COVID-19 pneumonia requiring intensive care unit admission. *Am J Obstet Gynecol MFM.* 2021;3(4):100373.

Saif K, Kevane B, Áinle FN, Rosovsky RP. The role of the PERT team in 2021. *Thromb Update.* 2022;6:100092.

Sakamoto J, Michels C, Eisfelder B, Joshi N. Trauma in pregnancy. *Emerg Med Clin.* 2019;37(2):317-338.

Shields A, de Assis V, Halscott T. Top 10 pearls for the recognition, evaluation, and management of maternal sepsis. *Obstet Gynecol.* 2021;138(2):289-304.

Varughese M, Patole S, Shama A, Whitehall J. Permissive hypercapnia in neonates: the case of the good, the bad, and the ugly. *Pediatr Pulmonol.* 2002;33(1):56-64.

Wang E, Glazer KB, Howell EA, Janevic TM. Social determinants of pregnancy-related mortality and morbidity in the United States: a systematic review. *Obstet Gynecol.* 2020;135(4):896.

Weiss SL, Peters MJ, Alhazzani W, et al. Surviving sepsis campaign international guidelines for the management of septic shock and sepsis-associated organ dysfunction in children. *Intensive Care Med.* 2020;46(1):10-67.

Wilcox SR, Wax RS, Meyer MT, et al. Interfacility transport of critically ill patients. *Crit Care Med.* 2022;50(10):1461-1476.

Zambrano LD, Ellington S, Strid P, et al. Update: characteristics of symptomatic women of reproductive age with laboratory-confirmed SARS-CoV-2 infection by pregnancy status—United States, January 22-October 3, 2020. *MMWR Morb Mortal Wkly Rep.* 2020;69(44):1641-1667.

CHAPTER 20

Burns

Tina Palmieri and Keturah M. Sloan

Patient Care Vignette

A 37-year-old male was involved in a house fire. He sustained inhalation injury of his airway and lungs, and a 50% total body surface area (TBSA) third-degree burn. The burns involved his head, neck, chest, abdomen, and his arms and legs. He required a breathing tube to be placed (i.e., intubated) at the scene, started on intravenous fluid, and transported to a burn center. He had longstanding high blood pressure, high cholesterol, as well as nicotine and alcohol dependence.

On admission to the Burn Center, he underwent large volume fluid resuscitation (18 L) in the first 24 hours. Fiberoptic bronchoscopy to examine his airway confirmed the presence of inhaled soot. Both arms developed compartment syndrome from muscle swelling (high pressure within an inelastic space that compromised blood flow and oxygen delivery) and required the full-thickness third-degree burns to be incised to allow the underlying tissue to expand. He remained on the ventilator due to his inhalation injury and required a tracheostomy for long-term ventilation.

He also needed his full-thickness burn wounds to be excised in the operating room followed by coverage with split-thickness skin grafting obtained from nonburned areas (donor sites). Areas of partial-thickness burn on his face, neck, and some parts of his legs did not require burn wound excision and healed with rigorous and specialized wound care. His hospital course was complicated by pneumonia, difficulty swallowing, alcohol withdrawal syndrome, and acute blood loss anemia; he required 40 units of red blood cells during hospitalization. As he recovered, his tracheostomy was removed, and he was discharged on hospital day 55 to an acute rehabilitation facility with nearly all wounds and donor sites healed.

■ ICU CARE CONSIDERATIONS FOR MAJOR BURN INJURY

Burns are typically characterized by "degree" into first, second, and third degree. Most are familiar with the first-degree burns as a minor sunburn. Second-degree burns are more intense, involve deeper layers of the skin, and are generally accompanied by blistering of the skin (aka "sun poisoning). Third-degree burns involve all layers of the skin, including the nerves, and are therefore painless. Despite being deeper and more severe, third-degree burns seem deceptive due to the lack of pain. Burns are also categorized as minor and major. Major burns are those that involve more that 20% of the body surface area, while minor burns involve a lesser total area. The initial management of such patients can challenge even the most capable intensivist. Burn pathophysiology is unique and requires modification of standard intensive care unit (ICU) algorithms to improve burn patient survival and subsequent quality of life. Such care is best delivered in a specialized burn center. Relatedly, burn injury is unique, in that the skin is the organ injured. As the largest organ in the body, the skin functions not just as a physical barrier against the environment, but also regulates body temperature, provides immune surveillance, senses pain, controls insensible fluid loss, and participates in vitamin synthesis. The skin is seldom involved in illnesses treated in the ICU, except life-threatening soft tissue infections (i.e., flesh-eating bacterial infection). Moreover, when patients develop septic shock, blood flow and perfusion of vital organs such as the brain and heart take priority compared to the skin. With burn injury, skin perfusion is a priority at every phase of illness.

If the burned skin does not heal, the patient is unlikely to survive. In addition, burn treatment has substantial and protracted ICU resource requirements, with an anticipated ICU length of stay of at least one day per percent burn. Therefore, patients with major burn injury are at high risk for the postintensive care syndrome (see Chapter 15). Specialized burn ICUs have been developed to meet these intense and sustained staffing, resource, and equipment needs. Relatedly, in the United States there is a national burn verification system in place to assure that quality care is delivered. As such, ICU care of the severely burned patient should be ideally delivered in specific centers with training, protocols, and resources uniquely crafted for the burn injured patient. Even if the initial care is rendered in a burn center, clinicians should be aware of the kinds of care the patient previously received as well

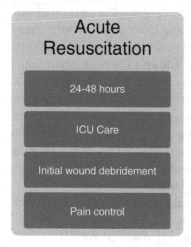
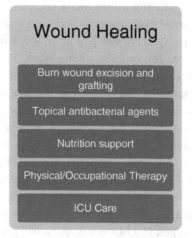
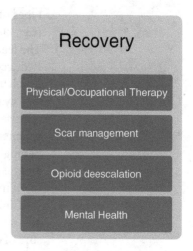

FIGURE 20-1. Phases of Major Burn Injury Care.

as common issues that occur during recovery. Patients and family members also benefit from such awareness as they will be the first to recognize that the patient needs additional care or even rescue for an emergency condition. Therefore, this chapter is divided into three care phases: acute resuscitation, wound healing, and recovery (Fig. 20-1).

■ RESUSCITATION PHASE

The acute burn resuscitation phase begins at the time of injury and ends when the patient no longer requires large volume intravenous fluid. This phase commonly lasts 24-48 hours after the initial injury. The initial treatment goals during acute burn resuscitation are similar to those for any acute injury—identifying and correcting life-threatening injuries or conditions. An approach that uses the alphabet is common and is as follows: A = airway, B = breathing, C = circulation, D = disability, and E = exposure of all injuries. It is important to ensure that all nonburn injuries are identified and addressed prior to burn center transfer. Following those evaluations, burn resuscitation is a primary concern during the first 24-48 hours. Some consequences of burn injury—such as inhalation injury—make resuscitation and management more challenging even at the specialized burn center.

Inhalation injury is common with major burns and is associated with increased mortality as well as long-term morbidity. Inhalation injury is not a single disease entity. Rather, inhalation injury is the term used to describe the different types of respiratory tract injury that result from specific injurants; treatment may be specific to the cause of the injury. For example, major types of inhalation injury include hypoxia (low oxygen), toxic gas inhalation (e.g., chlorine gas), upper airway heat injury, and lower airway smoke injury. The leading cause of death at a fire scene is hypoxia as fire consumes oxygen. Reduced oxygen can also create brain injury known as hypoxic brain injury unrelated to the skin burn. Toxic gases, such as carbon monoxide, ammonias, and cyanide, may be inhaled at the fire scene, especially if the fire is in an enclosed space. Carbon monoxide, among the most common inhaled gases, is generated from combustion of organic materials. Because its affinity for hemoglobin is 250 times that of oxygen it can cause tissue—including brain and heart—hypoxia. Therefore, burn victims and the clinicians who care for them must often address injuries besides the burn.

If inhalation injury is suspected, peripheral pulse oximeter–derived oxygen saturation should not be used as a surrogate for measuring partial pressure of oxygen in a blood gas, as carboxyhemoglobin will falsely elevate pulse oximeter saturation (hemoglobin is saturated with something, just not oxygen). The symptoms of carbon monoxide poisoning generally consist of a progressive decline in the level of alertness and mental acuity as well as exercise tolerance. In general, a face mask providing 100% oxygen is all that is required to treat carbon monoxide poisoning. The most severe cases, including those who lose consciousness, may benefit from a unique way of providing very high oxygen concentration in the bloodstream and the tissues. This approach is called hyperbaric oxygen (HBO) and delivers 100% oxygen at pressure similar to what is experienced at about 66 fppt (approximately 2 atmospheres or 2ATM) underwater while scuba diving; HBO session are often termed "dives." The pressure drives oxygen in very high concentration into tissues and helps to support wound healing. Moreover, the very high oxygen concentration may kill certain bacteria. HBO schedules (how many "dives" per day and for how long) may be unique to the patient as well as the approach used by each center. This is a specialized therapy that may be provided not only at a burn center but also at many major trauma centers and is quite staff labor-intensive.

Cyanide is generated from burning plastics and is another inhaled chemical that can influence resuscitation. The hallmark of cyanide toxicity is unremitting profound metabolic acidosis despite adequate resuscitation. Treatment for cyanide toxicity, hydroxocobalamin, causes orange/red discoloration of body fluids, including urine, and can interfere with certain lab tests as well as hemodialysis device sensors. Hydroxocobalamin use by prehospital providers and emergency department clinicians as an adjunct to treat fire-related inhalation injury is common.

The second type of inhalation injury, airway obstruction, is generally caused by airway edema from exposure to intense heat near the face, mouth, pharynx, and neck. When swelling occurs in these areas, it can rapidly worsen due to the administration of fluid required to resuscitate patients, which can leak from capillaries much more rapidly in the injured patient. Hence, monitoring for airway obstruction is important for those with severe burns. Most patients with burns more than half of their total body surface area (TBSA), especially those involving the face, benefit from having a breathing tube placed before airway edema becomes severe. Placing a rescue breathing tube is much more difficult once there is swelling around the airway, and sometimes it is impossible without placing a surgical airway through the front of the neck. When there are facial burns, the burn center uses a different approach to securing the breathing tube in place so that there is no tape on the burned skin. In general, airway edema is largely resolved after 3-5 days. A variety of tests are performed prior to breathing tube removal (extubation) to ensure that airway swelling has sufficiently decreased to make tube removal safe, and that the patient can breathe on their own. Safely extubating a burn patient becomes more challenging by the increased metabolic rate that occurs after burn injury. The increased metabolism requires the patient to breathe more than normal each minute to keep up with waste products such as carbon dioxide (CO_2) that are generated. Moreover, increased metabolism also consumes normal muscle mass—despite supplemental feeding—and makes the recovering burn patient weaker. Chest wall burns also make the chest wall stiff which makes breathing more difficult without the support of the ventilator. Therefore, early tracheostomy (within a week of injury) is often performed for burn patients with severe burn injury and anticipated prolonged mechanical ventilation needs. A tracheostomy is a breathing tube that goes in through the front of the neck instead of the mouth and requires a small surgical procedure to place. It is more readily tolerated by patients who require long periods of mechanical ventilation and also helps shorten overall time on the ventilator.

The final type of inhalation injury is one of the lower respiratory tract from inhaling the products of combustion. After exposure to smoke, the cells that line the airway sustain an injury and may separate from their underlying base. Those cells may then function like a plug and obstruct the airway leading to collapse of portions of the lung. Moreover, a required airway cell product called surfactant (it is a lot like soap) is produced in much smaller amounts. This product is essential in making it easy for the individual airway units called alveoli to open as gas flows into them. The best way to assess a lower airway inhalation injury is by flexible bronchoscopy that uses a small endoscope (similar to the much larger one used for colonoscopy) to look at the airways. It can also deliver and suction fluid, or take biopsies as needed. An integrated approach that maintains airway humidity and suctions out debris is used to treat this kind of injury; repeated bronchoscopy may be required for directed suctioning. Bronchodilators, similar to those used for asthma or chronic obstructive pulmonary disease (COPD), also help keep airways open. A variety of other medications have been tried to help improve outcomes after lower tract inhalation injury but seem less helpful than desired.

The prodigious fluid resuscitation acutely required after burn injury is a hallmark of burn intensive care. Formulas for intravenous resuscitation after major burn injury were created to provide practitioners with a guide, as the volume of fluid required after major burn injury far exceeds that of virtually any other condition. For example, the standard Parkland formula (4 mL per kilogram per percent burn) if applied to the patient in our vignette would estimate the starting intravenous fluid rate to be 4 mL × 80 kg (patient weight) × 50 (TBSA-burn size) = 16,000 mL fluid in the first 24 hours, with half being delivered in the first 8 hours. Formulas are only an estimate and only 20% of patients receive the fluid volume predicted by any formula. Fluid rates need to be adjusted based on patient response using a combination of urine output, laboratory evaluation, and monitoring of blood pressure in conjunction with a variety of other measures of perfusion. Heart rate is not used to help adjust fluid resuscitation after major burn injury as the injury and the increased metabolic rate lead to a high heart rate regardless of intravascular fluid. Family members should be aware of this, as in other circumstances, heart rate is rigorously tracked. Our vignette patient required more than his calculated resuscitation likely due to both inhalation injury and alcohol use that led to preburn injury dehydration. Finally, because major burn patients will develop massive total body edema from capillary leak, adjusting fluids based on patient edema is not appropriate after burn injury.

Once resuscitation is complete, the patient is transitioned to maintenance fluid that contains dextrose and a reduced amount of salt compared to resuscitation fluid. Maintenance fluids are administered at a much lower rate than resuscitation fluids. Nutritional support is started early after burn injury to help address the effects of hypermetabolism. A nutritional formulation (of which there are many) is delivered by a temporary feeding tube placed in the nose that ends in either the stomach, or further down in the small bowel. Similarly, physical and occupational therapy are started early to preserve range of motion, help preserve strength in unburned areas, and help decrease edema formation.

The other major area of concern in this phase, as well as throughout all phases, is the burn wound. After initial evaluation and stabilization, burn wounds are washed with soap and water just as with any wound. Then, already dead or dying tissue is removed and a topical antibiotic is applied. Since the skin is no longer intact and cannot serve as a barrier to bacterial invasion, the antibiotic helps decrease bacteria in the open wound. Burn wound infections are exceedingly rare in the first 48 hours after injury, but the risk increases thereafter. Intravenous antibiotics during this phase do not help decrease burn wound infection and should be reserved for documented infection in other sites.

Burn wound debridement (removal of dead or dying tissue) involves challenges that are common to any procedure, and also places a unique stress on the staff. This process requires a trained team of experienced wound care clinicians. During wound care, the burn team makes repeated searches for complications of the burn including compartment syndrome (see above) or muscle breakdown that can damage the kidneys (rhabdomyolysis). Rhabdomyolysis is more common after electrical injury, crush injury, and the more rare fourth-degree burn that involves muscle and/or bone. There are a variety of approaches to rhabdomyolysis that include a search for a reparable cause, additional intravenous fluid of a specific electrolyte composition, and some cases require dialysis for management.

Pain control in the acute phase is essential especially with the burn injury and the required debridements; sedation is much less frequent except for those who require invasive mechanical ventilation (see Chapter 21). Pain control may be challenging during the initial phase of burn injury, particularly during the initial debridement. Short-acting agents are ideal for acute pain control during debridements, but burn wound pain may be persistent in between those procedures. Therefore, a multimodal approach to pain control is ideal and in a unique way leverage long-acting opioids shortly after burn center admission. This approach is standard of care and reflects a unique aspect of burn injury management despite the highly publicized and durable efforts to reduce overall opioid use during and after acute hospitalization to avoid the risk of opioid dependence disorder.

■ WOUND-HEALING PHASE

After the resuscitation phase is complete, the wound-healing phase begins. The hypermetabolic response predominates in this phase, resulting in an elevated baseline temperature (38.5°C is normal), tachycardia, and increased nutritional requirements. Maneuvers to improve wound healing are the focus of this phase and coexist with ongoing critical care needs. Patients with anticipated invasive mechanical ventilation need for more than 2 weeks, as well as patients with severe face burns, benefit from early tracheostomy. The tracheostomy provides a stable airway, permits aggressive pulmonary toilet measures, and eases moving toward breathing independently. Therefore, especially in this patient population, tracheostomy should not be viewed as a failure or as a sign of poor outcome. Early burn wound excision and tissue coverage is the priority in this phase. Early tissue coverage is beneficial with respect to metabolism, infection, and protein loss across the wound. Since burn wound excision is generally accompanied by blood loss, transfusion is not uncommon with smaller wounds, and quite required with larger ones. Randomized transfusion trials in burn patients reported a mean blood transfusion need of 20-30 units of red blood cells for a burn wound that is more 20% TBSA.

Excision and autografting, in which the patient's unburned skin will be used to cover the open area of the excised burn wound, necessarily increases total wound size since the donor site must also heal. Cadaveric or artificial skin placement is used in patients who have insufficient donor sites to cover the entire burn wound. These modalities are temporizing measures until the already used donor sites have healed and can be used to provide a new graft (about 10-14 days after the initial graft was obtained). Excised and grafted wounds are usually covered with antimicrobial saturated or silver-based dressings to reduce bacterial or fungal colonization, invasion, and infection.

Major burn injury disrupts part of the immune system and increases a patient's infection risk. Certain cells that are key in recognizing and fighting infection do not function normally after a major burn. Standard markers of infection are also impacted making infection hard to diagnose in the burn patient. Temperature is often elevated from the increased metabolic rate, and laboratory markers of infection can vary around operations. Because all wounds become colonized, routine wound cultures are not helpful and should not be used to diagnose wound infection. Quantitative cultures may indicate infection above certain thresholds, but are not uniformly reliable. Intravenous agents that help raise blood pressure (vasopressors) often do so by creating vasoconstriction or narrowing of blood vessels even as they help the heart to pump more strongly. Excessive vasoconstriction can reduce skin blood flow and impede healing. Reduced blood flow also reduces the delivery of oxygen and other cells that help prevent or address infection. Therefore, avoiding vasopressors to the greatest extent possible helps support wound repair. Furthermore, tailoring antibiotics to only the bacteria or fungi that are causing infection at that moment helps reduce the driving pressure to create multidrug resistant organisms—a common event during prolonged burn wound care.

Early nutrition support is essential for wound healing and also decreases mortality, infection, and hospital length of stay. Since many major burn patients also require invasive mechanical ventilation, they need an alternate way of obtaining nutrition as they cannot eat around a breathing tube. Therefore, feeding tubes are placed through the mouth or the nose to deliver liquid nutrition. Postburn nutrition regimens provide much more protein than is required at baseline and are calculated using standard formulas. Adjustment of the nutritional prescription may use laboratory assessments as well as specialized equipment to assess whether what is being fed to the patient matches what they need. Despite these efforts, major burn patients will lose lean muscle mass due to the overwhelming catabolic response. Some centers also provide anabolic steroids to help maintain lean body mass (muscle). While a balanced diet during health typically supplies micronutrients and vitamins (copper, selenium, zinc, and vitamins A, B, C, D, E, and K), nutritional formulations may not provide enough of each of these for the major burn patient as they rebuild tissue and heal wounds. Therefore, regular supplementation is required.

Pain control remains an issue during this phase, especially around operative procedures and wound care. Moreover, many patients develop pain related to their nerves (neuropathic pain), particularly in areas with injury and later scarring. The multimodal approach to pain management can also provide specific agents to address neuropathic pain including gabapentin. Nonpharmacologic techniques for pain control, such as distraction, virtual reality, or guided imagery, can be used to decrease total opioid agent use. Physical and occupational therapy is essential to preserve range of motion and mobility which may create episodic pain that also needs to be addressed.

Patients with major burn injury should have therapy at least daily that includes early mobility, range of motion, strength training, and scar management plans. Early institution of therapy decreases scarring, improves strength, promotes wound healing, and helps to maintain muscle mass. Scars are tough and often inflexible, rendering therapy essential for maintaining movement especially around joints. Between therapy sessions every patient should be encouraged to continue movement, particularly for functional tasks, to accelerate physical recovery. Early ambulation in the ICU has been the standard of care for burn patients for more than three decades. When not active, patients with burn injury often require splints to maintain limbs in functional positions to prevent contracture. Importantly, splints maintain the patient's limb(s) in a position that supports use, but it is uncomfortable as the splints stretch the wounds. Nonetheless, splinting is a key part of the wound-healing process which helps ensure that patients get support for their activities of daily living such as bathing, dressing, and feeding during recovery.

■ RECOVERY PHASE

The recovery phase overlaps with the wound-healing phase as it begins when wounds are nearly, but not completely, healed. Patients with major burn injury have a prolonged stress response that often lasts for months after initial injury. That response has increased fight-of-flight hormones as well as the increased metabolism identified earlier. As a result, they often have a prolonged recovery phase. Although initial wound healing is almost completed, the wound continues to change in appearance for approximately 1-2 years. A wound that does not heal within 2 weeks has a nearly uniform likelihood of developing a thickened scar, known as hypertrophic scarring. Although grafts and wounds are initially flat, wounds with delayed healing begin to thicken in the months after grafting. This abnormal and maladaptive process continues over the majority of the first year and leads to a thick, red, and increasingly painful scar that is at increased risk of local infection. Custom-fit pressure garments are used to minimize scar thickening and to decrease scar height. These garments are designed to be extremely tight and can be difficult to put on as well as remove. Silicone sheeting beneath pressure garments can help flatten scars as well. Scar massage and moisturization helps with softening and may reduce scar thickening. These activities help engage patients and family members in care activities and provide an element of control during recovery. Wound care specialists are often involved in addressing hypertrophic scars that fail to respond to nonoperative treatment or those that partially respond but are disabling for patients.

Therapy continues and intensifies during recovery phase. Rebuilding muscle mass, strength, and range of motion is the goal of the therapy; each of these aspects also help increase endurance. Preventing contracture formation, especially around major joints is a major focus. While difficult and frequently time-consuming, scar management and range of motion are key aspects of recovery care that support return to independence. Failure to continue active therapy often requires operative management to release the contracture and includes another open wound, pain, and even more therapy. Patients often require substantial encouragement, as even after enduring months of painful acute wound care and dressing changes, pain continues during regular and repeated therapy sessions after hospital discharge. Ongoing therapy is helpful for patients with large burns in functional areas, particularly if the patient has difficulty with performing activities of daily living, ambulating, or speaking. Instead of requiring inpatient rehabilitation facility care, many burn patients receive outpatient physical or occupational therapy at home (limited travel ability) or at a local therapy center. Therapy should be ideally continued until maximum function is achieved, a process that generally requires months.

Other aspects of recovery care include monitoring for sequelae such as new and persistent itching within wounds as well as pain control agent de-escalation. Itching can generally be controlled using topical agents including moisturizers and oatmeal baths, but may benefit from medication management and should be guided by a clinician well versed in wound care. Opioid agents should be progressively weaned while maintaining nonopioid agents such as Tylenol, nonsteroidal anti-inflammatory drugs (NSAIDs), gabapentin, and topical lidocaine. This may be a prolonged process that benefits from including a pain specialist in the overall care plan. Pain specialists are often trained in anesthesiology and can offer a wide range of approaches to pain control. A pain medication contract between the patient and the clinician typically helps establish boundaries and expectations during the characteristically difficult weaning process.

The recovery phase is challenging for both patient and family. The patient has experienced intense physical and emotional stress during the wound-healing process and is often frustrated and exhausted by their lack of independence. Depression, grief, anger, and symptoms of the posttraumatic stress disorder are common. Burn wounds may be disfiguring even when they are well cared for, especially if they involve the face; patients may be unwilling or fearful of leaving their house as well as viewing themselves in a mirror. Compression garments may be visible, and assist devices such as a cane or a walker may be perceived by the patient as stigmatizing in public. They are also a constant reinforcer that the patient is now quite different compared to before their burn injury. Primary care clinicians are well positioned to surveil for and manage newly identified or acquired organ system complications that may occur after critical illness and, in particular, after major burn injury related to inhalation injury and hypermetabolism. Relatedly, concerns about quality of life, finances, pain, friends, work, and more may be debilitating as patients adjust to their new reality and the time required for recovery.

Family members, loved ones, or friends may be similarly exhausted in the recovery phase as they desire to help, but may be unsure how to do so. They may be similarly struggling to adjust changes in the patient's physical and mental capabilities that pervasively alter daily life. New schedules, new roles—especially for wound care and at home therapy—establish family members and others as uncompensated caregivers. The elderly, who may have underlying frailty, is a particularly vulnerable group who may never regain full independence and instead transition from an acute care facility such as a burn center to a long-term care facility. Prompt referral for psychiatric services is warranted for patients or family members exhibiting mental health difficulties. There is broad overlap with the post-intensive care syndrome as well (see Families, Chapters 14, 15, 16, and Support Groups). Due to vast changes in appearance, independence, and function, major burn injury survivors are at increased risk for suicide. Burn support groups, in which burn survivors meet to discuss their challenges, are a protective environment for burn survivors as well as family members. For example, The Phoenix Society, dedicated to improving outcomes for burn survivors, can provide valuable assistance to survivors and their families through recovery and beyond. Pursuing a life with quality, despite surviving critical illness coupled with injury, drives care improvements, continued assessments, and innovative approaches to care and recovery.

Unhomed individuals are especially vulnerable to undesired and poor outcomes due to the lack of a home and a support system. There is substantial interface with underlying cognitive, psychiatric, and addiction-related comorbidities during recovery. Frequent and repeated emergency department visits for care are common when there is no other venue within which to pursue burn aftercare. This may be especially true for those who are transferred to a regional burn center for acute care that is remote from where the burn occurred and the facility in which they received initial care. Social workers are a particularly valuable partner in helping to arrange aftercare for this unique population (see Chapter 12: Social Worker/Case Manager's Perspective). In an innovative way, street-level nursing programs have been developed to help address this care gap for the unhomed, but are far from widely represented across the United States.

Tips for Clinicians

1. Patients with major burn injury benefit from care in a Burn Center, but should have other injuries evaluated and addressed prior to transfer.
2. Inhalation injury drives airway edema and should prompt early endotracheal intubation using a sufficiently large tube to permit flexible bronchoscopy; preparation for a potential surgical airway is required when placing an oral endotracheal tube.
3. Resuscitation fluid formulae provide only estimates; adjust fluid volume to patient response.
4. If myoglobinuria is detected, evaluate for compartment syndrome, especially in those who have sustained an electrical injury. Myoglobinuria without an electrical injury raises concern for muscle injury as a direct result of the burn.
5. Establish an integrated pain management plan that uses nonpharmacologic, nonopioid, as well as opioid agents to decrease overall opioid exposure.
6. It is equally important to establish a structured approach to opioid de-escalation; certain patients may benefit from involving a pain management specialist.
7. Topical, instead of intravenous, antibiotics helps limit the development of multi-drug-resistant organisms.

8. Protein-rich nutritional support helps with wound repair and to address protein-loss across open wounds.
9. Early and sustained physical and occupational therapy are essential to prevent wound contracture and preserve function. Despite discomfort, splinting is a required approach to preventing contracture formation.
10. Planned surveillance for the post-intensive care syndrome as well as a variety of mental health disorders spanning depression, grief, anxiety, anger, fear, and the posttraumatic stress disorder should be conducted to identify patients—and family members—in need of rescue. Suicidality is a major risk, especially during the recovery phase of care. Every clinician who interfaces with the burn survivor should remain alert for these issues so that they can be addressed in a timely manner.
11. Remember that family members, loved ones, or friends may serve as uncompensated caregivers during the recovery phase and as such may also need mental health support.
12. Support groups as well as online resources may be particularly valuable for patients and family members as they adjust to postburn realities.
13. The elderly and the unhomed represent unique groups for whom additional resources may be required to support post-hospitalization recovery.

KEY REFERENCES

American Burn Association. *Advanced Burn Life Support Handbook*. https://ameriburn.org/education/advanced-burn-life-support-abls/. Accessed December 8, 2022.

Barrett LW, Fear VS, Waithman JC, et al. Understanding acute burn injury as a chronic disease. *Burns Trauma*. 2019;7.

Beckerman N, Leikin SM, Aitchinson R, et al. Laboratory interferences with the newer cyanide antidote: hydroxocobalamin. *Semin Diagn Pathol*. 2009;26(1):49-52.

Bergquist M, Hästbacka J, Glaumann C, et al. The time-course of the inflammatory response to major burn injury and its relation to organ failure and outcome. *Burns*. 2019;45(2):354-363.

Clark A, Imran J, Madni T, Wolf SE. Nutrition and metabolism in burn patients. *Burns Trauma*. 2017;5.

Duke JM, Boyd JH, Rea S, et al. Long-term mortality among older adults with burn injury: a population-based study in Australia. *Bull World Health Organ*. 2015;93:400-406.

Esselman PC. Burn rehabilitation: an overview. *Arch Phys Med Rehabil*. 2007;88(12):S3-S6.

Farny B, Fontaine M, Latarjet J, et al. Estimation of blood loss during adult burn surgery. *Burns*. 2018;44(6):1496-1501.

Finnerty CC, Jeschke MG, Branski LK, et al. Hypertrophic scarring: the greatest unmet challenge after burn injury. *Lancet*. 2016;388(10052):1427-1436.

Fowler E, Yosipovitch G. Post-burn pruritus and its management—current and new avenues for treatment. *Curr Trauma Rep*. 2019; 5(2):90-98.

Gardner PJ, Knittel-Keren D, Gomez M. The Posttraumatic Stress Disorder Checklist as a screening measure for posttraumatic stress disorder in rehabilitation after burn injuries. *Arch Phys Med Rehabil*. 2012;93(4):623-628.

Gittings PM, Grisbrook TL, Edgar DW, et al. Resistance training for rehabilitation after burn injury: a systematic literature review & meta-analysis. *Burns*. 2018;44(4):731-751.

Hall AH, Saiers J, Baud F. Which cyanide antidote? *Crit Rev Toxicol*. 2009;39(7):541-552.

Keating J, Kane-Gill SL, Kaplan LJ. Interaction of opioids with sedative practices in the ICU. In: *Opioid Use in Critical Care*. Cham: Springer; 2021:147-164.

Mercel A, Tsihlis ND, Maile R, Kibbe MR. Emerging therapies for smoke inhalation injury: a review. *J Transl Med*. 2020;18(1):1-6.

Moi AL, Haugsmyr E, Heisterkamp H. Long-term study of health and quality of life after burn injury. *Ann Burns Fire Disasters*. 2016;29(4):295.

Ong YS, Samuel M, Song C. Meta-analysis of early excision of burns. *Burns*. 2006;32(2):145-150.

Ozhathil DK, Wolf SE. Prevention and treatment of burn wound infections: the role of topical antimicrobials. *Expert Rev Anti Infect Ther*. 2022;32(2):1-6.

Palmieri TL, Holmes JH IV, Arnoldo B, et al. Transfusion requirement in burn care evaluation (TRIBE): a multicenter randomized prospective trial of blood transfusion in major burn injury. *Ann Surg*. 2017;266(4):595.

Palmieri TL, Molitor F, Chan G, et al. Long-term functional outcomes in the elderly after burn injury. *J Burn Care Res*. 2012;33(4):497-503.

Palmieri TL. Long term outcomes after inhalation injury. *J Burn Care Res*. 2009;30(1):201-203.

Romanowski K, Curtis E, Barsun A, et al. The frailty tipping point: determining which patients are targets for intervention in a burn population. *Burns*. 2019;45(5):1051-1056.

Romanowski KS, Carson J, Pape K, et al. American Burn Association guidelines on the management of acute pain in the adult burn patient: a review of the literature, a compilation of expert opinion, and next steps. *J Burn Care Res*. 2020;41(6):1129-1151.

Schwacha MG, Holland LT, Chaudry IH, Messina JL. Genetic variability in the immune-inflammatory response after major burn injury. *Shock*. 2005;23(2):123-128.

Spano S, Hanna S, Li Z, et al. Does bronchoscopic evaluation of inhalation injury severity predict outcome? *J Burn Care Res*. 2016;37(1):1-11.

Taylor SL, Lawless M, Curri T, et al. Predicting mortality from burns: the need for age-group specific models. *Burns*. 2014;40(6):1106-1115.

Taylor SL, Sen S, Greenhalgh DG, et al. Not all patients meet the 1 day per percent burn rule: a simple method for predicting hospital length of stay in patients with burn. *Burns*. 2017; 43(2):282-289.

Taylor SL, Sen S, Greenhalgh DG, et al. Real-time prediction for burn length of stay via median residual hospital length of stay methodology. *J Burn Care Res*. 2016;37(5):e476-482.

Walker PF, Buehner MF, Wood LA, et al. Diagnosis and management of inhalation injury: an updated review. *Crit Care*. 2015;19(1):1-2.

Weaver LK. Carbon monoxide poisoning. *N Engl J Med*. 2009;360(12):1217-1225.

Wick EC, Grant MC, Wu CL. Postoperative multimodal analgesia pain management with nonopioid analgesics and techniques: a review. *JAMA Surg.* 2017;152(7):691-697.

Williams FN, Herndon DN, Suman OE, et al. Changes in cardiac physiology after severe burn injury. *J Burn Care Res.* 2011;32(2):269-274.

Witt CE, Rowhani-Rahbar A, Rivara FP, et al. Long-term risk of mortality and pulmonary morbidity after inhalation injury among burn patients. *J Am Coll Surg.* 2017;225(4):S56-S57.

Trauma

Crisanto Torres, Jafar Haghshenas, and Joseph V. Sakran

Patient Care Vignette

A 28-year-old male was transported to the emergency department of a Level-1 trauma center as a victim of gun violence. He is alert and oriented, with a blood pressure of 98/64 mmHg. He has multiple gunshot wounds to the abdomen, flank, and back. Hypotension (88/60 mmHg) and tachycardia (HR = 124 bpm) develop rapidly. Massive blood transfusion is started followed by emergency and hopefully life-saving operation. Injuries to his liver and small intestine were managed by stopping bleeding and removing the section of the small bowel that was injured by bullets. Due to difficulty clotting, and the inability to clear waste products that were acids, the operation was converted to a damage control procedure. His abdomen was left open and covered with a device that provided both a temporary closure and a negative pressure across his abdomen, which controlled fluid leakage and protected his organs.

After 48 hours of complex ICU care, the patient returned to the OR to remove the temporary closure device, put his bowel back together, and close his abdomen. During this time, he received continuous infusions of an opioid analgesic (fentanyl) and an intravenous general anesthetic (propofol) interrupted by brief sedation holidays to assess his brain. At no point was he aware of the family that visited, and no family member had a meaningful interaction with him.

This patient is typical of those who sustain firearm injury and survive long enough to get to a hospital. Motor vehicle crashes, falls, and blunt assault have different kinds of injuries. Nonetheless, life-threatening injury can occur with all mechanisms of injury. This chapter uses firearm injury and subsequent care to illustrate how life-saving care can impact future recovery.

ICU CARE CONSIDERATION AFTER LIFE-THREATENING INJURY

Many of the ICU interventions required to rescue an injured patient who is at risk of death impact how patients perceive and interact with their care environment and those who provide care. The same concerns extend to how patients may interface with visitors including family members. Many of those interactions may be quite different from the patient's usual behavior. Brain injury, low blood flow followed by normal blood flow (reperfusion injury), edema, problems with blood flow within different spaces that function as compartments (brain, chest, abdomen), exposure to anesthetics and other medications that the patient does not usually receive, inadequate sleep, and infection may make patients either very sedated or inappropriately agitated. Some medications and conditions may induce temporary delirium, and may present a danger to patients who require care devices to remain in place such as catheters for monitoring blood pressure, infusing certain medications, or providing mechanical ventilation.

These behaviors may be profoundly disturbing for visitors, as may be the interventions required for patient and staff safety. Therefore, direct clear communication about what is happening—and what is likely to occur—is key in ensuring understanding and trust. Moreover, such communication supports patient- and family-centered care that may be derailed by the necessities of complex postinjury care in the critically ill and injured. It is equally important to recognize that abdominal injury (both penetrating and blunt) often occurs with other injuries including, but not limited to, spine fracture, traumatic brain injury, chest injury, as well as extremity injury and skin and soft tissue lacerations. Some of these other injuries may be less acutely life-threatening, but may be more substantially life-altering for those who survive. Survival of the patient in the vignette was aided by a damage control approach to his operation.

Damage Control Management

Life-threatening abdominal injury often requires a different approach than one that is used for elective operation. When patients sustain life-threatening injury or injuries, the length of operating room (OR) time required for definitive repair of all injuries may be quite long and places an avoidable stress on an already stressed patient. Longer OR time necessitates more anesthesia, a longer period of access through an open body cavity, more body heat loss, and more tissue handling. Furthermore, patients require more intravenous fluid during that time, much of which does not remain in the vascular system, but instead leaks into the extravascular space leading to both tissue and organ swelling known as edema. Importantly, the expanded organ size may create excessive pressure when trying to close the abdominal wall or thoracic cage since the organ now takes up more space. Each of those spaces are termed "compartments", and an increased pressure is also termed "hypertension." Compartment hypertension and organ injury will follow if one tries to force closure (see below). Such edema is often recognized by families as swollen feet, ankles, hands, and portions of the face, including most notably, the conjunctivae (chemosis).

In order to avoid much of the above, the damage control approach repairs only immediately life-threatening causes of bleeding, closes or removes portions of the gastrointestinal (GI) track that are perforated, often places temporary packs to control bleeding from raw surfaces, and creates a planned open body cavity that is commonly secured by a negative pressure wound therapy device (i.e., "vacuum" or "VAC" device). The abbreviated time in the OR is coupled with minimized crystalloid fluid (salt and water) and prioritizes component transfusion therapy (packed red blood cells, fresh frozen plasma, platelets) to reduce edema and enable clotting. Rapid transport to the ICU addresses hypothermia, acidosis, and clotting management and repairs abnormal salt concentrations (electrolytes) as well. Some electrolytes influence heart rhythms (as can a low temperature), making these therapies quite important after injury. Patients typically remain intubated (tube across their vocal cords) and receive invasive mechanical ventilation to control carbon dioxide clearance (metabolic waste product) and oxygenation, and to support the increased work of breathing imposed by an open abdomen or thoracic cage. Of necessity, analgesia and sedation are required for appropriate care, but also safety (see below).

When a damage control approach is required (~10-15% of injured patients), families should be counseled that the expected ICU and hospital length of stay will be lengthened, and that there are other considerations related to either injury or the ICU care that they should be aware of. Moreover, they should recognize that this approach is rooted in the 1980s and has been further refined to substantially increase survival. National and international organizations including the Eastern Association for the Surgery of Trauma (EAST), the Western Trauma Association (WTA), and the World Society of Emergency Surgery (WSES) have published comprehensive guidelines addressing the care of damage control surgery patients managed using an open abdomen approach. Therefore, the care that is being rendered is well established and will have a variety of anticipatable issues to manage.

Intra-Abdominal Hypertension and Abdominal Compartment Syndrome

Despite using an open abdomen approach with a damage control procedure, intra-abdominal hypertension (IAH) may still occur. When IAH is sufficiently high and is coupled with an attributable organ failure, the patient suffers the abdominal compartment syndrome (ACS). Patients at high risk for IAH and the ACS include those who: (1) require large volume component therapy transfusion or large volume fluid resuscitation (primarily those with thermal injury), (2) present in shock, (3) demonstrate organ-edema, (4) have retroperitoneal injury and hemorrhage, (5) require intra-abdominal packing, or (6) demonstrate ongoing or recurrent hemorrhage (Fig. 21-1). Both IAH and the ACS have standardized definitions developed by the Abdominal Compartment Society (formerly known as the World Society of the Abdominal Compartment Syndrome which was founded in 2004) and are presented in Fig. 21-2.

In general, IAH and ACS are similar to other forms of compartment syndrome (chest, limb, head) where increased pressure within an inflexible space can reduce tissue blood flow and oxygen delivery and create tissue ischemia (insufficient blood flow or oxygen delivery). While there are a variety of

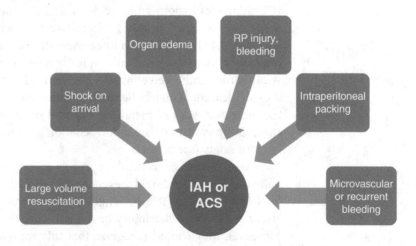

FIGURE 21-1. Patients at High Risk for IAH or the ACS. This graphic presents characteristics of patients who are at high risk for intra-abdominal hypertension (IAH) or the abdominal compartment syndrome (ACS). Large volume resuscitation includes component transfusion or normotonic crystalloid solutions. RP indicates the retroperitoneal space. Intraperitoneal packs are planned as temporary packs that are removed at a subsequent operation to help aid in bleeding control for acute injury.

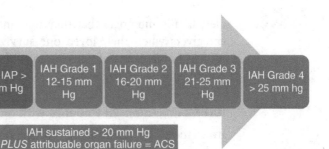

| IAH = IAP > 12 mm Hg | IAH Grade 1 12-15 mm Hg | IAH Grade 2 16-20 mm Hg | IAH Grade 3 21-25 mm Hg | IAH Grade 4 > 25 mm hg |

IAH sustained > 20 mm Hg
PLUS attributable organ failure = ACS

FIGURE 21-2. IAH and the ACS. This figure describes the grading of intra-abdominal hypertension (IAH) as measured by intra-abdominal pressure (IAP) as well as the abdominal compartment syndrome (ACS). IAP is typically measured by an indwelling bladder catheter using 25 mL of sterile 0.9% normal saline solution in line with a pressure transducer.

nonsurgical measures that may be used to address IAH and ACS, patients often require unplanned and repeated operation, especially in the setting of ongoing or recurrent bleeding; compartment syndromes like the ACS are surgical emergencies. Nonsurgical approaches to IAH may include sedation (which may be quite heavy), temporarily neuromuscular blockade (paralysis), GI track decompression with nasal or rectal tubes, and planned reduction in total body salt and water content using a diuretic agent or temporary dialysis. Many of these interventions may further derail family contact and interaction with the patient, and patients may not remember any of the events, unlike family who will remember it all. It is therefore critically important for family members to understand what is happening and why. IAH is present in 20-50% of critically ill or injured patients, and is associated with reduced survival over the course of the next 3 months. Some of that reduced survival may be related to a condition known as chronic critical illness.

Chronic critical illness has been well described, especially after injury. Such patients typically require ICU care for more than 14 days, have nonresolving organ dysfunction (ongoing organ failure), and develop recurrent infections. Furthermore, such patients demonstrate a persistently elevated metabolic rate such that they may progressively lose weight despite being fed an increased total amount of calories. Such ongoing illness is accompanied by weakness from muscle loss, despite commonly receiving double the usual amount of protein required for muscle mass maintenance in health. The impact of chronic critical illness may span an entire year, and is often punctuated by repeated admissions for acute care (as opposed to long-term acute care or rehabilitation). Accordingly, those with chronic critical illness have also been termed the "hospital dependent patient." Recognizing the vast increase in resources that are required for inpatient—as well as outpatient—care should alert family members that they may inadvertently become uncompensated caregivers when their loved one survives their life-threatening injury and returns home. Some of that care may be directly related to requiring an open body cavity for management.

ICU Management of Patients with an Open Abdomen

By virtue of the abdomen being left open, at least one repeat operation—and often more—is required. Although most such operations are performed within the OR, some such procedures, especially when the abdomen is not to be definitively closed, may be performed in the ICU. Operation may be safely undertaken in both locations, while operating in the ICU is often driven by the need for advanced approaches to mechanical ventilation that make transport less safe than desired. While the abdomen in open, there is a loss of protein in the fluid that drains across the surfaces of the abdominal organs, especially when there is a negative pressure wound therapy approach. Therefore, increased protein intake is required to help address protein loss, but to also support wound repair, including areas where hollow (bowel) or solid (e.g., liver) organs have required surgical repair.

Repeated operation has two significant potential complications—which families, consultants, and primary care clinicians should be aware of—fistula formation and ventral hernia formation. The more the bowel is handled, and the longer it takes to close the abdominal wall (fascial closure), the greater is the likelihood that an uninjured portion of bowel will develop an opening from which intestinal contents will leak. If it is the small bowel (more common), the fluid is termed "succus," and if it is the colon, the contents are termed "stool." Regardless of the site, fistula formation exists in two different fashions: (1) in connection to the air in an abdomen that is not and cannot be closed (enteroatmospheric fistula, EAF), and (2) in connection to the closed abdominal wall, often through the incision after closure (enterocutaneous fistula, ECF). The former is much more devastating than the latter.

EAFs are difficult to control; they often need multiple repeat operations to washout contents that have leaked around whatever control approach has been undertaken (there are many). Protein, enzymes, salts, and water will all be lost across the fistula. The closer the fistula is to the stomach, the higher the output, in general. EAFs are generally not amenable to additional surgery to excise them until inflammation and bowel wall edema has reduced—a process that takes months and sometimes up to a year. In the interim, the intestines may be covered with a split-thickness skin graft (STSG; similar to how burn patients get their wounds covered) with or without a dissolvable mesh to cover all of the bowel not involved in the EAF. This allows an ostomy bag to be placed over the EAF once the STSG has healed. During the first year, in particular, the healing STSG is more susceptible to sunburn than normal skin, and caution is essential with sun exposure. In addition, multiple hospitalizations are common, especially if the patient is unable to be fed orally or by a feeding tube that enters the bowel across the abdominal wall. Such patients must instead be fed intravenously using an indwelling long-term access catheter and total parenteral nutrition (TPN), a method that provides full nutritional support including protein, carbohydrates, and fats. Catheter infection is a common reason for readmission and requires catheter removal, therapeutic antibiotics, and new catheter insertion to resume TPN. Those who have an EAF are unable to achieve fascial closure and have an obligate ventral (surface of the body) hernia.

A ventral hernia is part of every EAF but may also develop in those who initially achieved fascial closure, but then develop a separation along the line of fascial closure; the skin, on the other hand, remains intact. This is much like a groin hernia where the intestines protrude into a space in which they do not belong but are contained by the subcutaneous fat and skin. Ventral hernias are not life-threatening in general, but are uncomfortable and unfavorably impact the patient's body image. Back pain is common as the hernia enlarges (there is no muscle to keep mobile organs like the small bowel contained in the peritoneal space, aka the abdomen proper). Infection underneath the lower portion of the hernia (especially fungal skin infections) are common, as are superficial abrasions from pants or belts. Therefore, ventral hernia repair is commonly desired; it is an elective procedure and may involve a plastic surgeon to help with reconstruction of the abdominal wall. On occasion, the bowel that protrudes through the defect in the fascia can get stuck (incarcerated) and lose its blood supply (strangulated). This is more likely to occur with small defects and is life threatening, warranting emergency operation.

Analgesia, Sedation, and Delirium

Unlike the medical ICU where procedure-related pain is much less common, the surgical ICU team must plan to manage pain. Multimodal analgesia (Figure 21-3) is now standard practice and is titrated to achieve an acceptable pain score for the patient when they can share their goals, and to physiologic indicators when they cannot (e.g., intubated and sedated immediately postoperatively, or with a serious traumatic brain injury). Nonpharmacologic aids (including topical ice) are coupled with nonopioid agents (Tylenol) and nonsteroidal anti-inflammatory agents (when safe; ketorolac, meloxicam, or ibuprofen) as an initial strategy with opioid analgesic therapy added as needed; topical lidocaine patches may be of value as well. Opioids may be delivered

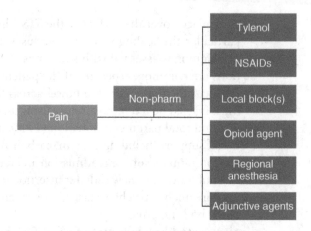

FIGURE 21-3. Postinjury or Postoperative Analgesia Approaches. This figure presents approaches to pain management after operation or injury. Non-pharm = nonpharmacologic therapies; NSAIDs = nonsteroid anti-inflammatory drugs.

as a continuous infusion in those who cannot manage an on-demand kind of delivery system, or an on-demand patient-controlled analgesia (i.e., PCA) system if they are awake but cannot receive medications by mouth or feeding tube. As patients improve, IV opioid analgesics are replaced with oral or feeding tube opioid analgesics but remain coupled with nonopioid therapy. When the GI track may be used, other analgesics such as gabapentin are added to expand multimodal therapy and reduce total opioid exposure. These practices may be accompanied by local or regional blocks using lidocaine or related agents, or may be coupled with neuraxial anesthesia such as an epidural catheter and infusion (commonly used during childbirth). Patients with chronic pain syndromes or opioid use disorder (OUD) or who are on maintenance therapy for prior OUD are more complex, may require a pain consultant, and are beyond the scope of this chapter.

Sedation is generally driven by the need for concomitant invasive mechanical ventilation. Short-acting agents that are readily titratable are preferred, and facilitate regular assessment of neurologic function and mental status. Propofol and dexmedetomidine are commonly used in this way and outperform other sedative agents such as benzodiazepines. Valium (diazepam), Ativan (lorazepam), Versed (midazolam), and others belong to the benzodiazepine class and are associated with delirium induction, in particular in the elderly. The goal of sedation is to alleviate anxiety and especially aid in tolerating invasive mechanical ventilation while allowing the patient to be engaged in their own care and interact with their family members or visitors. Those who are "out of synch" with the ventilator—assuming that the device is correctly set for the patient's lung—are at increased risk of ventilator-induced lung injury. In this case, more heavy sedation is required and the patient may not awaken or acknowledge a visitor; the patient can, on the other hand, hear visitors, and will benefit from a recognizable voice.

The ICU is an unfamiliar setting filled with uncommon sounds that functions around the clock—unlike what occurs at home. Therefore, ICU care may be quite disorienting regardless of age, an influence that is worsened by sleep deprivation. Noise reduction approaches are widespread, but care that is required often occurs on an hourly basis (and often more frequently) especially immediately after injury. Thus, the combined effects can lead to temporary delirium. Patients may not recall their experiences, but family members will do so with great clarity. Delirium may be quite disturbing, anxiety provoking, and fear inducing. While stopping deliriogenic influences is helpful, to family members, starting another medication (such as an antipsychotic agent like Seroquel [quetiapine] or Haldol [haloperidol]) seems counterintuitive. If familiar with either of those agents, family members may be concerned that the patient has psychosis. Education and reassurance is key, as is recognizing that the therapy is generally quite transient and not something to be continued after their ICU stay has ended.

Venous Thromboembolism (VTE) Prophylaxis

Critically ill patients are at a heightened risk for developing clots in deep (as opposed to superficial) veins as well as having those clots travel to and lodge in blood vessels in the lungs. This process is termed venous thromboembolism (VTE), and clots that lodge in lung blood vessels create a pulmonary embolism. Injured patients are highly susceptible to both of these undesirable events due to both the initial injury and the care that is required to manage the injury or injuries. Therefore, injured patients receive two kinds of therapy to prevent clots—mechanical and pharmacologic. Mechanoprophylaxis consists of sequential compression devices applied most commonly to the lower legs. Chemoprophylaxis consists of a low dose of an anticoagulant agent that is injected subcutaneously. The goal is not therapeutic or complete anticoagulation, but is instead to reduce the likelihood of clotting in veins where flow may be reduced due to immobility, local injury, or the presence of a catheter for example. Despite our best efforts, some injured patients develop both a DVT and a pulmonary embolus.

Therapy often consists of therapeutic anticoagulation, but it may be more complex, including therapy in the Interventional Radiology suite to aspirate (remove using suction) the clot when large. Many centers have specialized teams that address pulmonary embolism (i.e., Pulmonary Embolism Rescue

Team, PERT), adding to the number of different team members the family may meet, and for whom they will be asked to provide consent for procedures when the patient cannot. Pulmonary embolism may have transient effects on work of breathing as well as oxygenation, but can also exert long-lasting effects when the pulmonary vasculature clot burden is high. This impact may be disproportionate in the elderly and in those with preexisting pulmonary disease whether obstructive or restrictive. Secondary effects on the right ventricle (it must pump against a fixed obstruction) may be severe in those with preexisting heart failure as well. Follow-up evaluations to manage therapeutic anticoagulation as well as to assess lung and heart function are to be anticipated. Such care may require travel to a tertiary or quaternary care center if those management services are unavailable upon repatriation into the community.

Family Visitation and Participation

When not restricted by SARS-CoV-2 surges, family visitation is essential for patient- and family-centered care. This is very much like bond-centered care that is utilized by veterinarians when they treat the pet and the owner as a dyad. With regard to ICU care, family members—or at least one designated family spokesperson—should try to be present for daily bedside rounds. Since family members are indeed part of the team, their participation is ideal to ensure good communication around events, daily goals, planned future interventions, consultant findings, and goals of care. Having family members on rounds allows them to understand the thoroughness of the ICU team's care, the complexity of the patient's illness, and supports asking questions and gathering answers. The designated spokesperson can then interface with the rest of the family instead of having multiple members call the ICU at different times to secure information. This allows the nurse, the team member who fields most of these calls, to spend more time with the patient instead of the phone. Moreover, many ICUs encourage family members to participate in some care activities such as range of motion, stretching, bathing, and for some, ambulating.

When family members cannot be present, ICUs use digital communication platforms just as is done in the outpatient clinic to bring the ICU clinicians, the patient, and the family into the same virtual space. Finally, daily communication with the family is an excellent way to mitigate against conflict, especially when there is prognostication involved after serious injury, and the future is uncertain or quite grim. End-of-life care that may accompany injury in the elderly with serious comorbidities and devastating traumatic brain injury in the young are two common and quite potent triggers for conflict between family members and the ICU or admitting team. Having the family as a key member of the team on a daily basis helps establish rapport, trust, and a free exchange of findings, concerns, values, and perspectives.

■ CONSIDERATIONS FOR RECOVERY

Both young and elderly injured patients face challenges in recovering their normal function after injury that requires ICU care. These challenges span recovery of muscle strength, endurance, cognitive (thinking and reasoning) capability, and normal psychosocial dynamics (interacting with friends and family or pets) that impact restoring relationships and joy. Changes in body habitus may include those related to an open abdomen or other damage control techniques, but may also include limb loss or the loss of the use of a limb. Brain injury may lead to impaired short-term memory, speech, or coordination. Minor injury leads to rapid recovery but major injury often requires rehabilitation. The time frame for recovery may reach 2 years depending on injury severity and type. A collaborative effort involving the expertise of physical therapists, occupational therapists, speech-language pathologists, behavior therapists, social workers, and case managers is vital to evaluate the need for post-acute care, rehabilitation, or home-health services. A well-structured and safe discharge plan should be aimed at improving long-term outcomes, recovery, and minimizing readmissions. Thus, setting appropriate expectations and pathways to recovery for patients—and their family members—is essential.

Changes to living arrangements such as a first-floor bedroom, a ramp, or a caregiver may be required. Some accommodations disrupt normal family dynamics, and others happen alongside of them. Home services bring a steady stream of non-family members into the home and may be viewed as an intrusion or a burden. Patients may become depressed at being dependent or from being principally home confined during convalescence. An indwelling tracheostomy (tube into the airway in the neck) further impedes communication, and has an audible reminder of its presence, some of which may be frustrating for everyone in the home. Assistive devices occupy space, and serve as a reminder of lack of capacity. In this way, the primary care clinician who will see the patient and various family members in follow-up truly has an entire family to treat.

Repeated post-initial hospitalization discharge operative care is common for orthopedic (including chest wall) as well as soft tissue and GI track injury. Therefore, another hospital stay is generally involved and may trigger feelings of depression, anxiety, and, for some, symptoms like that of posttraumatic stress disorder. These kinds of consequences should be anticipated, especially after intentional violent injury, and addressed ahead of repeat operation or admission. Those who do survive their violent injuries are faced with lifelong physical, social, and psychological complications. In particular, those who have retained bullet fragments may be especially vulnerable to these issues. Moreover, surviving violent injury is a predictor of violent re-injury, arrest, and sometimes incarceration; this cycle has been termed the "revolving door phenomenon" and merits specific attention. Evidence-based hospital violent intervention programs have emerged to disrupt this cycle of violence and rescue care. To that end, ICU clinicians and primary care clinicians play a pivotal role in initiating and continuing interventions that restore life balance for patients and their family members.

Tips for Clinicians

1. Injury is not anticipated and may trigger anxiety, anger and fear—all affective (emotional) responses that should be anticipated.

2. Serious injury that requires ICU care generally has consequences for survivors that include the key features of the post-intensive care syndrome (PICS; see Introduction and Chapter 4) as well as the need for repeat operation to address both structural and functional elements of the initial injury (e.g., colostomy, ventral hernia, soft tissue defect, reconstructive undertakings).

3. Elements related to PICS may not be identified as such by the patient or the family. **Postdischarge evaluation should specifically inquire about strength, endurance, cognition, activities of daily living, and social dynamics.**

4. **Difficulties in each of the domains identified as part of PICS should prompt rehabilitation referral**, as well as discourse with the surgical team that cared for the patient—especially if the community to which the patient has been repatriated is remote from where they received complex care.

5. **Family members or close friends who accompany the patient to a follow-up appointment may be excellent sources of information**, as patients impacted by PICS may not recognize how they are impacted. These individuals are indeed part of the team helping care for the patient, many of whom may serve as uncompensated caregivers who may benefit from support services that they are unaware of. The office visit is a prime opportunity to provide direction and aid.

6. **Setting appropriate expectations for the rapidity of recovery is essential** with greater degrees of injury, in general, requiring longer periods of time. Those managed using an open abdomen approach for abdominal injury, or those with traumatic brain injury, may take 1-2 years for recovery to the greatest extent possible.

7. **Chronic pain may follow in the wake of multiple injuries** and efforts to mitigate against OUD start in the acute care facility, but benefit from being continued in the outpatient setting.
8. **The primary care clinician is encouraged to dialogue with the trauma team** regarding issues occurring in patients for whom they have provided care. Digital platforms readily enable such bidirectional communication to occur using a video link and not simply email or a phone conversation.

KEY REFERENCES

Anderson DR, Morgano GP, Bennett C, et al. American Society of Hematology 2019 guidelines for management of venous thromboembolism: prevention of venous thromboembolism in surgical hospitalized patients. *Blood Adv.* 2019;3:3898-3944.

Baksaas-Aasen K, Van Dieren S, Balvers K, et al. Data-driven development of ROTEM and TEG algorithms for the management of trauma hemorrhage. *Ann Surg.* 2019;270 (6):1178-1185.

Brohi K, Singh J, Heron M, Coats T. Acute traumatic coagulopathy. *J Trauma.* 2003;54 (6):1127-1130.

Burlew CC, Moore EE, Cuschieri J, et al. Who should we feed? Western Trauma Association multi-institutional study of enteral nutrition in the open abdomen after injury. *J Trauma Acute Care Surg.* 2012;73(6):1380-1388.

Byrne JP, Mason SA, Gomez D, et al. Timing of pharmacologic venous thromboembolism prophylaxis in severe traumatic brain injury: a propensity matched cohort study. *J Am Coll Surg.* 2016;223:621-631.e5.

Centers for Disease Control and Prevention, National Center for Health Statistics. Underlying Cause of Death 1999-2019 on CDC WONDER Online Database, released in 2020. Data are from the Multiple Cause of Death Files, 1999-2019, as compiled from data provided by the 57 vital statistics jurisdictions through the Vital Statistics Cooperative Program. Available at http://wonder.cdc.gov/ucd-icd10.html. Accessed on May 12, 2021.

Chabot E, Nirula R. Open abdomen critical care management principles: resuscitation, fluid balance, nutrition, and ventilator management. *Trauma Surg Acute Care Open.* 2017;2:e000063.

Chang R, Scerbo MH, Schmitt KM, et al. Early chemoprophylaxis is associated with decreased venous thromboembolism risk without concomitant increase in intraspinal hematoma expansion after traumatic spinal cord injury. *J Trauma Acute Care Surg.* 2017;83:1088-1094.

Christie S, Thibault-Halman G, Casha S. Acute pharmacological DVT prophylaxis after spinal cord injury. *J Neurotrauma.* 2011; 28:1509-1514.

Coccolini F, Ivatury R, Sugrue M, Ansaloni L, eds. *Open Abdomen: A Comprehensive Practical Manual.* Springer Nature; 2019.

Coccolini F, Roberts D, Ansaloni L, et al. The open abdomen in trauma and non-trauma patients: WSES guidelines. *World J Emerg Surg.* 2018;13:7. Published 2018 Feb 2.

Cook D, Crowther M, Meade M, et al. Deep venous thrombosis in medical surgical critically ill patients: prevalence, incidence, and risk factors. *Crit Care Med.* 2005;33:1565-1571.

Cooper C, Eslinger DM, Stolley PD. Hospital-based violence intervention programs work. *J Trauma Acute Care Surg.* 2006;61(3):534-540.

Coupez E, Timsit JF, Ruckly S, et al. Guidewire exchange vs new site placement for temporary dialysis catheter insertion in ICU patients: is there a greater risk of colonization or dysfunction? *Crit Care (London, England).* 2016;20(1):230.

Cryer H, Manley G, Adelson D, et al. ACS TQIP best practices in the management of traumatic brain injury. *J Am Coll Surg.* 2015;220(5):981-985.

Denson K, Morgan D, Cunningham R, et al. Incidence of venous thromboembolism in patients with traumatic brain injury. *Am J Surg.* 2007;193:380-383.

Diaz JJ Jr, Cullinane DC, Dutton WD, et al. The management of the open abdomen in trauma and emergency general surgery: part 1-damage control [published correction appears in J Trauma. 2010 Aug;69(2):470. Bilaniuk, Jarolslaw O [corrected to Bilaniuk, Jaroslaw W]]. *J Trauma.* 2010;68(6):1425-1438.

Diaz JJ Jr, Cullinane DC, Khwaja KA, et al. Eastern Association for the Surgery of Trauma: management of the open abdomen, part III-review of abdominal wall reconstruction. *J Trauma Acute Care Surg.* 2013;75(3):376-386.

Diaz JJ Jr, Dutton WD, Ott MM, et al. Eastern Association for the Surgery of Trauma: a review of the management of the open abdomen--part 2 "Management of the open abdomen". *J Trauma.* 2011;71(2):502-512.

Ditzel RM Jr, Anderson JL, Eisenhart WJ, et al. A review of transfusion- and trauma-induced hypocalcemia: is it time to change the lethal triad to the lethal diamond? *J Trauma Acute Care Surg.* 2020;88:434-439.

Dubose JJ, Scalea TM, Holcomb JB, et al. Open abdominal management after damage-control laparotomy for trauma: a prospective observational American Association for the Surgery of Trauma multicenter study [published correction appears in J Trauma Acute Care Surg. 2014 Mar;76(3):902. Erriksson, Evert [corrected to Eriksson, Evert]]. *J Trauma Acute Care Surg.* 2013;74(1):113-1122.

Duchesne JC, Kimonis K, Marr AB, et al. Damage control resuscitation in combination with damage control laparotomy: a survival advantage. *J Trauma.* 2010;69(1):46-52.

Eguia E, Cobb AN, Baker MS, et al. Risk factors for infection and evaluation of Sepsis-3 in patients with trauma. *Am J Surg.* 2019;218(5):851-857.

Fernández LG. Management of the open abdomen: clinical recommendations for the trauma/acute care surgeon and general surgeon. *Int Wound J.* 2016;13(Suppl 3):25-34.

Gabbe BJ, Braaf S, Fitzgerald M, et al. RESTORE: REcovery after Serious Trauma—Outcomes, Resource use and patient Experiences study protocol. *Inj Prev.* 2015;21:348-354.

Geerts WH, Code K, Jay RM, et al. A prospective study of venous thromboembolism after major trauma. *N Engl J Med.* 1994; 331:1601-1606.

Geerts WH, Jay R, Code K, et al. A comparison of low-dose heparin with low molecular-weight heparin as prophylaxis against venous thromboembolism after major trauma. *N Engl J Med.* 1996;335:701-707.

Gonzalez E, Moore EE, Moore HB, et al. Goal-directed hemostatic resuscitation of trauma-induced coagulopathy: a pragmatic randomized clinical trial comparing a viscoelastic assay to conventional coagulation assays. *Ann Surg.* 2016;263(6):1051-1059.

Heron M. Deaths: leading causes for 2017. *Natl Vital Stat Rep.* 2019;68(6). Hyattsville, MD: National Center for Health Statistics.

Hess JR, Brohi K, Dutton RP, et al. The coagulopathy of trauma: a review of mechanisms. *J Trauma.* 2008;65(4):748-754.

Holcomb JB, Tilley BC, Baraniuk S, et al. Transfusion of plasma, platelets, and red blood cells in a 1:1:1 vs a 1:1:2 ratio and mortality in patients with severe trauma: the PROPPR randomized clinical trial. *JAMA.* 2015;313(5):471-482.

Jacobs BN, Cain-Nielsen A, Jakubus JL, et al. Unfractionated heparin versus low-molecular-weight heparin for venous thromboembolism prophylaxis in trauma. *J Trauma Acute Care Surg.* 2017;83:151.

Jensen SD, Cotton BA. Damage control laparotomy in trauma. *Br J Surg.* 2017;104(8):959-961.

Johansson PI, Stensballe J, Vindeløv N, Perner A, Espersen K.Hypocoagulability, as evaluated by thrombelastography, at admission to the ICU is associated with increased 30-day mortality. *Blood Coagul Fibrinolysis.* 2010;21(2):168-174.

Kao AM, Schlosser KA, Arnold MR, et al. Trauma recidivism and mortality following violent injuries in young adults. *J Surg Res.* 2019;237:140-147.

Kaufman EJ, Wiebe DJ, Xiong RA, Morrison CN, Seamon MJ, Delgado MK. Epidemiologic trends in fatal and nonfatal firearm injuries in the US, 2009-2017. *JAMA Intern Med.* 2021;181(2):237-244.

Kirkpatrick AW, Roberts DJ, De Waele J, et al. Intra-abdominal hypertension and the abdominal compartment syndrome: updated consensus definitions and clinical practice guidelines from the World Society of the Abdominal Compartment Syndrome. *Intensive Care Med.* 2013;39(7):1190-1206.

Lane-Fall MB, Kuza CM, Fakhry S, Kaplan LJ. The lifetime effects of injury: postintensive care syndrome and posttraumatic stress disorder. *Anesthesiol Clin.* 2019;37(1):135-150.

Lee JC, Peitzman AB. Damage-control laparotomy. *Curr Opin Crit Care.* 2006;12(4):346-350.

Livingston DH, Tripp T, Biggs C, Lavery RF. A fate worse than death? Long-term outcome of trauma patients admitted to the surgical intensive care unit. *J Trauma.* 2009;67(2):341-348.

Lucas CE, Ledgerwood AM. Prospective evaluation of hemostatic techniques for liver injuries. *J Trauma.* 1976;16:442-451.

Maluso P, Olson J, Sarani B. Abdominal compartment hypertension and abdominal compartment syndrome. *Crit Care Clin.* 2016;32(2):213-222.

Muckart DJ, Bhagwanjee S. American College of Chest Physicians/Society of Critical Care Medicine Consensus Conference definitions of the systemic inflammatory response syndrome and allied disorders in relation to critically injured patients. *Crit Care Med.* 1997;25:1789-1795.

Napolitano LM, Ferrer T, McCarter RJ Jr, Scalea TM. Systemic inflammatory response syndrome score at admission independently predicts mortality and length of stay in trauma patients. *J Trauma Acute Care Surg.* 2000;49(4):647-653.

Napolitano LM. Intra-abdominal hypertension in the ICU: who to measure? How to prevent? *Crit Care Med.* 2019;47(4):608-609.

Osborn TM, Tracy JK, Dunne JR, Pasquale M, Napolitano LM. Epidemiology of sepsis in patients with traumatic injury. *Crit Care Med.* 2004;32(11):2234-2240.

Pereira BM. Abdominal compartment syndrome and intra-abdominal hypertension. *Curr Opin Crit Care.* 2019;25(6):688-696.

Rotondo MF, Schwab CW, McGonigal MD, et al. "Damage control": an approach for improved survival in exsanguinating penetrating abdominal injury. *J Trauma.* 1993;35(3):375-383.

Sava J, Alam HB, Vercruysse G, et al. Western Trauma Association critical decisions in trauma: management of the open abdomen after damage control surgery. *J Trauma Acute Care Surg.* 2019;87(5):1232-1238.

Stone HH, Strom PR, Mullins RJ. Management of the major coagulopathy with onset during laparotomy. *Ann Surg.* 1983;197:532-535.

Taveras LR, Imran JB, Cunningham HB, et al. Trauma and emergency general surgery patients should be extubated with an open abdomen. *J Trauma Acute Care Surg.* 2018;85(6):1043-1047.

Tisherman SA, Schmicker RH, Brasel KJ, et al. Detailed description of all deaths in both the shock and traumatic brain injury hypertonic saline trials of the Resuscitation Outcomes Consortium. *Ann Surg.* 2015;261(3):586-590.

Trunkey DD, Lim RC. Analysis of 425 consecutive trauma fatalities: an autopsy study. *J Am Coll Emerg Phys.* 1974;3(6):368-371.

Wafaisade A, Lefering R, Bouillon B, et al. Epidemiology and risk factors of sepsis after multiple trauma: an analysis of 30,420 patients from the Trauma Registry of the German Society for Trauma Surgery*. *Crit Care Med.* 2011;39(4):621-628.

Neurodiverse Patients

Gary Alan Bass, Caoimhe Carmel Duffy, Gloria M. Satriale, and Lewis J. Kaplan

Patient Care Vignette

MT, an adult female rear-seat passenger, was involved in a motor vehicle crash. The car was impacted on the passenger's side by a pick-up truck with 1-2 feet of intrusion. EMS found a wildly agitated, screaming, tearful, and non-cooperative patient with an open right femur fracture. The driver was comatose and subsequently intubated for airway control. MT actively resisted interventions precluding easy extrication. Medical Command gave permission for IM sedation and then airway control as needed.

MT arrived in the Trauma Bay intubated. Her injuries included isolated rib fractures (ribs 5-7) and an open midshaft femur (thigh) fracture on the right. No brain injury was noted. Acute operative intervention was undertaken for the femur fracture. While in the operating room (OR), MT's family was contacted. They disclosed that MT had autism and was principally nonverbal. The driver was transporting her to an adult day program and was not part of the family.

The OR team was unaware of the diagnosis and pursued routine liberation from mechanical ventilation at the end of the case. Non-redirectable agitation led to reintubation and sedation with transport to the ICU for care. Consideration of substance withdrawal was communicated at the patient handoff to explain unexpected and non-redirectable agitation that prompted reintubation. The ICU team explained the new information about MT's autism to the OR team, and both teams considered the implications of this diagnosis for ongoing care.

The neurodiverse patient population, which includes individuals with dyspraxia, dyslexia, attention-deficit hyperactivity disorder, dyscalculia, autism spectrum, and Tourette syndrome, is rapidly growing globally. While specialized pediatric acute care inpatient facilities are well-equipped to address the medical, surgical, psychiatric, emotional, and psychosocial needs of typical children and adolescents, they may not be equally well-prepared for those with neurodiversity. At even greater risk for being unprepared are adult acute inpatient care facilities. As the neurodiverse patient population ages and crests into adulthood, they are no longer entirely appropriate for pediatric or adolescent-focused facilities. Of necessity, they will require care in an adult acute care hospital (Fig. 22-1). To that end, this chapter explores the unique needs of the neurodiverse population with acute illness to aid facilities in planning, organization, and training to meet anticipated current and future care requirements as well as to support post-ICU recovery. Unlike neurotypical individuals, enabling successful post-ICU recovery critically depends on planning for a successful ICU and acute inpatient course.

The term "neurodiverse" has supplanted the nonspecific and all-encompassing term "special needs." The latter term included those with physical limitations and those with cognitive or behavioral disability. It is the latter of these two groups that present more challenge for facilities, as many physical limitation support elements have been addressed under the auspices of the Americans with Disabilities Act (ADA). At present, both cognitive and behavioral patient needs continue to impede care. The neurodiverse may have both needs, which will be the focus of this chapter. Many terms have been previously used to describe the array of cognitive and behavioral disabilities, some of which are viewed as pejorative, including "mental retardation" which persists in legal documents and court of law adjudicative procedures. Nonetheless, there are preferred terms that identify the specific disability

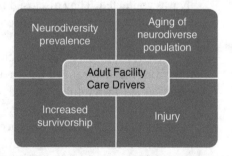

FIGURE 22-1. Factors Driving Adult Facility Care for Neurodiverse Patients. This figure presents four key factors that are increasing the number of neurodiverse patients within adult facilities, many of whom would have been previously cared for in a pediatric facility. Peds = pediatric acute care facility.

(i.e., cognitive, intellectual, or developmental disability), whose use may be less deleteriously labeling for parents, children, and stakeholders alike. Similarly, those with physical disabilities may be noted to have functional needs.

Current Centers for Disease Control and Prevention (CDC) estimates as well as those of the American Academy of Pediatrics place 1 in 54 children with autism (boys four times greater than girls) and 1 in 6 between the ages of 3 and 17 years with some kind of developmental disability including, but not limited to, autism, attention-deficit/hyperactivity disorder, blindness, and cerebral palsy. It is estimated that about 5.4 million US citizens over the age of 18 have autism spectrum disorder, with males continuing to be overrepresented compared to females. The CDC data also documents both geographic and racial/ethnic group differences in autism diagnosis prevalence spanning 2002-2016. Relatedly, access to routine care, social agency advocacy, and habilitation for the neurodiverse is disparate and appears strongly influenced by region, socioeconomic capability (including parental employment), and race/ethnicity. When admission to an acute care facility is planned, the institution and the care team is afforded the opportunity to address gaps in care preparedness and caregiver skill sets. To this end, an acute care facility needs to be prepared for unplanned evaluation and admission, as this group of disabled individuals presents unique challenges for the entire adult healthcare team.

Among the most common reasons for unplanned acute care facility evaluation and admission are injury or infection. Injury occurs across the age spectrum including both blunt and penetrating injury patterns. Certain factors may make injury more likely in this group than their typical age-matched peers. These factors include, but are not limited to, lack of situational awareness, lack of protective reflexes, medication-induced gait disturbance, inability to read social cues, lack of responsivity to warning signs, and self-injurious behavior that satisfies a sensory stimulation need or compulsion. More recently, children and young adults with autism have been the victims of intentional interpersonal violence as chronicled in the lay press. As there is a spectrum of disability, some may be present in the community unaccompanied by a therapeutic support staff (TSS) partner who may discourage such predatory events.

Regardless of the reason for admission to an ICU, the acute care team needs to have a working understanding of some of the key differences in the presentation of the neurodiverse. Developing an understanding of potential presenting issues and careful planning by the care team to minimize them can avoid suboptimal care, etiological confusion, and delay in therapy. Despite the unique presentation of the neurodiverse, there are some general guidelines that can assist in caring for this population within acute care settings. Collecting relevant information regarding the nature of the patient's neurodiversity can be critical to development of a plan of care and effective care delivery.

Indeed, such a tool has been created in a detailed fashion to facilitate information sharing that enhances care. Comprehensive preparation requires staff training as well as emplacing specific accommodations relevant for that individual's neurodiversity.

Unintentional injury, to both patient and staff, may also occur if restraints are utilized to facilitate emergency care. In general, this type of restrictive management should be avoidable with appropriate planning and care team engagement, including education that embraces first responders. Noninjury-related drivers of acute emergency department (ED) evaluation and inpatient care are not different from those of neurotypical individuals. However, given difficulties in communication for many neurodiverse individuals, such patients may present at a more advanced stage of disease or illness. Moreover, participation in health maintenance may be more difficult for the neurodiverse individuals due to challenges in transportation, reliance on others for scheduling, and for many, an inability to engage in clear interactive discourse with a healthcare professional. Certain neurodiverse individuals demonstrate speech patterns that can decrease a listener's ability to understand what the individual is trying to convey due to specific patterns such as echolalia, lack of differentiation in response (may respond yes to all questions), and an inability to convey nuance even when clear speech is present. Functional communication deficits present significant barriers to patient care. If a neurodiverse individual demonstrates expressive capabilities, proceed to gather as much information as possible from the individual regarding appropriate supports for their neurodiversity (see Appendix A). Should the patient present with limited expressive communicative ability, consider additional consultation such as Occupational Therapy to address sensory needs, Speech Therapy to address augmentative communication supports, and a Registered Dietitian to establish food preferences. Label room objects with words and explanatory pictures as individuals with limited expressive abilities may point to pictures to communicate.

Many neurodiverse individuals rely on hewing to an established routine that includes places, people, activities, and when utilized, therapeutic agent delivery. For some, even meal selections can be an important part of their usual daily activities. Acute care derails the normal routine and fills that space with few, if any, elements to which the neurodiverse patient may anchor. Relatedly, many seem to benefit from specific, and often repetitive, sensory stimulation activities. By definition, the events that necessitate acute care fall outside of these established routines, and this type of disruption can lead to agitation, and even destructive levels of challenging behavior. Acute care clinicians should recognize that the need for sensory stimulation does not indicate sensory tolerance. Indeed, unusual sounds, lights, and the usual "noise" that permeates the hospital environment (especially the ED and the ICU) may be poorly endured. Maladaptive responses may be ensuing, and may be readily misinterpreted for medical conditions other than sensory overload. Noise cancelling earbuds or headphones may be particularly effective at dampening undesirable stimuli.

Preferred activities may not be available during acute inpatient care, leading to further disruption of the daily routine and potential agitation. Other available preferred activities, such as viewing or listening to digital media on electronic devices, should be specifically provided if they play prominent roles in maintaining balance. Since many neurodiverse individuals are accompanied by a paraprofessional (aka therapeutic support staff [TSS]) during out-of-home or residence activities, their absence during inpatient care can present challenges for both the patient and the ICU team. Nuances of individual patterns of behavior, and successful management approaches, and the like are well known to caregivers and other stakeholders, but may not be readily apparent to the acute care team. Moreover, typical behavioral and environmental approaches to neurodiverse behaviors are uncommonly employed by adult facility teams, because such patients are infrequently encountered. Accordingly, patients exhibiting such behaviors may be instead sedated, instead of having the underlying trigger(s) addressed. Such sedation may increase the aversiveness of the acute care environment and in some cases could lead to exaggerated stress responses, or the recall phenomenon, both of which are associated with posttraumatic stress disorder. Of course, clinical conditions such as sepsis or septic shock, stroke, and acute intoxications can also derange baseline neurologic function in those who are neurotypical. Unfortunately, such derangements demonstrate some overlap with neurodiverse maladaptive behavior and may delay diagnosis of life-altering or life-threatening conditions. This specific aspect merits focused investigation and will likely be aided by evolving technology that facilitates identifying infection on the basis of a molecular signature in sampled body fluid.

■ CONSIDERATIONS FOR RECOVERY

Unlike neurotypical individuals, the neurodiverse patient population enjoys the best opportunity for recovery by avoiding the need to pursue recovery. Therefore, preparing the ICU environment—including team members—for neurodiverse care is essential. Resources and adaptations to mitigate against needing to be treated for post-intensive care syndrome (PICS) after an episode of ICU care may be conveniently divided into five interlinked domains: physical plant, team-structure and training, external partners, care environment, therapeutic agent management (Fig. 22-2). Each of these are explored in the following sections.

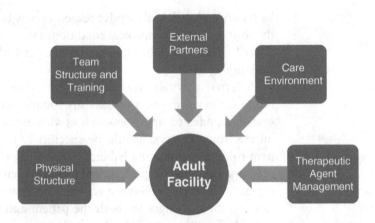

FIGURE 22-2. Preparing Adult Acute Care Facilities for Neurodiverse Care. These five elements are likely to be significantly helpful in preparing adult acute care facilities to provide high-quality and effective care for those with neurodiversity.

Physical Structure

Space is a key consideration as those with neurodiversity are likely to benefit from a larger rather than a smaller space. The room footprint should ideally support equipment movement and care activities within the room to avoid transport to other locations within the facility. Sufficient space to include a cot or bed for a parent, guardian, or paraprofessional to remain overnight is essential to maintaining patient stability. Furniture such as a reclining chair and table for the accompanying individual is also appropriate. Service animal presence is supported by the Americans with Disabilities Act (ADA), and such animals (limited to dogs and miniature horses) serve both task-based and psychological support-based roles. Animal care, including feeding, watering, and toileting, will need to be addressed—but not by ICU staff. Often, service animal organizations are able to assist with care. Of course, animal presence may trigger some conflict for those who are fearful of dogs, those with dog-related allergy, and for those who are concerned about safety during emergency procedures, should they need to occur. Hence, preplanning for such an eventuality is important for neurotypical and neurodiverse patients. Of note, emotional support animals are not embraced by the ADA.

Ramps, handrails, and mobility assist devices that match or replace the function of those used outside of the facility should be available or at least acquirable. Video surveillance capability should be emplaced akin to what is used for tele-critical care, whenever practical to help ensure safety and recognize early indicators of danger. Wiring for Wi-Fi-based digital device access supports video conferencing with family, caregivers, and perhaps, equally importantly, the patient's outpatient care team. That team may include staff at an adult day program as well as clinicians. Such access helps support the patient's normal daily flow and routine. Rooms with natural light and views of the outside world are preferred to those with only walls as an open view helps avoid feeling confined. This element and those that support nature and balance in structure, color, and function appear as key design features in ICU guidelines.

Team-Structure and Training

Team membership will, of necessity, be broad, and generally benefits from a larger roster than for neurotypical patients to address the breadth of behavioral, pharmacologic, and social support needs. The individual's primary care provider may be invaluable as a resource for the inpatient team; their presence in the inpatient setting may be beneficial to the patient if there is a preexisting and trusting relationship. Therefore, the usual critical care team may be supplemented by a paraprofessional(s), a community support coordinator, a psychopharmacologist, a behavioral health specialist, as well as a child life specialist. For patients who require elective admission, a preadmission planning conference using a digital platform may help identify best practices and opportunities for improvement to craft a successful stay. Much akin to elective admissions to the ICU after certain kinds of surgery, a video tour, narration of expectations, as well as a review of kinds of people and their roles may help prepare the neurodiverse for inpatient care. Capturing such an introduction using a point-of-view (POV) approach presents the information as if it were occurring from a first-person perspective.

While the neurodiverse individual may be chronologically aged as an adult, their behavioral needs—including preferred activities—may be rooted in activities more typically associated with younger individuals. These activities may include cartoons, figurines, coloring, painting, and other activities usually associated with childhood. A child life specialist is instrumental in meeting such needs, but are not typically present in adult facilities. Therefore, developing a relationship with such a specialist should be part of a plan to care for the neurodiverse. Such activities are not the rule, but preparation to meet such needs when present enables a much less disruptive stay and supports a successful transition out of the acute care facility.

Despite the usual rotation of bedside caregivers—especially nurses—the facility should consider approaches to minimize the number of unfamiliar faces who interface with the patient, e.g., nurses and specialists. Engaging a 1:1 "sitter" may also help provide stability, but benefits from that individual serving as a facilitator and not just a monitor. Specific training may be required to fulfill such a role. Simulation training is a superb method of developing and retaining such skills especially in low-frequency settings. Every team member who may interface with a neurodiverse patient will benefit from such training, spanning the radiology technician to the phlebotomist. Conflict management training dovetails nicely with this kind of education and is suitable for the entire ICU team. These skills may be particularly helpful in addressing the concerns of other patients, visitors, or team members when there is a neurodiverse patient on the unit.

External Partners

Partners that may enhance the inpatient experience include agencies that source therapy animals, as well as places of employment or schools or day programs that may bring familiar faces to the hospital. Postdischarge relevant agencies such as the community support agency can help address unique needs prior to discharge instead of having to address problems that arise after discharge. Some relevant planning may include education or training of rehabilitation specialists, visiting nurses, as well as EMS personnel engaged in transport between the facility and home or vice versa. The ability to include a paraprofessional during transport may require policy or procedure modification.

Care Environment

Deliberate environment management and adaptation minimizes stress during planned and unplanned acute care. Actions that help mimic the patient's preexisting and comfortable environment aid in achieving that goal. Temperature preferences, fan use, personal blankets (especially comfort aids) or pillows, preferred toys, and personal electronic devices are readily pursued adaptations. Personal electronic devices such as i-Phones, i-Pads, and computers are commonly used for reinforcing activities such as watching videos and listening to music as well as to structure the individual's expectations in the environment (linear scheduling of events, i.e., wake up, get dressed, breakfast, etc.). The use of timers to count down duration of an event, followed by reinforcement, may increase tolerance to the environment or activity. Noise cancelling earbuds or headphones can also help insulate the neurodiverse patient from typical ICU sounds and noise levels. Maintaining a day-night sleep cycle support is also essential. Door closure (provided it does not impede line-of-sight) helps in this regard as well. Natural lighting benefits have been previously addressed, but day-night sleep cycle support is essential. In-room alarm volume may be reduced (but not disabled or muted) while preserving out-of-room external monitoring alarm volume.

Environmental safety is a major concern, and a few approaches may be useful. Low bed height and routine bed alarms may be coupled with floor mat alarms as well. Assessing for smooth edges to countertops and corners may help prevent inadvertent injury. Limiting IV tubing helps prevent undesirable tangling or dislodgement. Avoiding arterial access of central venous access when feasible helps limit the potential for external blood loss related to catheter dislodgement. Wireless monitoring is preferred to tethering wires and is likely to be perceived as less confining. Motion sensor lighting at the floor level may be key in enhancing safety during nighttime movement especially for toileting. An in-room toilet is essential, and an in-room shower for hygiene is highly desirable. For many, the morning routine of hygiene is an anchor for the rest of the day. Caregivers should not assume that self-care devices including patient-controlled anesthesia (PCA) pumps, nurse call bell, and others cannot or will not be independently utilized even if it would be appropriate to do so. Participation in care may be difficult or impossible for many neurodiverse patients, even if provided clear instructions and context. Therefore, constant supervision is recommended.

Therapeutic Agent Management

Given the likelihood that neurodiverse individuals are receiving one or more medications for behavior control from different classes, drug–drug interactions should be anticipated during an inpatient critical illness care episode. Moreover, many are on a specific schedule of therapeutic agent intake—a series of events that frame daily activities and expectations. Medications relevant for critical care may have untoward interactions, or the patient's clinical condition may preclude oral medication intake. Therefore, such patients are at high risk of withdrawal symptomatology, or escape from well-established control of aspects of their specific behavioral condition(s). A dedicated and unit-based Doctor of Pharmacy (PharmD) can serve as an essential team member. In certain facilities, a daytime PharmD is present but evenings and nights (as well as weekends) are covered by a remote PharmD in the clinical pharmacy. A management plan to establish daytime support as well as evening and night outreach to a specifically skilled individual with psychopharmacology training appears optimal. Medication dose adjustments should be discussed with the outpatient clinician to anticipate likely responses and to ensure care continuity.

Since mood and mind-altering substances are often utilized in the perprocedure period, an internally consistent plan is required to avoid undesirable effects such as disinhibition and inappropriate pain sensing. Therefore, avoiding opioids to the greatest extent possible is ideal and may be addressed using alternatives including acetaminophen, gabapentin, topical lidocaine, lidocaine infusion, ketamine, and meloxicam (or other NSAIDs). Intraprocedure agents should also include the use of regional anesthesia, local anesthesia, and the specific avoidance of long-acting benzodiazepines unless they represent continuation therapy or anxiety is the major disorder being addressed. Sleep aids should be planned and may include melatonin or L-arginine with confidence, but the use of other agents should be informed by a discussion with a clinician well-versed in psychopharmacology to avoid iatrogenesis.

Tips for Clinicians (see also Tables 22-1 to 22-4)

1. Caring for the neurodiverse in a well-orchestrated fashion during planned or unplanned critical illness care is the best method of helping them avoid PICS. This population is quite difficult to assess for cognitive dysfunction, weakness, and disordered relationships as many have preexisting and disabling issues with social interactions and communication; some have preexisting physical disabilities as well.
2. Therefore, planned discourse with the team that provides outpatient care helps establish a baseline set of expectations for the inpatient care team, and engages the team that knows the patient and their response(s) to change, new environments, and altered medication regimens the best. Accordingly, the ICU team may gain new insights that directly impact neurodiverse patient care.
3. Conflict management and de-escalation are different for neurodiverse adults, especially those with autism, and is generally aided by fewer people in place instead of more. Understanding triggers helps avoid conflict and unnecessary stress. Moreover, logical reasoning is typically ineffective for conflict management, and alternative strategies should be used. Parents and the external team often understand what works best, and those should be employed even when counterintuitive—they use those strategies on a daily basis.
4. Routine room visits (pastoral care, etc.) that are not tied to that patient's specific care needs should be scrupulously avoided as they add individuals to an already unknown environment.
5. Coordinating with a pediatric facility to leverage their best practices and detail a plan that has been deployed, tested, and refined, but may be further refined for the unique elements found in an adult facility.
6. Humanizing the care in the ICU is supremely important for the neurodiverse who bring unique needs into a complex environment.

■ TABLE 22-1. Lack of Responsiveness to Questions

Presenting Issue: Lack of Responsiveness to Questions or Directions from Medical Professional

Potential Misinterpretation: Combative Patient

Potential ICU Response Based on Misinformation: Attempt to Obtain/Evaluate Without Input from Individual/Stakeholder Thereby Eliminating Potential Symptoms/Critical Information Resulting in Unsafe, Suboptimal Patient Care and Health Outcomes

Assessment Recommendations	Communication Strategies	Treatment Considerations
– Obtaining accurate, complete, patient-specific information is critical to quality care; this information can be obtained during assessment if properly executed – Limit to "Yes" or "No" responses whenever possible; individuals can also be hyper/hyposensitive to pain and therefore may not accurately identify pain responses – Individuals may "rote" respond and select an answer from the options rather than appropriately discriminating. Others may engage in echoic responses and repeat the last word or choice given, therefore avoid being suggestive in your speech (e.g., avoid "does your tooth hurt" and instead "touch where it hurts" – Allow for additional time in responding; this can be anywhere from 5 seconds to 1 minute in order for an individual to process the request and begin to respond accordingly	– If available, ask caregiver the individual's communication modality (one- to two-word answers, conversational, an augmentative device, sign language, picture exchange system) – If unavailable, ask three establishing questions to assess responding level (e.g., what is this *hold up a pen*, can you touch your nose, can you do this *raise hand in air*); always focus on language ability, not deficits and disability – Asking a question that requires a verbal response will determine if the staff will be able to interpret the individual's vocal/verbal behavior (e.g., may be verbal but inappropriate in tone, cadence, or intelligibility) – Giving a simple directive like touching your nose establishes their ability to follow single-step direction – Asking the individual to model your body movements establishes their imitation skills which may assist when needing to deliver more complex medical directives	– Ensure you have properly obtained the individual's attention prior to making a request or asking a question (say their name, pause [processing time may be increased], and allow them to focus), it may be difficult to ascertain when attention has been gained, as individuals may refrain from eye contact, engage in self-talk, or other forms of stereotypy – Individuals respond to different tones, affect, and interaction styles based on preference or hyper/hyposensitivity; therefore, staff should attend to the individuals' responses to each approach type – Use concise, literal, direct language free of superfluous information, metaphors, or figures of speech; consider first/then statements (first listen heart, then listen back; first wipe cut, then Band-Aid), or delivering requests in stages (e.g., stand up [wait], raise your arm like this [wait and hold model], now I'm going to touch your arm)

■ TABLE 22-2. Dangerous of Self-destructive Behavior

Presenting Issue: Dangerous or Destructive Behavior: Self-Injury, Aggression, or Destruction of Property (e.g., throwing, breaking of objects/items)

Potential Misinterpretation: Psychosis, Alcohol or Substance Abuse, or Acute Psychiatric Disorder

Potential ICU Response Based on Misinformation: Chemical or Physical Restraint, Referral to Psychiatric Treatment Unnecessarily

Assessment Recommendations	Communication Strategies	Treatment Considerations
– Attend to what occurred immediately before the behavior and attempt to remove evocative stimuli (e.g., if you asked the individual to disrobe, tell them they can remain clothed) – Move/offer the individual the ability to move to a safer, less stimulating environment or an environment absent of presumed medical procedures (e.g., instead of lying on the bed, sitting in the chair, instead of sitting in the chair, allow them to stand) – Avoid quick movements or positioning self out of the view of the individual and be cautious and intentional with sharp objects or medical materials; reduce clutter and items within reach	– Limit your verbal and physical interactions with the individual to only those that you presume will reduce risk of injury to themselves or others during challenging behaviors – Repeat simple phrases without varying speech (e.g., sit down please, *10 second silent count*, sit down please) until compliance is achieved in a low, calm tone – In a highly agitated state individuals are often unavailable to treatment or redirection until they have sufficiently de-escalated and re-engaged in the current environment	– All behavior has a function; and that behavior is communicative. The behavior may be a result of pain or discomfort, confusion or uncertainty, or in response to past negative medical experience (e.g., trauma responding) – Default to trauma informed care; remove all objects and items that could result in risk to harm of self and others, create space if possible/safe, refrain from "trapping" or "closing in" on the individual and escalating/creating panic responses (e.g., opening the door, putting down any medical items in your hand at that moment) – Reduce variation in staffing whenever possible, once trust is gained having multiple nurses and staff treating the individual may reduce success

■ TABLE 22-3. Repetitive Behaviors

Presenting Issue: Loud, Nonsensical, or Repetitive Vocalizations or Body Movements
Potential Misinterpretation: Psychosis, Stroke, Tremors, or Other Acute Neurological Insult
Potential ICU Response Based on Misinformation: Focus on Scanning/Imaging and Singular, Directed Treatment

Assessment Recommendations	Communication Strategies	Treatment Considerations
– Present as nonthreatening, using direct and accurate verbal description of what needs to be completed (e.g., hold up stethoscope and state "I need to put this on your heart under your shirt" while modeling placing the disk against your chest) – Obtain individual's attention prior to initiating assessment protocols, direct gaze, and reduce rapid movements to allow individual time to process and follow directives	– Often verbal communication can become overly complex and unnecessary, particularly when an individual is in an overloaded state – Focus on brief, simple directives, reduce unnecessary explanations, and use nonverbal, discrete, direct communication whenever possible (e.g., holding up items, modeling, gestures)	– Be prepared to proceed slowly through even simplistic assessments to gain compliance and trust of the individual (e.g., allow them to hold the stethoscope to ascertain its safety—it is not sharp, it is cold, or touch it first to their palm, then arm before moving to more invasive under the shirt) – Increases in stereotypy may correlate to sensory overload and attention should be given to the frequency of monitoring noise and sensations present in the ICU (e.g., new articles of clothing, hospital bracelets, novel smells such as soaps or cleansers)

■ TABLE 22-4. Refusal of Participation or Contact

Presenting Issue: Refusal to Permit or Participate in Medical Procedures, Tests, Refusal to Allow Physical Contact
Potential Misinterpretation: Refuse to Treat, Declining Treatment
Potential ICU Response Based on Misinformation: Unnecessary Sedation or Physical Restraint

Assessment Recommendations	Communication Strategies	Treatment Considerations
– Present as nonthreatening, using direct and accurate verbal description of what needs to be completed (e.g., hold up stethoscope and state "I need to put this on your heart under your shirt" while modeling placing the disk against your chest – Be prepared to give the individual time to process, accept, and participate in the assessment or treatment; forced participation (e.g., chemical or mechanical restraint) should be considered as a last resort under only emergent circumstances as both result in lack of trust	– These individuals may be concrete thinkers, and not able to understand or translate abstract concepts; therefore, use clear exemplars and concrete statements whenever possible – Be as direct as possible without providing unnecessary or untrue statements in order to obtain compliance (e.g., it will only hurt a little, it isn't a shot it's just a prick) – Be prepared that honest statements are critical to obtaining trust, but to refrain from discussing potential or future assessment or treatment unnecessarily to reduce potential fixation, anxiety, or further refusal responses	– Be prepared to proceed slowly through even simplistic assessments to gain compliance and trust of the individual (e.g., allow them to hold the stethoscope to ascertain its safety—it is not sharp, it is cold, or touch it first to their palm, then arm before moving to more invasive under the shirt) – Prioritize best practice standards with most critical and necessary processes to optimize success (e.g., is continuous pulse oximeter or blood pressure monitoring critically necessary if individual is continuing to remove the device or are other procedures of more critical relevance)

KEY REFERENCES

Anderson DC, Halpern NA. Contemporary ICU design. In: Martin ND, Kaplan LJ, eds. *Principles of Adult Surgical Critical Care*. Cham: Springer; 2016:539-549.

Appropriate Terms to Use About Disability. National Disability Authority. Nda.ie/Publications/Attitudes/Appropriate-Terms-To-Use-About-Disability. Accessed August 11, 2021.

Bracq MS, Michinov E, Jannin P. Virtual reality simulation in nontechnical skills training for healthcare professionals: a systematic review. *Simul Healthc*. 2019;14(3):188-194.

Carter J, Broder-Fingert S, Neumeyer A, et al. Brief report: meeting the needs of medically hospitalized adults with autism: a provider and patient toolkit. *J Autism Dev Disord*. 2017;47(5):1510-1529.

Colombo-Dougovito AM, Dillon SR, Mpofu E. The wellbeing of people with neurodiverse conditions. In: *Sustainable Community Health*. Cham: Palgrave Macmillan; 2020:499-535.

Data & Statistics on Autism Spectrum Disorder. Centers for Disease Control and Prevention. www.cdc.gov/ncbddd/autism/data.html. Accessed August 11, 2021.

Dietz PM, Rose CE, McArthur D, Maenner M. National and state estimates of adults with autism spectrum disorder. *J Autism Dev Disord*. 2020;50:4258-4266.

Folostina R, Dragomir AA. Autism spectrum disorder and the paradigm of neurodiversity. In: *Interventions for Improving Adaptive Behaviors in Children With Autism Spectrum Disorders*. IGI Global; 2022:39-51.

Heras G, Zimmerman J, Hidalgo J. Humanizing critical care. In: *Critical Care Administration*. Cham: Springer; 2020:189-197.

Hosey MM, Jaskulski J, Wegener ST, et al. Animal-assisted intervention in the ICU: a tool for humanization. *Crit Care*. 2018;22. https://doi.org/10.1186/s13054-018-1946-8.

Johnson NL, Rodriguez D. Children with autism spectrum disorder at a pediatric hospital: A systematic review of the literature. *Pediatr Nurs*. 2013;39(3):131-141.

Jolly AA. Handle with care: Top ten tips a nurse should know before caring for a hospitalized child with autism spectrum disorder. *Pediatr Nurs*. 2015; 41(1):11-16.

Karpur A, Lello A, Frazier T, et al. Health disparities among children with autism spectrum disorders: analysis of the national survey of children's health 2016. *J Autism Dev Disord*. 2019;46:1652-1664.

Kayser JB, Kaplan LJ. Conflict management in the ICU. *Crit Care Med*. 2020;48(9):1349-1357.

Lane-Fall MB, Kuza CM, Fakhry S, Kaplan LJ. The lifetime effects of injury: postintensive care syndrome and posttraumatic stress disorder. *Anesthesiol Clin*. 2019;37(1):135-150.

Mandal I, Basu I, De M. Role of nursing professionals in making hospital stay effective and less stressful for patients with ASD: a brief overview. *Int J Adv Life Sci Res*. 2020;3(1):1-9.

Martin N, Pascual JL, Crowe DT Jr, et al. Comfort at the crossroads: service, therapy and emotional support animals in the intensive care unit and at the end-of-life. *J Trauma Acute Care Surg*. 2018;84(6):978-984.

McLaughlin CJ, Childress P, Armen SB, Allen SR. Adult trauma patients with autism spectrum disorder: a case-control study to evaluate disparities after injury. *Injury*. 2021;52(11):3327-3333.

Schopf D, Stark S, Chiappetta L, et al. An alternative admission process for patients with an autism spectrum disorder and/or an intellectual disability. *Learn Disabil Pract.* 2020;23(1):26-32.

Subramanian S, Pamplin JC, Hravnak M, et al. Tele-critical care: an update from the society of critical care medicine tele-ICU committee. *Crit Care Med.* 2020;48(4):553-561.

Thompson DR, Hamilton DK, Cadenhead CD, et al. Guidelines for intensive care unit design. *Crit Care Med.* 2012;40(5):1586-1600.

Trowbridge R, Landaverde B. Autistic man assaulted more than once at Ware park. *Western Mass News*; May 13, 2021. https://www.westernmassnews.com/news/autistic-man-assaulted-more-than-once-at-ware-park/article_316ed664-b429-11eb-bdb1-7bb4e78daf3d.html. Accessed August 12, 2021.

Vaeza NN, Delgado MC, La Calle GH. Humanizing intensive care: toward a human-centered care ICU model. *Crit Care Med.* 2020;48(3):385-290.

Werner S, Yalon-Chamovitz S, Tenne Rinde M, Heymann AD. Principles of effective communication with patients who have intellectual disability among primary care physicians. *Patient Educ Coun.* 2017;100(7):1314-1321.

LGBTQIA+ Patients and Families

David S. Shapiro, Garret Garbo, and Alexis Moren

Patient Care Vignette

A 64-year-old patient presented to the emergency department with dyspnea, fever, and malaise 1 week following a motor vehicle collision resulting in six right-sided rib fractures and a pulmonary contusion. Discharged from an outside facility, the patient presented to the hospital yesterday, and rapidly progressed to demonstrating septic shock with a diagnosis of an ipsilateral pneumonia and worsening hypoxia. Though unaccompanied on arrival by private vehicle, the patient reports being in a long-term relationship with a partner of 26 years. The patient did not come with documentation from the outside facility but was able to report that he is a transgender man and is taking gender-affirming hormone therapy in the form of topical testosterone. The patient quickly became obtunded in the emergency department and was intubated.

The last 24 hours have resulted in intubation and mechanical ventilation, broad-spectrum antimicrobial coverage, multiple vasoactive agents, and worsening hemodynamics, leading to multiple organ system dysfunction. His partner arrived at the hospital with more documentation, including home medications for hypertension and Type II diabetes mellitus, which he reported to be in good control. The patient's partner identified himself as the patient's husband, but also reported that they never married legally. The patient has adult children from his previous marriage, and is estranged from his adult son, but does communicate with his adult daughter periodically. The other father of his children died 3 years ago following a prolonged intensive care stay, resulting from an intracranial hemorrhage, where he lingered with a tracheostomy for 10 days before succumbing. The adult children are his only other relatives. After 3 days in the hospital, the patient is proving challenging to liberate from the ventilator, and a family meeting is requested to discuss further future measures, including possible tracheostomy. The patient's partner says, "he would never want that," citing that watching his first husband's death was terrifying for the patient. The patient's daughter, however, feels that he would want everything done after all that was put in to medically and socially affirming his gender. He eventually undergoes tracheostomy and recovers sufficiently to return home from rehabilitation. He demonstrates signs of significant cognitive decline and may be depressed, leading to a lack of interest in improvement.

Patients in the lesbian, gay, bisexual, transgender, queer, intersex, asexual, "plus" (LGBTQIA+) community have historically encountered challenges in the healthcare system that undermine care, weaken trust, and compromise outcomes. Given this, it is important to understand the concerns of patients and families who identify with this community, as these concerns influence critical illness recovery from both clinical and social perspectives. In this chapter, we present some considerations unique to LGBTQIA+ care and support during critical illness recovery, starting with a discussion of stigma and language, then discussing transgender people, preexisting health status in specific LGBTQIA+ subgroups, and social and family needs for LGBTQIA+ patients. The chapter concludes with post-ICU care considerations for LGBTQIA+ patients. Key terms relevant to the LGBTQIA+ community are presented at the end of the chapter and underlined on first use in this chapter. The considerations in this chapter are most relevant in the United States, but these concepts are important around the world.

■ STIGMA AND LANGUAGE

When navigating the medical system, people in the LGBTQIA+ community may face stigma stemming from social expectations and stereotypes that confer preferred status to *cisgender heterosexual* people. Such stigma is culture- and community-specific; some localities are welcoming, perhaps viewing identification with the LGBTQIA+ community as just another descriptor like educational attainment. In other places, acknowledging one's identification with this community brings risks of alienation and deliberate lack of acknowledgment of one's preferences for how to be addressed (e.g., preferred *gender pronouns*) and the involvement of *chosen family* in one's care.

Unsurprisingly then, LGBTQIA+ patients sometimes avoid seeking healthcare due to a fear of discrimination. They may be reluctant to divulge information over an understandable worry about judgment. This may influence both ICU admission and recovery. For example, avoiding primary care for chronic conditions like hypertension, asthma, and diabetes may lead to clinical exacerbations that require ICU treatment. In the recovery phase, patients may similarly avoid follow-up care to minimize discomfort on interaction with the medical establishment.

Using appropriate terminology with LGBTQIA+ patients and their families can help strengthen trust and promote follow-up that can support optimal recovery after critical illness. For example, when medical professionals affirm *sexual orientation*, including considering the perspectives of partners, friends, and other loved ones, the therapeutic relationship between the team, patient, and family is strengthened. When medical professionals affirm a patient's *gender identity* (including using appropriate pronouns), it creates a pathway to efficient and competent care for that patient. Ideas for how to use open questions to facilitate conversation are presented in "Tips for Clinicians" at the end of this chapter, and in Table 23.1.

Transgender People

Transgender people comprise a diverse group of individuals whose gender identity differs from that originally assigned at birth. *Sex assigned at birth* is determined primarily based on the appearance of genitals; however, chromosomal and hormonal makeup and secondary sex characteristics may also be used. Transgender patients may have a "dead name," or birth name, that has not been used since transitioning. Due to the exorbitant cost, time, restrictions, and complexity of changing a name on a state and federal level, an individual's birth name may be their legal name, and therefore appear on the medical chart.

There is no one way to look or be transgender; there is tremendous heterogeneity in how people experience and express being transgender. Many transgender individuals will not medically affirm their gender, while others will employ gender-affirming hormone therapy (GAHT) and/or gender-affirming surgery (GAS).

Transgender people face multiple barriers to optimal healthcare, partially explaining higher rates of chronic illness in this group. For example, higher rates of depression, anxiety, suicidality, substance abuse, and HIV can be attributed to gender minority status and the societal oppression that transgender people experience. Structural, interpersonal, and individual forms of stigma are highly prevalent among transgender folks and have been linked to these and other adverse health outcomes.

Structural stigma manifests in disparate access to affirming medical, social, and financial resources, and legal protection from harassment and discrimination. In the United States, laws denying gender-affirming care for transgender people, especially transgender youth, are an example of structural barriers to optimal health.

Interpersonal stigma can play out in medical settings and undermine therapeutic patient–provider relationships. For example, many transgender adults report experiencing harassment or refusal of care in medical settings, and a small number have actually experienced violence in medical settings.

There are societal efforts to increase protection for transgender people and other marginalized groups. In February 2021, the U.S. Equality Act was passed. This is a bill that bans discrimination against people based on sexual orientation and identity. It amends the Civil Rights Act of 1964, acknowledging the inequities experienced by groups including the LGBTQIA + community, women, people of color and faith. The bill attempts to minimize the prejudice faced regarding employment, housing, credit, jury service, federally funded programs, and public spaces and services. Despite this, access to healthcare continues to remain a challenge for LGBTQIA+ people, with a higher rate of discrimination in hiring, exorbitant deductibles, and insurance exclusions for gender-affirming medicine.

From a clinical perspective, it is important to note that some transgender patients choose to transition socially, changing their names and pronouns, while others transition medically with GAHT and/or GAS. GAHT causes either feminization or virilization. Assigned male at birth transgender women may be on GAHT including an androgen blocker, estrogen, and progesterone. The most common androgen blockers are spironolactone (a potassium sparing diuretic), or the 5α-reductase inhibitors finasteride or dutasteride. Estrogens may include oral, transdermal, or intramuscular estradiol. Progesterone supplementation may include medroxyprogesterone or micronized progesterone. Assigned female at birth transgender men may be on GAHT including testosterone. Testosterone is administered by intramuscular or subcutaneous injection, transdermally through a gel, patch, or cream, or through inserted subcutaneous pellets. The long-term risks of hormone therapy are unclear, given the paucity of research on this subject, but some concern has been raised about a somewhat increased risk for breast cancer and venous thromboembolism in transgender women compared to cisgender women.

A comprehensive discussion of GAS is beyond the scope of this chapter; more information is provided in Key References. An important consideration for trans women is that GAS for these patients generally does not include prostatectomy; prostate cancer screening is therefore warranted between the ages of 51 and 71 or for 13 years after orchiectomy. Transgender male patients may still have their uterus and therefore menstruate (though testosterone usually stops menses within 6 months of initiation). Cervical and other uterine cancers are therefore plausible diagnoses in these patients. Testosterone is not a form of birth control, and transgender men who have sex with people who produce sperm are still at risk for pregnancy.

Preexisting Health Status in Specific LGBTQIA+ Subgroups

LGBTQIA+ patients are part of a historically marginalized group, which confers elevated risk for conditions related to social status. Such conditions include mood and anxiety disorders including depression with or without suicidality; obesity, eating disorders, and body image disorders; human immunodeficiency virus (HIV) and other sexually transmitted infections (STI); tobacco and other substance use disorders; and peer bullying/assault, intimate partner violence, and homelessness. Related to the stigma discussed earlier, LGBTQIA+ patients may present without prior primary, secondary, or tertiary medical care. The following are considerations when working with some specific groups within this population:

Lesbian/bisexual women: Cardiovascular disease is an important cause of morbidity for all women. This issue is even more prevalent among cisgender lesbians, who have elevated rates of obesity, smoking, and stress. These conditions are themselves risks for other diseases like cancers of the uterus, ovary, and colon. Lesbian cisgender women, particularly those who are "masculine presenting" have been shown to avoid primary care such as mammograms and PAP smears, and so may present with advanced forms of primary care–sensitive conditions. Undiagnosed chronic disease can complicate clinical care and recovery, so it may be prudent to maintain a low threshold for appropriate screening. The post-ICU recovery period may offer an opportunity to diagnose and treat chronic conditions like those mentioned here, improving overall health.

Gay/bisexual/pansexual men and men who have sex with men (MSM): Although there are multiple viral infection risk factors unrelated to sexual orientation and gender identity (e.g., injection drug use, sex without barrier use), MSM and people with penises are at higher than typical risk for HIV infection and Hepatitis A, B, and C. They are also at elevated risk of cancers of the colon, anus, testes, and prostate. Post-ICU care should include screening and treatment for these conditions as clinically appropriate.

■ SOCIAL AND FAMILY NEEDS FOR LGBTQIA+ PATIENTS

Family structure, formal supports, and informal supports in the LGBTQIA+ community exhibit a great deal of diversity. Many LGBTQIA+ individuals have strong relationships with their biological families, whereas others experience familial rejection and/or harassment. For this latter group, "chosen family" becomes very important, as these individuals may be more familiar with a patient's medical history, needs, and preferences. In the clinical vignette above, the patient's partner constitutes part of the patient's chosen family.

Relevant to the concept of chosen family, there is heterogeneity in local, state, and federal laws about who may serve as a healthcare proxy or surrogate decision-maker in the absence of an advanced directive or healthcare power of attorney. Without such documentation, local laws may require that the decision makers for incapacitated patients be part of a legal hierarchy that places spouses at the top followed by biological children and other biological relatives. This can prove problematic for patients who are estranged from their biological families. When possible, chosen family should be allowed to make decisions for patients. At the very least, chosen family should be part of the clinical care discussion to the extent possible and allowed by law and healthcare facility policy. Social workers, chaplains, and ethics consultants can be helpful in these discussions, especially if the patient's chosen and biological families are not acquainted or on good terms. Care should be taken not to "out" patients whose LGBTQIA+ identity may not be known to biological family members.

In the recovery period, patients may need to access multiple social services to facilitate recovery. Related to social stigma and marginalization, some LGBTQIA+ patients lack social supports and may therefore be ineligible for services. Case managers and social workers can be particularly helpful in navigating social services for these patients. Obtaining an advanced directive or healthcare power of attorney (if not already done) may be useful in the recovery period as patients contemplate future interactions with the healthcare system. Completing changes in legal documents (e.g., updating the name on identification documents) may be useful to ensure unfettered access to services.

Religious and spiritual care are just as important for LGBTQIA+ patients as they are for patients not in this community. LGBTQIA+ patients are less likely than others to belong to formal religious groups, many of whom have exclusionary attitudes toward LGBTQIA+ people. These patients, therefore, may need assistance in finding religious and spiritual care communities that are welcoming and affirming.

Finally, as with any caregivers, the caregivers of LGBTQIA+ patients may need support as well, which will enable them to be more effective in their support of recovering patients. These caregivers may have experienced specific trauma during the patient's ICU admission related to exclusion from clinical care and decision making.

Post-ICU Care Considerations for LGBTQIA+ Patients

1. *Anatomical considerations and the physical exam*: The physical exam should be respectful and relevant to the patient's anatomy regardless of gender identity. One should examine without assumption or bias. Be sensitive when taking a history and include only relevant questions about GAHT and/or GAS. The University of California San Francisco has a great

resource for clinicians on the physical exam of transgender patients (see Key References). Transgender patients may have secondary sex characteristics of their natal and/or affirmed sex, depending on whether a patient uses GAHT as part of their transition. A very important anatomical consideration for physical exams is the presence or absence of reproductive organs. For organ-specific exams, consider what reproductive organs a patient may/may not possess, and the effect that GAHT has on that tissue. For example, testosterone can lead to vaginal atrophy, making pelvic exams on assigned female at birth patients particularly challenging, while 5α-reductase inhibitors can lead to an atrophied prostate in people assigned male at birth, making prostate exams difficult. Invasive physical exams should only be performed when absolutely necessary, keeping in mind that these exams may be significantly more traumatic for transgender patients. The harm-reduction model of care must be utilized, which may necessitate leaving this exam out in favor of maintaining a therapeutic alliance.

2. *Gender-affirming care*: Both hormonal therapy and possible postsurgical changes in anatomy (for patients undergoing surgery during ICU admission) should be addressed in the ICU recovery period. In general, a patient should not be taken off GAHT unless there is a clinical contraindication, including interactions with other medications. Before ceasing (or opting not to restart) a transgender person's GAHT, consider whether a cisgender person's endogenous hormones would be blocked in the same situation. Suspending GAHT may also have an influence on mental health and other systems. In our clinical vignette above, our patient's depression and lack of interest could be compounded by the effects of discontinuing GAHT.

3. *Antiviral therapy*: Antiviral therapy for HIV (either prophylaxis or treatment) and for hepatitis B and C may have been stopped in the ICU. If these therapies are restarted, interactions with new medications started in the ICU should be evaluated, as should the risk for exacerbating organ failure. For example, HIV medication Truvada (emtricitabine/tenofovir) can cause hepatotoxicity, nephrotoxicity, osteoporosis, and lactic acidosis. In a patient recovering from kidney injury or liver failure, a different regimen may need to be considered. In patients previously receiving prophylaxis for opportunistic infections (OI) like Pneumocystis pneumonia, these medications may have been stopped. If a patient continues on antibiotic therapy after ICU discharge, OI prophylaxis could be redundant; consultation with an infectious disease specialist may be prudent.

4. *Perioperative care*: Patients recovering from critical illness may need ongoing surgical intervention to optimize recovery. LGBTQIA+ patients may need assistance in seeking out surgical teams with cultural competency,

sensitivity, and a lack of judgment. Given that surgery often entails repeated contacts (e.g., preoperative evaluation, surgery, postoperative evaluation), measures should be taken to ensure that LGBTQIA+ patients are cared for in a respectful way. For example, if postsurgical care is provided in sex-segregated rooms or wards, transgender patients should be placed in private rooms or on the ward that matches their gender. Such affirming care is likely to improve outcomes and satisfaction with care.

Additional Considerations for Recovery

- Transitions in care across settings may be fraught for LGBTQIA+ patients for several reasons. First, handovers may be complicated or undermined by references to a person's dead name or misgendering a patient with incorrect pronouns. Returning a patient from the critical care setting to the post-acute environment may be fraught with concerns for resumption of gender-affirming therapies, and the physiological and/or emotional ramifications of their interruption.
- It is important to affirm a patient's gender identity while acknowledging clinical concerns relevant to each patient's assigned sex at birth. For example, some transgender men can become pregnant or develop uterine cancer, while transgender women with an intact prostate gland will need prostate cancer screening

Tips for Clinicians

When working with LGBTQIA+ patients and caregivers, take steps to establish and maintain trust. Even when the patient's sexual orientation and/or gender identity are known to you (e.g., documented in the medical record), it can be useful to approach conversations with LGBTQIA+ patients in a way that lets them tell their own stories. Specific useful approaches include:

1. **Take steps to educate yourself about LGBTQIA+ issues.** Note that patients may opt to help you develop understanding, but this should not be considered their responsibility.
2. **If you are an ally, identify yourself as such.** Nonverbal approaches to such identification include wearing your pronouns badge indicator or a pin on one's uniform or lab coat.
3. **Ask about preferences for how the patient would like to be addressed.** Example questions include "How would you like me to address you?" "What pronouns do you use?"

4. **Ask about family and proxy decision-makers without assuming relationships.** Useful questions include "Who helps you make decisions? With whom do you live? Who is that person to you?" Ask who their social network is and who they trust in case of emergency, as there are sometimes strained relationships between LGBTQIA+ patients and their families of origin.

5. **Ensure confidentiality.** Assure patients of confidentiality, reiterating as needed, to engender trust and to facilitate open communication. If a patient indicates hesitation in discussing a particular matter, ask for permission to discuss it: "With your permission I'd like to discuss this matter."

6. **Exhibit humility.** If you make a mistake (e.g., misgendering a patient), acknowledge it, apologize, move on, and try to ensure that mistake isn't made again. Be respectful and hold others in your workplace accountable. If an error is made in use of an incorrect name, gender identity, or pronoun, offer the patient the opportunity to educate you as a provider if they desire, acknowledging that our patients do not owe us any emotional or educational labor.

■ TERMINOLOGY

Language about sexual orientation and gender identity is culturally specific and evolves over time. It is important to familiarize oneself with LGBTQIA+ related language, understanding that terms used will change over time. Sample scripts for conversing with patients and families are provided in Table 23-1.

General Terms

- *Chosen family*: Also referred to as "family of choice" or "found family," the chosen family refers to those people who, while not blood relatives, fulfill roles of support, teaching, comfort, and kinship, and can be sibling-like, parental, or any variety of relation.
- *Drag*: Often used with a regal descriptor, as in "drag king" or "drag queen." The performance of masculinity or femininity as a form of art. This is a performance unrelated to gender identity.
- *LGBTQIA+*: Lesbian, gay, bisexual, transgender, queer, intersex, asexual, "plus." This initialism describes a community of people identifying with diverse sexual orientations and gender identities.
- *Queer*: A reclaimed slur, Queer is an identity term for those who do not conform to the norms of heterosexuality and/or the gender binary. Queer should not be a label applied to any individual unless they identify themselves with this term first.

■ **TABLE 23-1. Sample Scripts for Interaction with Patients Identifying as LGBTQIA+**

Best Practice	Sample Script
Avoid using gender terms, such as "sir" or "ma'am," when addressing patients.	"How may I help you?" "May I ask for your pronoun? Mine are 'he/him'." (Self-identifying pronouns can introduce comfort without requiring uncertain inquiry.)
Avoid wrong pronouns and other gender terms when talking with coworkers about patients. Alternatively, mirror terms the patients use for themselves. Alternatively, use gender neutral terms such as "they" until identified. Never use impersonal terms such as "it." Use the patient's name.	"Your patient is here in the waiting room." "They are here for their appointment." "Jay is here, and uses the pronouns she/her."
Avoid assumptions of gender for patient, partner, or spouse.	"Are you in a relationship?" "Who shall I contact after your procedure?" "Do you prefer to have your spouse or partner present during this discussion?"
Use the same terms people use to describe themselves or their clinical scenario.	If someone calls themself, "gay," do not use the term "homosexual." If a woman refers to her "wife," use the same term, and avoid references such as "your friend," etc.
Ask respectfully about names or other details if they do not match your existing medical record.	"Were you known as another name in the past?" "Could your medical record be under a former name?" "Can we update your name in our records?" Have an existing process to do this.
Offer a sincere apology if a mistake in communication happens.	"I apologize for using the wrong pronoun—please correct me and I will help assure the team uses the proper pronouns as well."
Ask only for information required by the clinical interaction.	Ask yourself: What do I know? What do I need to know? How can I ask in a plain but sensitive way?
When you don't know something, be honest, and ask.	

Sexual Orientation

Sexual orientation describes the gender identity of one's desired romantic partners in relationship to one's own gender identity. Specific sexual orientations include:

- *Asexual*: A person who falls along the spectrum of not experiencing sexual attraction. This term is sometimes shortened to "ace."
- *Bisexual*: An identity label sometimes claimed by people who are sexually attracted to the same and other genders, not necessarily equally or simultaneously.

- *Gay*: An identity label sometimes claimed by man/male-identified people who form their primary romantic and sexual relationships with other man/male-identified people. This label may also be used as an alternative to lesbian (i.e., may be claimed by women/female-identified people who form their primary romantic and sexual relationships with other women/female-identified people).
- *Heterosexual*: An identity label describing people who identify as either female or male and who form their primary romantic and sexual relationships with people who identify as the "opposite" gender descriptor. This label infers that gender is binary.
- *Lesbian*: An identity label sometimes claimed by woman/female-identified people who form their primary romantic and sexual relationships with other women/female-identified people.
- *MSM*: Men who have sex with men. A descriptor for cisgender men who have sex with cisgender men—the label MSM names *activity* and not necessarily *identity*. Straight men may be MSM, and still identify as straight.
- *Pansexual*: People who experience sexual attraction regardless of gender identity or sex.

Gender Identity Terms

- *Agender*: Individuals who identify as having no gender, or who do not experience gender as a primary identity component.
- *Assigned sex at birth (ASAB)*: The phenotypic designation assigned to an infant, based on external genitalia. Also simply called "Sex." Assigned female at birth (AFAB) and assigned male at birth (AMAB) are also used.
- *Binary*: The concept of dividing sex or gender into two clear categories. According to this concept, sex is either male or female, gender either is man or woman. This is considered by many to be an artificial dichotomy.
- *Cisgender*: A person whose gender identity aligns with the sex they were assigned at birth.
- *Gender-expansive*: An umbrella term used to refer to people, often youth, who don't identify with traditional gender roles.
- *Gender expression*: The way a person communicates their gender to the world through mannerisms, clothing, speech, behavior, etc. Gender expression varies depending on culture, context, and historical period and is independent of gender identity.
- *Gender fluid (also "genderfluid")*: Not identifying with a single, fixed gender. This may also describe a person whose gender identity may shift.
- *Gender identity*: One's internal definition of self as male, female, both, or neither. A person's gender identity may not align with their sex assigned at birth, and may or may not be outwardly visible.

- *Gender nonconforming*: People who don't conform to traditional expectations of their gender. Gender nonconforming people may be cisgender or transgender.
- *Gender pronouns*: Words people use when they refer to an individual without using their name. Examples are "she/her/hers, they/them/theirs, he/him/his, ze/hir/hirs."
- *Gender queer (also "genderqueer")*: An umbrella term that describes a person whose gender identity falls outside of the traditional gender binary of man/woman.
- *Gender role*: The societal constructs that are assigned to men and women. When people talk about "gender stereotypes" they are referring to the ways we expect men/boys and women/girls to act/behave.
- *Intersex*: Describes a group of congenital conditions in which the reproductive organs, genitals, and/or other sexual anatomy do not develop according to historical expectations for males or females.
- *Mx*: An honorific prefix similar to Mr., Ms., and Mrs. that is gender neutral. It is often the option of choice for folks who do not identify within the gender binary: *Mx. Smith is a great teacher.*
- *Nonbinary*: Someone who doesn't identify exclusively as a man/woman. This may overlap with a genderqueer identity.
- *Transgender*: A person whose gender identity differs from the sex they were assigned at birth
- *Transgender man*: A man who was assigned female at birth.
- *Transgender woman*: A woman who was assigned male at birth.

KEY REFERENCES

Guidelines for Care of Lesbian, Gay, Bisexual and Transgender Patients 2006 [cited March 23, 2021]:1-35. Available at http://glma.org/_data/n_0001/resources/live/GLMA%20guidelines%202006%20FINAL.pdf.

Injustice at every turn: A report of the National Transgender Discrimination Survey. Washington, DC: National Center for Transgender Equality and National Gay and Lesbian Task Force; 2011.

Institute of Medicine (US) Committee on Lesbian, Gay, Bisexual, and Transgender Health Issues and Research Gaps and Opportunities. *The Health of Lesbian, Gay, Bisexual, and Transgender People: Building a Foundation for Better Understanding*. National Academies Press; 2011.

Linda Wesp M, NP-C. Transgender patients and the physical examination. University of California San Francisco UCSF; 2016 [updated June 2016; cited May 1, 2021].

Unger CA. Hormone therapy for transgender patients. *Transl Androl Urol*. 2016;5(6):877-884.

White Hughto JM, Reisner SL, Pachankis JE. Transgender stigma and health: a critical review of stigma determinants, mechanisms, and interventions. *Soc Sci Med*. 2015;147:222-231.

Patients with Limited English Proficiency

Toba Bolaji, Asanthi Ratnasekera, and Paula Ferrada

Patient Care Vignette

Mrs. Obayemi is a 78-year-old female who you've been caring for in your intensive care unit. Her hospital course has been complicated and her health is slowly deteriorating. Mrs. Obayemi came to the United States from Nigeria last year, initially to visit her adult children, but after realizing that many of her chronic medical issues had not been controlled, she now permanently lives with her children.

She initially presented after a fall, sustaining a severe traumatic brain injury, but her course has been complicated by the incidental discovery of ovarian cancer and subsequently underwent a placement of a tracheostomy and a feeding tube. Mrs. Obayemi is non-English speaking and was born and lived all her life in a small village in northern Nigeria. She speaks an uncommon dialect of Yoruba and because of that, all of your communication with her has been accomplished with her children as intermediaries. Using her children as de facto interpreters has led to misunderstanding and miscommunication about her prognosis and ultimately the goals of her care.

■ INTRODUCTION

For the majority of US residents, English is the only language spoken in the home. However, the composition of the United States makes it clear that we are represented by residents who speak many different languages and dialects. Indeed, 21.6% of US residents report that they speak a language other than English at home and the proportion of non-English-speaking and limited English proficient (LEP) people is rapidly growing. This presents a challenging issue for healthcare systems and clinicians in the coming decades as communication regarding treatments, options, informed consent, and goals of care may require skilled interpretation to achieve with fidelity. Our task will be to trying to deliver standardized, patient-centered care to an increasingly diverse population. Over the last 30 years, the largest group of migrants into the United States have been individuals who are primarily—or exclusively—Spanish speaking. By 2060, this population is expected to reach 111 million, making up close to 30% of the country's population by that time. Yet, Hispanics are among the least represented within the healthcare industry, creating additional need for medical interpreters as that role cannot be borne by a native, Spanish-speaking healthcare professional. This specific stressor is magnified by the breadth of languages spoken by US residents, and the lack of competence in unique dialects among medical interpretation professionals.

The impact of language barriers on patient outcome has been recently receiving greater attention. There is evidence to support that adverse outcomes that affect LEP patients are most frequently attributed to errors in communication and are more likely to result in serious harm compared to harms related to communication in English-fluent patients. An avoidable 3-day increase in length of stay when an interpreter isn't used at admission or discharge increases the risk of falls and nosocomial infection in LEP patients. Also, future care is affected as there is a decreased chance of preventive screening for these patients based on lack of understanding of necessity or lack of access. An increased frequency of avoidable harm may be anticipated unless system-based remedies can be emplaced in the hospital as well as within the broader context of the medical community.

Clear and understandable communication also supports high-quality post-acute care once patients return home. In the outpatient setting, language barriers have been found to contribute to gaps in health access, lower rates of preventive services, decreased comprehension, poorer adherence, and decreased satisfaction with care. New medications or new medications regimens, wound care, mobility, and at-home rehabilitation exercises all need to be readily understood. The same goes for follow-up visits and the triggers for an unscheduled call of return to the emergency department. Without clear communication, potentially avoidable complications, including readmissions are likely to ensue. For example, in 2018, there was an average of 3.8 million adult hospital readmissions within 30 days, and in 2019, the cost of hospital readmission was estimated to be approximately 26 billion dollars.

Tackling language barriers are only one aspect of delivering comprehensive care for our diverse communities. Cultural competency is our ability as clinicians to offer care that addresses the cultural, social, and spiritual needs of our patients. Delivering culturally competent care improves patient quality care outcomes and patient satisfaction. As we look toward an always changing future, the changing demographic of the country will encourage healthcare systems to build infrastructure and provide resources that are inclusive and equitable. Much of that diversity is expressed during an episode of critical illness or injury when complex care is required, the patient cannot participate in their own care, and their surrogate(s) must help provide substituted judgment to help guide clinicians.

■ ICU CARE CONSIDERATIONS FOR PATIENTS WITH LIMITED ENGLISH PROFICIENCY (LEP)

Adverse events in non-English-speaking or LEP patients are usually a result of errors in communication between patient and clinician. The presence of language barriers or the lack of available clear communication between patient and clinician leaves ample room for misunderstanding, dissatisfaction, and even distrust within a patient–clinician or family–clinician relationship. This untoward effect is magnified when there are multiple teams involved in care compared to when there is only one clinician. There are a variety of prototypical scenarios where erroneous communication may occur with patients with LEP, and offer opportunities to prepare for them to help ensure robust and clear communication. These scenarios may be conveniently grouped into four domains that are explored as follows (Fig. 24-1):

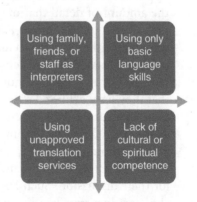

FIGURE 24-1. Drivers of Erroneous Communication with Patients of Limited English Proficiency.

1. Using family members, friends, or nonqualified staff as medical interpreters

The convenience of having loved ones or friends, or even nonqualified but language-fluent staff (i.e., lay interpreters) at the bedside as a bridge for communication with the patient can be tempting, especially when no suitable medical interpreter is available. However, this approach is fraught with peril. Nonmedially sophisticated family members or friends may not be sufficiently familiar with specifics to accurately convey relevant detail, and may not even have the correct words to convey a specific diagnosis or therapy. This can lead to the misrepresentation of disease processes and the under- or over-emphasizing of likely events. Moreover, lay interpreters are likely subject to optimism bias, especially since the patient is a loved one. This relationship may make it difficult for the lay interpreter to share difficult or devastating diagnoses or prognoses. Since it is often younger members of the family who could serve as a lay interpreter, asking them to do so often adds another care-taker role for them within their family structure. Unsurprisingly, such individuals report moderate to high stress due to the complexities of navigating the health system, difficulty in understanding the challenging medical needs of their loved ones, and then serving as the link between their family and the clinical team. Regardless of how you explore the use of lay interpreters, the prevailing standard is to use a trained, qualified medical interpreter to ensure high-quality communication.

2. Clinicians who possess only basic non-native language skills

Staff members who have basic language skills may attempt to use their limited skills as their sole method of communication with a patient or their family. This practice is also error-prone as fluency, not basic skill, is required for effective communication. If only basic language skill is used, the amount of detail that may be provided to the patient about their care plan is also quite limited. Patient- or family-generated questions may be difficult for the clinician to understand, and the ability to answer them in a complete fashion remains compromised. In such circumstances, clinicians may heavily rely on their nonverbal communication skills, often believing that they have achieved a degree of understanding from the patient that is quite inaccurate. This practice is to be avoided and should never be used as the basis for providing informed consent or establishing goals of care. Social communication may be well supported by basic skills including daily greetings, name, specialty, and that the clinician will be using an interpreter for their discussion. Such language skills may benefit from practice if the clinician does not already possess sufficient knowledge to carry on a social conversation.

3. Use of unapproved translator services in the ICU

Medical interpreters are an essential resource in breaking the language barrier in patient–clinician communication. They are trained to understand and translate medical terminology and phrasing in a culturally relevant and parallel manner. Accordingly, they implicitly break the culture barrier related to language and communication style and norm. Therefore, their presence can help facilitate an environment of trust. Medical interpreters are trained through the National Council on Interpreting in Health Care which has curriculum standards that have been created to provide formal training opportunities. Participants who successfully complete the course receive certification and are then eligible to take a national exam, becoming a board-certified medical interpreter. Moreover, most complex care centers have access to in-house medical interpreters and third-party verified and high-quality telephone or technology-based translator services. The robustness of these resources is usually linked to the needs of the community they serve. These resources provide an easily accessible means for having important conversations and discussions with non-English-speaking and LEP patients and family members. Problems may readily arise when unapproved and perhaps web-based services are used instead of licensed and qualified medical interpreters or interpretations services.

Inappropriate translation most commonly arises from the use of nonvalidated translation applications. The use of these methods is usually only good for the translation of short, concrete questions and similarly terse and often binary (yes/no) responses. Such approaches are typically incapable of translating the technical aspect of medical terminology or procedural plans, and therefore put both clinicians and institutions at high liability risk. Importantly, culturally relevant nuances are not included in such programs and may erode trust—even if the intent is to help build trust by trying to bridge a communication gap. Finally, most such applications are not compliant with the provisions of the Health Insurance Portability and Accountability Act (HIPAA).

4. Failing to understand the effects of cultural and religious identity on comprehensive ICU care

Providing culturally competent care is a key goal of modern healthcare delivery systems. With an increasingly dynamic and diverse population, the implications of an individual's culture, beliefs, and values on the care they want and receive has never been more apparent. Culturally competent care aims to provide equitable care regardless of cultural, ethnic, racial, or spiritual identity. Besides using approved medical interpreters, including culturally diverse staff in the ICU helps reinforce the ICU as a culturally sensitive and appropriate care environment. It is key to recall that the four pillars of

Western ethics that permeate native US ethics (autonomy, beneficence, justice, and non-maleficence) may not apply to other cultures. Specific spiritual tenets may also shape how medical or surgical care is provided. For example, Buddhism holds that mind-altering medications should be avoided in death, and that the state of mind at death influences rebirth. Therefore, the medications that providers usually administer during the late stages of life may be prohibited. Patients who follow Islam may require that female patients are cared for only by a female physician, and that a handshake or other contact between genders is prohibited. Spiritual identity may also influence medical decision-making in other anticipatable ways such as the Jehovah's Witness prohibition against receiving blood products or therapeutics that have come from outside their body. These influences are likely to be highly—but not exclusively—represented in patients and families with LEP. These very limited examples show that every religion is unique and our ability to provide care for those with a faith-based existence may be directly and indirectly impacted by their unique beliefs and tenets. It is therefore incumbent upon clinicians to understand key aspects of different cultures and religions to provide culturally and spiritually competent care. LEP patients present a unique challenge to doing so, as the common platform—language—must be bridged by an individual or series of individuals (medical interpreters)—not directly engaged in care delivery.

◼ WORKING WITH AN INTERPRETER

Most clinicians are not taught how to best work with a professional medial interpreter. However, being able to do so in a seamless fashion is critical to ensure that what the clinician needs to have interpreted is done so in a clear and well-understood fashion. *First*, once the need for interpretation is established, it is best to meet with the interpreter ahead of meeting with the patient or family. This allows the clinician and the interpreter to review the context of the discussion, and to explore any unique words or concepts with which the interpreter must be familiar during the conversation. *Second*, while tempted to look at the interpreter, the clinician must instead always look at the patient and family. This supports having the patient and family feel engaged. It also helps the clinician to read nonverbal cues that serve as a guide to how the conversation is being received. *Third*, instead of speaking in full sentences that flow into one another as one would do with a native English speaker, information should be divided into easily translatable chunks. This allows the interpreter to readily translate and share discrete information without having to "store" all of it in their head while waiting for the clinician to finish speaking. It also allows the patient and family to process sequential but low-volume pieces of information. This point cannot be overemphasized and benefits from practice. Recall that the clinician often has no idea what is being said by the interpreter and therefore completely relies on the interpreter having a clear understanding of what needs to be shared. *Fourth*, remember that many languages require more words to say the same as fewer words may in standard English. Therefore, patience is required during this process. *Fifth*, encourage patients and families to ask questions to ensure that they clearly understand each point before moving on to the next one. *Sixth*, the clinician should ask the interpreter for feedback on their work together, and what the clinician could improve during the next session.

■ CONSIDERATIONS FOR RECOVERY

When a patient is discharged from the acute care hospital, a transition of care occurs. Similar to a transition of care in the hospital from an ICU to an acute care unit, a thorough handoff enables safe patient care, and decreases medical errors. In the transition during discharge to home, the patient or their family member(s) become responsible for medication administration, creating and keeping follow-up appointments, and following medical advice during recovery. Each of these aspects benefits from being explained using medical interpretation services. Since instructions may be quite voluminous, they are also provided as printed discharge instructions. It is critical that these are also provided in the patient and family member's primary language as well as English. The former is for the patient and family, and the latter is for any other clinicians who will see the patient outside of the hospital. It is important to note that the discharge process is, of necessity, longer than the process for patients with English language proficiency. Several studies have demonstrated that outpatient adverse drug events occur due to a lack of patient education and specialist management which in turn increases hospital readmissions. Patients with LEP had a decreased knowledge of drug type and the reason that they are prescribed that specific medication. This directly reduces compliance, but also places the patient at risk of inappropriate medication use. Clearly, explaining discharge instructions, including medication directions, using a professional interpreter (rather than family members) improves medication understanding and safe medication use. A pharmacist (PharmD) may be ideally involved in this process as well, especially if the patient is to be discharged home or to another care facility directly from the ICU. The socioeconomic status of the patient also impacts the transition from the ICU to discharge. A lower literacy level correlates with a lower comprehension of medical advice and discharge instructions which increases medication errors, medication toxicity, and impaired postdischarge follow-up.

■ ESTABLISHING FOLLOW-UP CARE

After discharge, access to preventive care and health maintenance care is another area of healthcare disparity that impacts patients with LEP. Since LEP patients benefit from medical interpreter services during their inpatient care, it is of little surprise that the same would be required for outpatient care. Outpatient telephone conversations are particularly difficult as they typically occur without medical interpretation—unless three-way calling using an approved interpreter service is engaged. This process increases the amount of time—and perhaps the cost—of the phone call if the service is not provided free-of-charge to the outpatient clinician's office. Clear instructions and follow-up conversations are essential to gauge progress (or lack thereof), assess medication efficacy, and help support health aspects including mobility exercise, tobacco cessation, and dietary modification that may have been started during inpatient care. Access to healthcare may be limited by under- or uninsured status and may drive the need for regular transportation to sites of free healthcare, or a return to the complex care center for follow-up in the perioperative period. All of this coordination is complex and quite difficult without clear understanding. Some facilities use a nurse navigator who is fluent in the patient's native language to provide follow-up and deliver clear instructions, answer questions, and support medical literacy and health maintenance for those with LEP. This may be considered a best practice in many ways. The nurse navigator can also serve as a bridge between patients and their families and social workers or social work–related services spanning everything from medical assistance, energy bill forbearance, medical transportation and supplies, to homemakers' services. Caring for patients with LEP requires a comprehensive approach to care that may be considered as a form of community outreach in the postdischarge time frame.

■ CONCLUSIONS

Patients with LEP are at high risk for a variety of medical errors related to failed or inadequate communication. Ensuring effective communication starts with recognizing patients with LEP and emplacing processes to help address communication. One of those key processes is ensuring professional medical interpretation using appropriately trained interpreters or approved phone or web-based interpreter services. Family members, friends, or staff who are not professionally trained and credentialed should not serve in this capacity. Learning to work with a medical interpreter is an essential skill for all clinicians. The transition from inpatient acute care to outpatient care is a highly vulnerable period for patients and family members who demonstrate LEP. Discharge instructions should be provided in a bilingual fashion and attention should be paid to communicating discharge instructions using a medical interpreter. Outpatient follow-up and care requires the same diligence to communication and is at highest risk for communication failure during telephone conversations if an interpreter is not employed. Clinicians should avoid using only basic non-native language skills and arrange for expert medical interpretation to provide high-quality communication and care.

Tips for Clinicians

1. **Support the routine identification of LEP patients** upon hospital admission or introduction to a new healthcare setting using quality improvement, implementation science, or other change management approach.
2. **When possible, use in-person professional interpreters** for interactions with patients and family caregivers. Remote services, even when employing professional interpreters, are less personal and may be perceived as less effective.
3. **Use professional interpreters to communicate important information** (e.g., medication changes, medical recommendations, referrals, etc.) rather than relying on family or friends to ensure clear, precise, and effective communication.
4. **Provide verbal and written instructions in the patient's preferred language** and ensure that they understand what is being shared with regard to medications, home care, and follow-up.
5. **Limit polypharmacy where possible** to reduce medication errors and medication toxicity which contributes to higher hospital readmissions.
6. **Learn to seamlessly work with a professional medical interpreter** to enhance effective communication.

KEY REFERENCES

Alvarez-Arango S, Tolson T, Knight A, et al. Juntos: a model for language congruent care to better serve Spanish-speaking patients with COVID-19. *Health Equity*. 2021;5(1):826-833.

Background on Patient Safety and LEP Populations. Agency for Healthcare Research and Quality. Available at https://www.ahrq.gov/health-literacy/professional-training/lep-guide/chapter1.html. Accessed February 4, 2022.

Brooks LA, Bloomer MJ, Manias E. Culturally sensitive communication at the end-of-life in the intensive care unit: a systematic review. *Australian Crit Care*. 2019;32(6):516-523.

Budnitz D, Pollock D, Weidenbach K, et al. National surveillance of emergency department visits for outpatient adverse drug events. *JAMA*. 2006;296(15):1858-1866.

DuBard CA, Gizlice Z. Language spoken and differences in health status, access to care, and receipt of preventative services among US Hispanics. *Am J Public Health*. 2008; 98(11):2021-2028.

Ferdinand KC, Nasser SA. African-American COVID-19 mortality: a sentinel event. *J Am Coll Cardiol*. 2020;75:2746-2748.

Fiscella K, Franks P, Doescher MP, Saver BG. Disparities in health care by race, ethnicity, and language among the insured: findings from a national sample. *Med Care*. 2002;40(1):52-59.

Improving patient safety systems for patients with limited English proficiency. Agency for Healthcare Research and Quality. Available at https://www.ahrq.gov/health-literacy/professional-training/lepguide/index.html. Accessed November 22, 2022.

John-Baptiste A, Naglie G, Tomlinson G, et al. The effect of English language proficiency on length of stay and in-hospital mortality. *J Gen Intern Med*. 2004;19(3):221-228.

Karliner L, Auerbach A, Napoles A, et al. Language barriers and understanding of hospital discharge instructions. *Med Care*. 2012;50(4):283-289.

Karliner LS, Kim SE, Meltzer DO, Auerbach AD. Language barriers and hospital care. *J Hosp Med*. 2010;5:276-282.

Language Use in the United States: 2019. Unites States Census Bureau. Available at https://www.census.gov/library/publications/2022/acs/acs-50.html. Accessed November 22, 2022.

Martinez DA, Hinson JS, Klein EY, et al. SARS-CoV-2 positivity rate for Latinos in the Baltimore-Washington, DC Region. *JAMA*. 2020;324:392-395.

National standards for healthcare interpreter training programs. National Council on Interpreting in Health Care. Available at https://www.ncihc.org/ethics-and-standards-of-practice. Accessed November 22, 2022.

Price-Haywood EG, Burton J, Fort D, Seoane L. Hospitalization and mortality among Black patients and White patients with Covid-19. *N Engl J Med*. 2020;382(26):2534-2543.

Semere W, Napoles A, Gregorich S, et al. Caregiving for older adults with limited English proficiency: Transitioning from hospital to home. *J Gen Intern Med*. 2019;34(9):1744-1750.

Schenker Y, Perez-Stable EJ, Nickleach D, Karliner LS. Patterns of interpreter use for hospitalized patients with limited English proficiency. *J Gen Int Med*. 2011;26(7):712-717.

Squires A. Evidence-based approaches to breaking down language barriers. *Nursing*. 2017; 47(9):34-40.

Squires, Allison PhD, RN, FAAN Strategies for overcoming language barriers in healthcare. *Nurs Manage*. 2018;49(4):20-27.

Van Dorn A, Cooney RE, Sabin ML. COVID-19 exacerbating inequalities in the US. *Lancet*. 2020;395:1243-1244.

Wilson E, Chen AH, Grumbach K, et al. Effects of limited English proficiency and physician language on health care comprehension. *J Gen Int Med*. 2005;20(9):800-806.

Woloshin S, Schwartz LM, Katz SJ, Welch HG. Is language a barrier to the use of preventive services? *J Gen Intern Med*. 1997;12(8):472-477.

COVID-19

Deborah Stein, Camille Lineberry, Nina Raoof, and Neil Halpern

Patient Care Vignette

A Patient's Personal Account of COVID-19 (produced with patient's permission).

I became infected with COVID-19 early April 2020, when I was 68 years old. I had recently retired after 38 years of service as a pharmacist, and was in good health, although I had type 2 diabetes.

In mid-March, my son became sick, but his COVID result came back negative and I let my guard down—my mask came off. After 2 weeks, my son felt better, but I had a fever and was bedridden. By day 3, I could not breathe, and was diagnosed with COVID-19 at a local ER. I was to be sent to a nursing home, but my daughter was able to arrange a transfer to my former hospital of employment. I was admitted to a COVID ward; however, before intake was complete, I needed to go to the ICU because I couldn't breathe. I vaguely remember a voice telling me my numbers were dropping and that they would have to intubate me. I said, "do what you have to do...."

When I woke up in the ICU, I was told 5 weeks had passed. I was on a ventilator with very high-dose sedation. I slowly began to survey my surroundings and realized that I was connected to oxygen, multiple monitors, IV access, and that I had a tracheotomy and G-tube. It is a strange feeling waking up after a medically induced coma, and it took me a while to grasp my bearings and deal with the weird dreams that I experienced.

After 2 more weeks of excellent ICU care, I was transferred to the inpatient ward. To my surprise and delight, I had lost 23 pounds, but my legs and thighs had become painfully thin and I felt very weak. It was a huge challenge to stand up and ambulate daily with physical therapist (PT) and occupational therapist (OT). Besides my tracheostomy and G-tube, I also had bed sores on my lower back, and a discolored chin (black).

My trach tube was removed while on the ward, and I was eventually transferred to Kessler Acute Rehab and underwent intense physical and occupational therapy. I was sent home with a walker, wheelchair, and commode; at home, visiting nurse services saw me for one month. I was not able to climb stairs, so I slept in a bed in my living room. I continued to receive PT and OT at home, and then as an outpatient for 6 months. Thankfully, my daughter stayed with me for 2 months, helping me with dressing changes and G-tube irrigation. I have never felt so helpless in my life.

COVID-19 left me weak, with increased heart rate and blood pressure, and no appetite. A hypertensive crisis landed me in the ER in September, and I was placed on medication. I had to force myself to eat, gradually increasing my protein intake. Despite being on a regular diet, my G-tube could not be removed for a while. Thankfully, the trach opening closed quickly, and my bed sores and chin healed after several months, but I developed Telogen effluvium and clumps of my hair started to fall off. Eventually, it grew back.

The most challenging and annoying symptom is a persistent cough. COVID-19 left me with fibrosis in both lungs, and there is no medication my pulmonologist can prescribe, only lozenges. At times, I get a dull ache in my chest cavity if I lie in bed in a certain way—it is quite scary to be able to feel one's damaged lungs. Coughing at night also disturbs my sleep and I have resorted to taking melatonin.

It has been over a year since my hospital discharge, and my cough and chronic fatigue persist. Overall, I have improved a lot and am quite functional, and I can say that I have come a long way.

■ INTRODUCTION

In 2019, the virus that causes COVID-19 infection, severe acute respiratory syndrome-coronavirus 2 (SARS-CoV-2), emerged and evolved into a worldwide pandemic. As of December 2022, there have been upwards of 645 million COVID-19 infections worldwide, leading to an estimated 6.6 million deaths. In the United States alone, there have been more than 100 million confirmed cases, with over 1 million deaths. Up to 40% of patients with COVID-19 infection required hospitalization during the pandemic, and intensive care unit (ICU) admission was dependent upon underlying health conditions.

In the first year of the pandemic, rates of infection, hospitalization, and deaths surged intermittently, likely due to suboptimal vaccination success and noncompliance with social distancing guidelines. Subsequently, the overall hospitalization rate is on the decline.

More than 2 years after the start of the pandemic, patients recovering from COVID-19, particularly those with more severe infections, were noted to have unique issues during recovery. In addition to post-hospitalization and critical illness syndromes that are becoming more familiar, a new framework for post-COVID illness is being delineated. These include post-acute COVID syndrome (PACS) and "Long COVID." While many COVID-19 survivors experience few post-hospital symptoms, others suffer severe and persistent debilitating physical and mental symptoms. As yet, there are no internationally accepted standards for the definition of the entirety of the COVID-19 syndrome or for the individual systemic effects, but clusters of symptoms and signs persist. Efforts at codification are under way to codify the diagnosis. In the schema outlined in Fig. 25-1, the course of illness is divided into acute COVID-19 (weeks 1-4) and post-acute COVID-19 (>week 4). The latter phase is further divided into subacute or ongoing COVID-19 (weeks 4-12) and chronic or post-COVID-19 (>12 weeks; aka long-COVID). Of note, even in the post-acute COVID phase, nasopharyngeal swabs may still be polymerase chain reaction (PCR) positive; however, such positivity does not often correlate with transmissibility.

ICU CARE CONSIDERATIONS FOR PATIENTS WITH COVID-19-ASSOCIATED CRITICAL ILLNESS

The goal of this chapter is to summarize acute COVID illness and its treatment, delineate the transition to post-COVID illness with its attendant pathophysiology, and summarize the limited treatment options that have been identified. We will focus on each organ system separately to provide clarity of information.

Pandemic-Related Modifiers

When caring for patients with acute or post-COVID infection, it is of vital importance to consider the cultural milieu in which this care must be rendered. The psychological effects of prolonged isolation, clinical short- and long-term uncertainty, and economic anxiety have affected patients with COVID, their families, and healthcare clinicians. In fact, the rates of posttraumatic stress disorders and major depressive disorders are higher in frontline medical staff than in their peers, even among those without underlying

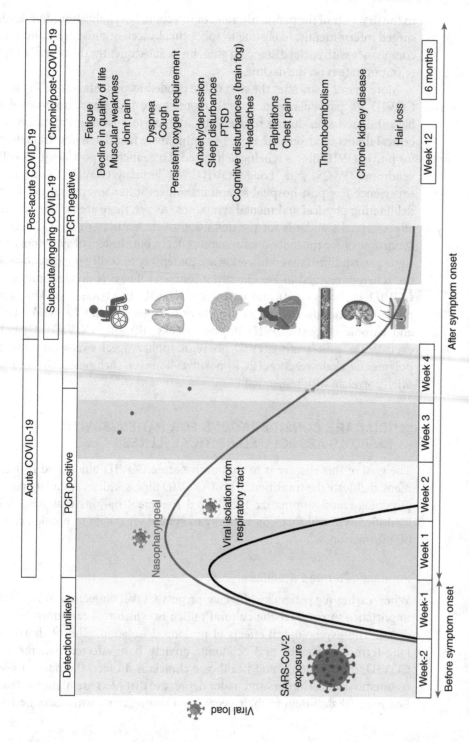

FIGURE 25-1. Changes in PCR Testing and Symptoms after Exposure to SARS-CoV-2 Virus. This figure demonstrates how exposure and infection with SARS-CoV-2 virus influences polymerase chain reaction (PCR) testing in the context of acute versus post-acute COVID-19 infection. (Reproduced with permission from Nalbandian A, Sehgal K, Gupta A, et al. Post-acute COVID-19 syndrome. *Nature Med.* 2021;27(4):601-615.)

psychiatric disorders. Moreover, 40% of US adults without COVID-19 have reported delaying their general medical care (including emergency care) due to pandemic-related fears. In fact, 35% of excess deaths early in the pandemic in the United States were attributed to non-COVID illnesses such as diabetes and heart disease. Providing comprehensive care in the post-COVID era requires consideration of how patients with and without COVID-19 may have been affected by these unprecedented events, and will no doubt have repercussions for years.

Non-COVID Illness Modifiers

Survivors of hospitalization and of critical illness are known to develop post-hospital discharge morbidities across a broad range of organ systems, with significant impact on quality of life. Among COVID-19 survivors, there is a great deal of overlap with standard post-hospitalization (PHS), post-intensive care syndrome (PICS), and persistently symptomatic, nonhospitalized presentations. Primary care clinicians can expect to see a spectrum of symptoms among COVID-19 survivors that may differ by race, gender, comorbid conditions, and other factors, with expectations and treatment options changing as our understanding improves.

Data from a large US health plan was analyzed to compare outcome of patients with COVID-19 across a spectrum of severity as well as to compare them with survivors of other lower respiratory tract viral-based infections. Among the group with SARS-CoV-2 infection, 14% had one or more sequelae that required medical care. Time to development of sequelae was up to 4 months for some types of events and risk factors included gender (certain sequelae were more common in women, others in men), older age, preexisting medical conditions, and hospitalization status (Fig. 25-2). It is important to remember that sequela can be found even among young patients and those with a mild course of disease for whom we might not initially have considered post-COVID illness as a cause of their presenting complaints because they were not hospitalized. Interestingly, when compared to survivors of other viral illnesses, the relative risk of developing certain sequela was not notably higher. The scale of infection is quite different, however, and may contribute to the perception that sequelae from SARS-CoV-2 infection are more common.

Neuropsychiatric

Neuropsychiatric manifestations of COVID-19 infection are common and range from migraine headaches and anosmia (loss of smell) to cerebrovascular accident (CVA, stroke), Guillain-Barré syndrome, and seizure.

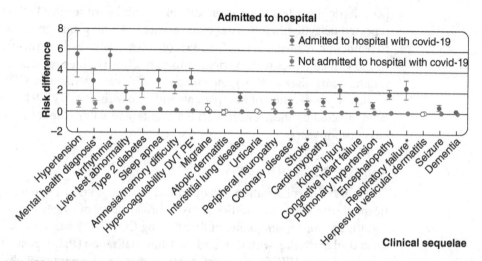

FIGURE 25-2. Risk of Developing Post-Hospitalization Complications With and Without COVID-19. This figure demonstrates that a wide variety of post-hospitalization complications are more common after requiring hospital care with COVID-19 infection compared to those who did not have COVID-19 infection. DVT = deep vein thrombosis; PE = pulmonary embolus.
*Includes multiple subdiagnoses. DVT = deep vein thrombosis; PE = pulmonary embolism (Reproduced with permission from Daugherty SE, Guo Y, Heath K, et al. Risk of clinical sequelae after the acute phase of SARS-CoV-2 infection: retrospective cohort study. *BMJ.* 2021;373:n1098.)

Small studies have documented the presence of neurologic symptoms in 36% of patients with COVID-19 overall, with symptoms increasing to 84% in those who survive the acute respiratory distress syndrome (see Chapter 5). The main psychiatric manifestation of COVID-19 infection is delirium. Delirium rates among critically ill, mechanically ventilated patients had been decreasing prepandemic from 80% down to 17-33%. Unfortunately, delirium became much more common during the pandemic and increased to 65% in those cared for in the ICU.

Possible explanations for the increased prevalence of delirium among COVID-19 patients include limitations in resources, prolonged periods of sedation, invasive mechanical ventilation with strict isolation, and direct neurologic injury from the SARS-CoV-2 virus. Inpatient management is similar to other patients with delirium—evaluate for underlying directly treatable causes such as sepsis while ensuring patient and staff safety during periods of agitation.

The pathophysiology behind the neurologic manifestations is thought to include direct viral invasion of the central nervous system (CNS), generalized inflammation leading to neuroinflammation, and the general consequences of critical illness such as hypoxia (low oxygen) and impaired cerebral perfusion (reduced blood flow) due to hypotension (low blood pressure). Clotting on a large and microvascular scale has been well described with COVID-19 infection. Anosmia (impaired sense of smell) and dysgeusia (impaired sense of taste) are prevalent, affecting up to 88% of patients, with a female predominance, and an early olfactory recovery rate of 44%. Some of these symptoms change as the virus mutates, leading to a confusing array of "typical" symptoms.

Post-COVID neuropsychiatric dysfunction is quite common as a consequence of acute events such as CVA but also due to PICS (see Chapter 3, Considerations for Recovery). These symptoms include fatigue, cognitive impairment, weakness, psychosocial difficulties, depression, and insomnia. Up to 50% of post-COVID patients will also be diagnosed with a new psychiatric disorder such as posttraumatic stress disorder, depression, or obsessive-compulsive disorder. Of note, cognitive difficulties and mood alterations are increasingly described among nonhospitalized COVID-19 survivors as well. Because of the high prevalence across classes of disease severity, it is vital to ensure that outpatient follow-up includes thorough screening for neurologic and psychiatric sequelae. Family members can be particularly helpful in identifying that their loved one has not quite returned to their baseline, especially at follow-up visit with a primary care clinician or in a post-ICU clinic (see Chapter 15).

Pulmonary

The hallmark of pulmonary infection with SARS-CoV-2 is profound hypoxemia, impacting about two-thirds of patients admitted to the ICU. Initial management included early intubation and invasive mechanical ventilation. As the pandemic progressed, noninvasive ventilation and prone position therapy became much more common as we learned how to best match patient needs with provided therapy, and as the spectrum of disease began to shift (see Chapter 5). Some of those shifts reflect virus mutation as well as novel therapies that have now become standard. Those therapies seemed to have reduced viral infection severity and include the COVID vaccines as well as steroids. Therapy with dexamethasone (a steroid) reduces mortality for patients with COVID pneumonia, particularly in those with more severe disease and has remained a mainstay of therapy. Therapies such as monoclonal antibodies and other immune modulators that are more appropriate for outpatient care continue to evolve in parallel with virus mutation.

Post-COVID pulmonary sequelae are unfortunately quite common in survivors of severe disease. The incidence of a range of symptoms increases with the severity of the acute illness and with higher levels of inflammatory markers measured in the bloodstream. Up to two-thirds of survivors report prolonged shortness of breath even 6 months after hospital discharge.

While specific testing of pulmonary function or imaging of lung abnormalities can be pursued, they do not change outcome as they do not guide the selection of specific therapies other than pulmonary rehabilitation—a program that existed well before the onset of COVID. It is clear that rapid resolution—as opposed to slower resolution—of severe COVID symptoms that require hospitalization does not reduce the potential for the long-term sequelae known as "long-COVID."

■ CARDIAC

Myocardial injury occurs in 20-30% of COVID-19 patients, increasing to 55% in patients with preexisting cardiac disease. Direct viral-mediated injury may result in myocarditis or myositis, while indirect injury can result in myocardial infarction (MI), atrial and ventricular arrhythmias, QTc prolongation, and stress cardiomyopathy. Steroids and time are most commonly used to address COVID-associated myositis. No association has been found between using a specific kind of antihypertensive agent (angiotensin-converting enzyme inhibitors) and COVID risk or myocardial injury. Persistent myocardial inflammation may be detected using cardiac magnetic resonance imaging in up to 60% of survivors. The significance of this finding remains to be discovered. However, given the possibility of sequelae even in those with mild disease, primary care clinicians should have a high index of suspicion and screen for cardiac manifestations even with unusual symptoms. Long-term follow-up will help define what identified abnormalities mean for survivors.

■ HEMATOLOGIC

The most significant hematologic abnormality associated with COVID-19 infection is hypercoagulability—an abnormal likelihood of clotting in an abnormal way and in sites where there is no need for a clot to stop bleeding. In fact, this may have the most significant contribution to the dysfunction of other organ systems as micro- and macrothrombosis are common autopsy findings (up to 34% of cases) in various organs. One of the most hotly debated topics has been the advisability of providing routine anticoagulation for all hospitalized patients with acute COVID infection. Current recommendations support administering only the routinely used prophylactic (lower) dose of an anticoagulant in the absence of deep vein thrombosis or pulmonary embolism for which therapeutic (higher) dose anticoagulation is appropriate. Post-COVID clotting risk is uncertain and therefore no recommendation for postdischarge thromboprophylaxis has been made.

■ RENAL

Acute kidney injury (AKI) is common in the acute phase of illness. Of patients admitted to the ICU, 31% need some form of dialysis, termed "renal replacement therapy (RRT)." At least half of the patients who require RRT recover kidney function within 3 weeks. For those who continue to need dialysis after their COVID hospitalization, care is largely supportive while clinicians watch for evidence of renal recovery including an increase in urine volume and an improvement in lab tests of kidney function. Similar to any patient who requires RRT during hospitalization, follow up with a nephrologist—in addition to a primary care clinician—is recommended. The causes of acute COVID-related AKI are many and are difficult to separate from those common to all patients with critical illness or injury. However, a specific COVID-associated nephropathy (COVAN) has been identified in a minority of patients and is characterized by a localized inflammatory and scarring process termed "sclerosis" that impacts the functional units of the kidney.

■ PEDIATRIC CONSIDERATIONS

It has been generally accepted that most COVID-19 infections in children and adolescents are more likely to be mild in comparison to infection in adults. Proportionately fewer children with an acute COVID infection have needed ICU care compared to adults. However, like adults, children and teens with preexisting comorbidities are more likely to develop symptomatic or severe COVID. Nonetheless, one way in which COVID-19 in children differs from that in adults is the development of multisystem inflammatory syndrome (MIS-C). This syndrome is diagnosed most often in children with resolved COVID-19 and elevated inflammatory markers who present with fever, diarrhea, hypotension (low blood pressure), and skin lesions. Severe cases rapidly progress to shock, neurologic compromise, AKI, and respiratory failure. Full details of diagnostic criteria can be found on the CDC website: https://www.cdc.gov/mis/about.html. Treatment is complex and is delivered during inpatient care; outpatient options which are common for mild adult COVID are not appropriate for this potentially life-threatening condition. Long-term outcome of children with MIS-C, decreased left ventricular ejection fraction (LVEF), and neurologic compromise is as yet unclear.

■ OBSTETRIC CONSIDERATIONS

Vertical transmission rates of SARS-CoV-2 (i.e., from mother to baby pre- and postdelivery) appear to be quite low (<4%), with likelihood increasing if infection occurs in the third trimester. It appears more likely that neonates diagnosed with COVID-19 infection have been infected by caregivers through respiratory droplet transmission. Relatedly, an international study recently demonstrated a substantial increase in maternal morbidity (complications) and mortality (death) as well as neonatal complications in women with symptomatic COVID-19 infections. In comparison, asymptomatic mothers with COVID-19 were at increased risk for maternal morbidity but not mortality. Therefore all pregnancies during which the mother is found to have an acute COVID-19 infection should be referred for high-risk obstetrical care regardless of infection severity.

■ ENDOCRINE

Endocrine manifestations of acute COVID infection include diabetic ketoacidosis (DKA; high glucoses with an increase in bloodstream acid) in the absence of known diabetes, refractory hyperglycemia (high glucose), thyroiditis (thyroid inflammation), bone demineralization, and hair loss. While bone demineralization and hair loss are known complications of critical illness, COVID-related glycemic abnormalities and thyroid abnormalities have important consequences in COVID patients. Patients with diabetes have demonstrated a quite high mortality rate compared to those without diabetes. Moreover, the development of new post-COVID diabetes is well described (Fig. 25-2). It is not clear yet if this will be a long-term comorbidity for COVID-19 survivors, but if it is, it is anticipated to have significant long-term health impacts identical to other patients with diabetes. Patients who develop thyroiditis have a small but important risk (5%) of developing hypothyroidism (decreased thyroid function). For all of these endocrine complications, outpatient follow-up with an endocrinologist is required.

■ MISCELLANEOUS

Ocular (eye) manifestations of COVID-19 infection are varied and include conjunctivitis, retinitis, and optic neuritis—all linked by inflammation. These manifestations are more common in patients who have more severe disease. While more data is needed regarding visual impairments in survivors of COVID-19, symptoms should not be overlooked, and appropriate referral to an ophthalmologist undertaken. Short-term abnormalities of hepatic function generally resolve but also merit outpatient laboratory evaluation during recovery; failure to return to normal should prompt referral to a liver disease specialist (hepatologist). Finally, a disorder similar to MIS-C in children has also been described in adults, but this is uncommon.

■ CARE DELIVERY MODELS POST-ACUTE ILLNESS

Multiprofessional clinics specifically designed to identify and address the sequelae of severe COVID infection in ICU survivors are springing up around the United States. Most of these clinics are concentrated in urban areas and within academic medical centers based on resource and clinician availability. While care can be safely and comprehensively provided by individual primary care clinicians in the community, the need for an organized and thorough screening approach with availability of specialist referral is increasingly being recognized. Recently, the *British Medical Journal* (BMJ) published an infographic that provides a very clear path for outpatient evaluation and escalation of care (Fig. 25-3). It is recommended that all patients with ongoing symptoms of three or more weeks after a COVID diagnosis undergo clinical, laboratory, and radiologic screening to identify post-COVID sequelae. This evaluation begins with a clear understanding of the acute disease course and any significant inpatient events. The BMJ infographic emphasizes medical management as well as self-management with lifestyle changes and specialist care. Primary care clinicians should utilize available tools including telemedicine and home monitoring to expand the reach of their care. We have also included recommendations for assessment and evaluation following hospital discharge for surviving critical care COVID-19 patients (Table 25-1).

■ GRIEF AND COPING

It is increasingly clear how the lack of contact with family, friends, and bedside clinicians during ICU and hospital admission has impacted patients' long-term emotional states. Significant alterations in ICU care delivery were deemed necessary due to strict and unique COVID-19 isolation requirements that were intended to limit staff exposure and spread of illness. Layers of personal protective equipment (PPE) render patient–caregiver interactions confusing and impersonal. In addition, other aspects of care were altered to support staff protection and PPE preservation during periods of shortage. These included, but were not limited to, patient care rounds conducted from the hallway and over videoconferences with patients, and strict visitor restrictions in the midst of crisis situations when patients most need their support systems. Each of these "adaptations" created additional and unique stressors for critically ill or injured patients, their loved ones, as well as healthcare clinicians. Complicated grief is an anticipated outcome as a result of all of the above protective measures taken throughout the various waves of the pandemic and may need to be addressed by primary care clinicians and post-ICU

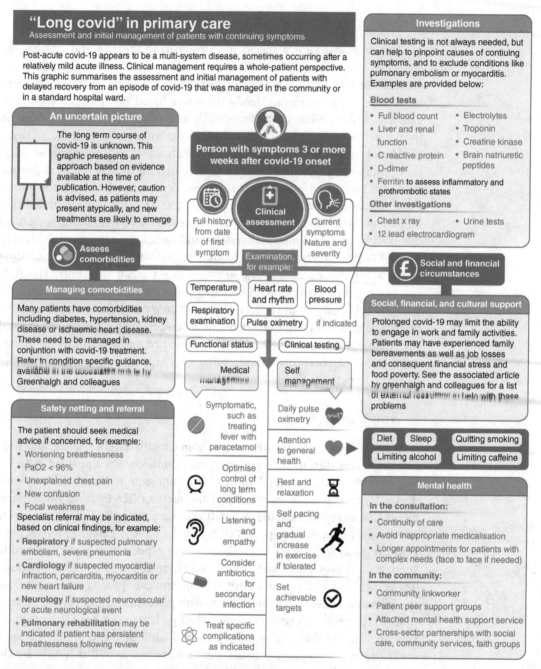

"Long covid" in primary care
Assessment and initial management of patients with continuing symptoms

Post-acute covid-19 appears to be a multi-system disease, sometimes occurring after a relatively mild acute illness. Clinical management requires a whole-patient perspective. This graphic summarises the assessment and initial management of patients with delayed recovery from an episode of covid-19 that was managed in the community or in a standard hospital ward.

An uncertain picture
The long term course of covid-19 is unknown. This graphic presesents an approach based on evidence available at the time of publication. However, caution is advised, as patients may present atypically, and new treatments are likely to emerge

Assess comorbidities

Managing comorbidities
Many patients have comorbidities including diabetes, hypertension, kidney disease or ischaemic heart disease. These need to be managed in conjunction with covid-19 treatment. Refer to condition specific guidance, available in the associated article by Greenhalgh and colleagues

Safety netting and referral
The patient should seek medical advice if concerned, for example:
- Worsening breathlessness
- PaO2 < 96%
- Unexplained chest pain
- New confusion
- Focal weakness

Specialist referral may be indicated, based on clinical findings, for example:
- **Respiratory** if suspected pulmonary embolism, severe pneumonia
- **Cardiology** if suspected myocardial infraction, pericarditis, myocarditis or new heart failure
- **Neurology** if suspected neurovascular or acute neurological event
- **Pulmonary rehabilitation** may be indicated if patient has persistent breathlessness following review

Person with symptoms 3 or more weeks after covid-19 onset

Clinical assessment

Full history from date of first symptom

Current symptoms Nature and severity

Examination, for example:

Temperature

Heart rate and rhythm

Blood pressure

Respiratory examination

Pulse oximetry   if indicated

Functional status

Clinical testing

Medical management

Self management

Symptomatic, such as treating fever with paracetamol

Optimise control of long term conditions

Listening and empathy

Consider antibiotics for secondary infection

Treat specific complications as indicated

Daily pulse oximetry

Attention to general health

Rest and relaxation

Self pacing and gradual increase in exercise if tolerated

Set achievable targets

Investigations
Clinical testing is not always needed, but can help to pinpoint causes of contiuing symptoms, and to exclude conditions like pulmonary embolism or myocarditis. Examples are provided below:

Blood tests
- Full blood count
- Liver and renal function
- C reactive protein
- D-dimer
- Ferritin to assess inflammatory and prothrombotic states
- Electrolytes
- Troponin
- Creatine kinase
- Brain natriuretic peptides

Other investigations
- Chest x ray
- 12 lead electrocardiogram
- Urine tests

Social and financial circumstances

Social, financial, and cultural support
Prolonged covid-19 may limit the ability to engage in work and family activities. Patients may have experienced family bereavements as well as job losses and consequent financial stress and food poverty. See the associated article by greenhalgh and colleagues for a list of external resources to help with these problems

Diet   Sleep   Quitting smoking
Limiting alcohol   Limiting caffeine

Mental health
In the consultation:
- Continuity of care
- Avoid inappropriate medicalisation
- Longer appointments for patients with complex needs (face to face if needed)

In the community:
- Community linkworker
- Patient peer support groups
- Attached mental health support service
- Cross-sector partnerships with social care, community services, faith groups

FIGURE 25-3. A Schematic to Evaluate and Manage Post-COVID Symptoms within Primary Care. This infographic presents an integrated approach to evaluating and managing post-COVID symptoms within primary care as opposed to a resource-rich inpatient space. (Reproduced with permission from Greenhalgh T, Knight M, Buxton M, Husain L. Management of post-acute covid-19 in primary care. *BMJ.* 2020; 370:m3026.)

■ **TABLE 25-1. Screening and Management Recommendations for Post-ICU COVID-19 Survivors**

System	Assessment	Clinical Concern	Diagnostic Workup	Management Considerations
General Impression	Comprehensive physical exam Screen for Post-COVID syndromes	Postdischarge follow-up between 1 and 2 weeks of hospital discharge. Follow-up determined by severity of symptoms	CBC, BMP, possibly LFTs, TSH, and T4 Targeted to reported symptoms especially if persistent >12 weeks	Multidisciplinary post-ICU COVID-19 clinic referral
General	Fever Fatigue Pain	Chronic fatigue or pain syndromes	Infectious evaluation, as indicated	Supportive care
Neurologic	New-onset confusion or focal deficits Delirium (among older adults) Cognitive blunting, "brain fog" Headaches	Long-term neurologic sequelae Executive and functional impairments Impact on QOL	Mini-Mental Status Examination	Neurology referral Supportive management
Psychiatric	Anxiety Depression **PTSD** Sleep disturbances Behavioral changes	Suicide Homicide Executive and functional impairments Impact on QOL	PTSD Symptom Scale Patient Health Questionnaire-9 Insomnia Severity Index Assessment	Emergency referral for severe psychiatric symptoms Psychology or psychiatry consult Education/focus on mindfulness and self-care: Peer & social support Outreach mental health services
Pulmonary	Dyspnea Chronic cough (>8 weeks) Exertional dyspnea Pleuritic chest pain	Anemia Impaired lung function Exercise tolerance level	Modified Medical Research Council Dyspnea Scale 1-minute sit-to-stand CXR at 12 weeks for nonhospitalized patient	Breathing exercises Home pulse oximetry self-monitoring Pulmonary consultation Pulmonary rehab (clinic-based or telehealth)

(Continued)

■ **TABLE 25-1. Screening and Management Recommendations for Post-ICU COVID-19 Survivors (*Continued*)**

Cardiac	Chest pain ECG abnormalities Palpitations Positional tachycardia, syncope	Heart failure Dysrhythmias Heart blocks Cardiomyopathy Myositis/myocarditis Orthostatic intolerance syndromes	Serial ECG Cardiac MRI CXR Tilt-table test Troponin, BNP	Emergency care for cardiac chest pain Specialty cardiology referral Avoid intense exercise regimens (pericarditis/myocarditis) For orthostatic syndromes: • Cautious standing • Compression garments • Midodrine or fludrocortisone
Hematologic	VTE during hospitalization Easy bruising or bleeding	Deep vein thrombosis Pulmonary embolism ITP HIT	Lower extremity Doppler studies CT chest with contrast CBC, D-Dimer Fibrinogen	Hematology specialty referral
Renal	AKI History of RRT during hospitalization	Permanent organ damage Progression of renal impairment Electrolyte disturbances Acid-base disturbances	Urine studies Labs: BMP ABG	Renal specialty referral
Special Groups	Multisystem inflammatory syndrome—child (MIS-C) Pregnant women	Rapid decompensation if MIS-C Maternal and fetal morbidity		If MIS-C suspected urgent hospital admission High-risk obstetrician specialty referral
Musculoskeletal	Debilitation Weakness Joint or muscle pain Inability to perform ADLs	ICU-acquired myopathy or neuropathy Functional impairments Impact of QOL	BERG Balance Scale Nutrition evaluation	Rehabilitation specialty referral Occupational therapy Consider equipment needs and home environment assessment Telehealth-guided exercise programs for homebound

■ TABLE 25-1. Screening and Management Recommendations for Post-ICU COVID-19 Survivors (*Continued*)

Social	PICS or PICS-F
	Financial toxicity
	Child/Intimate
	  partner abuse
	Job loss
	Multiple deaths in
	  family unit
	Caregiver strain
	Member of
	  underserved
	  or vulnerable
	  group
		Increased risk for
		  stress-induced
		  health events
		Dysfunctional grieving
		Impaired executive or
		  cognitive function
		Impaired QOL
		Caregiver burnout
		Mental health
		  disorders
			EuroQol-5D Mental
			  health screening
			Solicit caregiver
			  input
				Child/Adult protective
				  services referral as
				  indicated
				Online support
				  groups/resources
				Community support
				  programs
				Spiritual/Faith
				  support groups
				Social work/
				  counseling referral
				Grief/Bereavement
				  counseling

ABG, arterial blood gas; BMP, basal metabolic panel; BNP, brain-type natriuretic peptide; CBC, complete blood count; CRP, c-reactive protein; CT, computed tomography scan; CXR, chest x-ray; ECG, electrocardiogram; GI, gastrointestinal; HIT, heparin-induced thrombocy-topenia; INR, international normalized ratio; ITP, idiopathic thrombocytopenia purpura; LMWH, low-molecular-weight heparin; MI, myocar-dial infarction; MRI, magnetic resonance imaging; PCR, polymerase chain reaction; PFT, pulmonary function test; PT, prothrombin time; PTSD, posttraumatic stress disorder; PTT, partial thromboplastin time; QOL, quality of life; VTE, venous thromboembolism.
Modified from https://www.cdc.gov/coronavirus/2019-ncov/hcp/clinical-care/post-covid-index.html (Accessed July 02, 2021)

care clinics alike. Similarly, the lack of family members, surrogates, or other loved ones at the bedside during critical illness means that the narrative of what happened during the ICU stay may not be able to be reconstructed for the ICU survivor. Many find the lack of recall of events—as well as the abnormal recall of sometimes frightening care events—quite disturbing. ICU diaries (see Chapter 14) help with event and care course reconstruction, but are conspicuously absent for patients whose care occurred during periods of lockdown and substantial visitor restriction.

Formal guidelines have not yet been fully developed and disseminated by professional medical societies for the follow-up care and surveillance of post-ICU COVID-19 patients. Current recommendations are largely based on incomplete data, prior experience with viral diseases thought to be similar (i.e., MERS or SARS-CoV), as well as expert consensus. However, a consensus is developing that care for this population should be multidisciplinary, holis-tic, and patient and family centered.

■ SOCIAL MEDIA, PATIENT SUPPORT, AND LARGE DATA SETS

In the face of the pandemic, the online community has provided a medium for support and advocacy for both medical professionals and

COVID-19 survivors. During the first wave of the pandemic, a number of internet and social media networks of medical providers were developed to facilitate the rapid sharing of medical information and treatment suggestions. Similarly, online networks and communities of COVID-19 survivors such as *survivorcorps.com* and *longcovidsos.org* and the twitter hashtag *#longcovid* provide peer-to-peer validation, resources, and psychosocial support. It is valuable for primary care clinicians to be aware of these resources in order to better understand the concerns of this patient cohort, available resources that patients may access, and a global perspective on COVID-19 infection consequence management during recovery.

During the first year of the pandemic, over four million people in the United Kingdom, United States, and Sweden downloaded the Zoe COVID Symptom Study APP which collected voluntarily self-reported information. This contributed to the identification of anosmia and delirium as key symptoms in patients with COVID-19 infection. It has also charted geographic distribution of infection, the impact of smoking on hospitalization rates, and the impact of population density on disease prevalence. This is the first large-scale evidence of the utility and feasibility of public data gathering and participation in research for a newly identified infectious agent. More importantly, it also underscores the importance of the public as key partners in discovery and care.

■ FUTURE RESEARCH AND RECOMMENDATIONS

Recommendations for future research centers on populations of interest including post-ICU discharge COVID-19 patients and their nonhospitalized post-COVID counterparts who will be seen in the primary care setting. Baseline data about extent, duration, and severity of common symptoms is needed, along with a better understanding and characterization of all symptoms that persist in COVID-19 survivors—both post-ICU and chronically among nonhospitalized groups. It is vital that primary care clinicians maintain awareness of new recommendations as they are disseminated. Finally, the role of technology, telehealth, and creatively designed remote medicine, rehabilitation, and mental health support programs in improving and expanding care delivery to all patients, including post-ICU COVID-19 survivors, is of increasing interest, relevance, and inspiration.

Tips for Clinicians

1. **Survivors of acute COVID-19 infection may demonstrate long-lasting symptoms** that impact quality of life and activities of daily living (Box 25-1).

2. **Some post-COVID symptoms overlap** with the post-intensive care syndrome symptoms.

3. **Primary care clinicians should specifically inquire about post-COVID sequelae** during the initial office visit after acute care facility discharge or following acute infection that resolved at home.

4. For hospitalized patients, in particular, **both the patient and their family member(s) should be interviewed** about the patient's cognition, strength, and psychosocial function as patients may not recognize when they are not at their baseline.

5. As the SARS-CoV-2 virus mutates, **primary care clinicians have the difficult task of keeping up to date with evolving recommendations for therapy.** Since patients and family members have preexisting relationships with the primary care clinicians they may turn to the primary care clinician for guidance as well as clarity regarding outpatient and inpatient care.

6. **A variety of resources exist** that may help both patients and primary care clinicians to identify key information and utilize best practices that include the globally connected medical community across social media, but also sites that are specifically focused on patients and family members.

Box 25-1—Post-COVID Sequelae

"My Father's Fight with COVID-19: A Nurse Practitioner's Story"

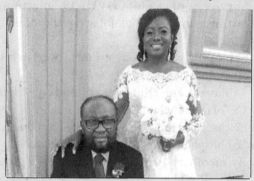

Personal recollection provided by Kenny Mikita LaCossiere, Nurse Practitioner in New York City. Images reproduced with permission.

My family's life took a turn for the worse when my father was diagnosed with COVID-19 in April 2020.

When COVID-19 first came on the horizon, I thought it would never enter our home, let alone almost take my father's life. He presented with a mild cough that was worse after a week. On Tuesday, April 7th, 2020, I decided the cough had lasted too long and took him to the local urgent care center. As soon as we arrived, the doctor checked his pulse oximetry, which was 87%. He was diagnosed with COVID-19 and needed to go to the hospital right away.

My heart dropped, and my mind immediately flashed to the hospital situation in New York City, how overwhelmed they were, with dozens of people dying every day from COVID-19. When we arrived in the ER, the nurses admitted him right away, and I was told to wait outside. That separation was exceedingly difficult, especially knowing how scared he was and how little English he spoke. As I waited, the seriousness of his diagnosis started to sink in, and memories flashed through my mind. The possibility that he might not live to walk me down the aisle on my wedding day brought tears to my eyes.

He needed to be admitted, and on Thursday, April 9th, 2020, I received a phone call at 12:10 pm that would forever change my life—he had taken a turn for the worse: he was short of breath, sweating profusely, with a sudden drop in his blood pressure, and had to go to the ICU. I received another call that he would need to be intubated. I spoke with him briefly in Creole through the speaker phone to tell him that he would be placed on the breathing machine.

This was the beginning of a long hospital stay that would be further complicated by hemorrhagic shock from an internal bleed, and liver and kidney failure. He was finally discharged on May 1st, 2020. No words can describe how my mother felt not being able to see him for almost a month.

He was readmitted two other times for gallbladder and kidney infections, and deep vein thrombosis in both his legs. His recovery since discharge has been long, slow, heart-wrenching and humbling. He was severely debilitated and had to learn again to talk, walk, sit, stand, eat, and do simple things. With intense in-home physical therapy, he was able to walk me down the aisle on my wedding day on September 27th, 2020.

As we approach the one-year anniversary of my father's battle with COVID-19, he is about 75% recovered. He's more forgetful, his ability to comprehend things has decreased, and he has problems climbing stairs. Although he is grateful to have survived COVID-19, he wonders when he is going to be back to his former self.

KEY REFERENCES

Aemaz Ur Rehman M, Farooq H, et al. The association of subacute thyroiditis with COVID-19: a systematic review. *SN Compr Clin Med*. 2021;3(7):1515-1527.

Bertoli F, Veritti D, Danese C, et al. Ocular findings in COVID-19 patients: a review of direct manifestations and indirect effects on the eye. *J Ophthalmol*. 2020; doi:10.1155/2020/4827304.

Bhattacharjee S, Banerjee M. Immune thrombocytopenia secondary to COVID-19: a systematic review. *SN Compr Clin Med*. 2020;2(11):2048-2058.

Birkin LJ, Vasileiou E, Stagg HR. Citizen science in the time of COVID-19. *Thorax*. 2021; 76(7):636-637.

Callard F, Perego E. How and why patients made Long Covid. *Soc Sci Med*. 2021;268:113426.

Carfi A, Bernabei R, Landi F. Persistent symptoms in patients after acute COVID-19. *JAMA*. 2020;324(6):603-605.

Centers for Disease Control and Prevention. Clinical Questions about COVID-19: Questions and Answers (updated Sept 26, 2022). Available at https://www.cdc.gov/coronavirus/2019-ncov/hcp/faq.html. Accessed December 5, 2022.

Chew NW, Lee GK, Tan BY, et al. A multinational, multicentre study on the psychological outcomes and associated physical symptoms amongst healthcare workers during COVID-19 outbreak. *Brain Behav Immunol*. 2020;88:559-565.

Chiu M, Goldberg A, Moses S, et al. Developing and implementing a dedicated prone positioning team for mechanically ventilated ARDS patients during the COVID-19 crisis. *Jt Comm J Qual Patient Saf*. 2021;47(6):347-353.

CDC COVID-19 Response Team. Severe outcomes among patients with coronavirus disease 2019 (COVID-19)—United States, February 12–March 16, 2020. *MMWR Morb Mortal Wkly Rep*. 2020;69(12):343-346.

Cuker A, Tseng EK, Nieuwlaat R, et al. American Society of Hematology living guidelines on the use of anticoagulation for thromboprophylaxis in patients with COVID-19: May 2021 update on the use of intermediate-intensity anticoagulation in critically ill patients. *Blood Adv*. 2021;5(20):3951-3959.

Daugherty SE, Guo Y, Heath K, et al. Risk of clinical sequelae after the acute phase of SARS-CoV-2 infection: retrospective cohort study. *BMJ*. 2021;373:n1098.

Doyen D, Dupland P, Morand L, et al. Characteristics of cardiac injury in critically ill patients with coronavirus disease 2019. *Chest*. 2021;159(5):1974-1985.

Gavriatopoulou M, Korompoki E, Fotiou D, et al. Organ-specific manifestations of COVID-19 infection. *Clin Exp Med*. 2020;20(4):493-506.

Gertz AH, Pollack CC, Schultheiss MD, Brownstein JS. Delayed medical care and underlying health in the United States during the COVID-19 pandemic: a cross-sectional study. *Prev Med Rep*. 2022;28:101882.

Gesi C, Carmassi C, Cerveri G, et al. Complicated grief: what to expect after the coronavirus pandemic. *Front Psychiatry*. 2020;11:489.

Gottlieb RL, Vaca CE, Paredes R, et al. Early remdesivir to prevent progression to severe Covid-19 in outpatients. *N Engl J Med*. 2022;386(4):305-315.

Graham EL, Clark JR, Orban ZS, et al. Persistent neurologic symptoms and cognitive dysfunction in non-hospitalized Covid-19 "long haulers". *Ann Clin Transl Neurol.* 2021;8(5):1073-1085.

Greenhalgh T, Knight M, Buxton M, Husain L. Management of post-acute Covid-19 in primary care. *BMJ.* 2020;370:m3026.

Gupta A, Madhavan MV, Sehgal K, et al. Extrapulmonary manifestations of COVID-19. *Nat Med.* 2020;26(7):1017-1032.

Henderson LA, Canna SW, Friedman KG, et al. American College of Rheumatology clinical guidance for multisystem inflammatory syndrome in children associated with SARS-CoV-2 and hyperinflammation in pediatric COVID-19: version 1. *Arthritis Rheumatol.* 2020;72(11):1791-1805.

Hirsch JS, Ng JH, Ross DW, et al. Acute kidney injury in patients hospitalized with COVID-19. *Kidney Int.* 2020;98(1):209-218.

Hosey MM, Needham DM. Survivorship after COVID-19 ICU stay. *Nat Rev Dis Primers.* 2020;6(1):1-2.

Johns Hopkins University of Medicine Coronavirus Resource Center. Home—Johns Hopkins Coronavirus Resource Center (jhu.edu). Accessed December 5, 2022.

Khan SH, Lindroth H, Perkins AJ, et al. Delirium incidence, duration, and severity in critically ill patients with coronavirus disease 2019. *Crit Care Explor.* 2020;2(12):e0290.

Kotlyar AM, Grechukhina O, Chen A, et al. Vertical transmission of coronavirus disease 2019: a systematic review and meta-analysis. *Am J Obstet Gynecol.* 2021;224(1):35-53.

Mandal S, Barnett J, Brill SE, et al. "Long-COVID": a cross-sectional study of persisting symptoms, biomarker and imaging abnormalities following hospitalisation for COVID-19. *Thorax.* 2021;76(4):396-398.

Mazza MG, De Lorenzo R, Conte C, et al. Anxiety and depression in COVID-19 survivors: role of inflammatory and clinical predictors. *Brain Behav Immun.* 2020;89:594-600.

Morris SB, Schwartz NG, Patel P, et al. Case series of multisystem inflammatory syndrome in adults associated with SARS-CoV-2 infection—United Kingdom and United States, March–August 2020. *MMWR Morb Mortal Wkly Rep.* 2020;69(40):1450-1456.

Nalbandian A, Sehgal K, Gupta A, et al. Post-acute COVID-19 syndrome. *Nat Med.* 2021; 27(4):601-615.

Nasiri N, Sharifi H, Bazrafshan A, et al. Ocular manifestations of COVID-19: a systematic review and meta-analysis. *J Ophthalmic Vis Res.* 2021;16(1):103-112.

National Institute of Health. Coronavirus Disease 2019 (COVID-19) Treatment Guidelines. Available at https://www.covid19treatmentguidelines.nih.gov/. Accessed December 6, 2022.

Puntmann VO, Carerj ML, Wieters I, et al. Outcomes of cardiovascular magnetic resonance imaging in patients recently recovered from coronavirus disease 2019 (COVID-19). *JAMA Cardiol.* 2020;5(11):1265-1273.

RECOVERY Collaborative Group. Dexamethasone in hospitalized patients with Covid-19. *N Engl J Med.* 2021;384(8):693-704.

Roth NC, Kim A, Vitkovski T, et al. Post–COVID-19 cholangiopathy: a novel entity. *Am J Gastroenterol.* 2021;116(5):1077-1082.

Rubino F, Amiel SA, Zimmet P, et al. New-onset diabetes in Covid-19. *N Engl J Med.* 2020;383(8):789-790.

Sawalha K, Abozenah M, Kadado AJ, et al. Systematic review of COVID-19 related myocarditis: insights on management and outcome. *Cardiovasc Revasc Med.* 2021;23:107-113.

Sivan M, Taylor S. NICE guideline on long covid. *BMJ.* 2020;371:m4938.

Stevens JS, King KL, Robbins-Juarez SY, et al. High rate of renal recovery in survivors of COVID-19 associated acute renal failure requiring renal replacement therapy. *PLoS One.* 2020;15(12):e0244131.

Tsankov BK, Allaire JM, Irvine MA, et al. Severe COVID-19 infection and pediatric comorbidities: a systematic review and meta-analysis. *Int J Infect Dis.* 2021;103:246-256.

Villar J, Ariff S, Gunier RB, et al. Maternal and neonatal morbidity and mortality among pregnant women with and without COVID-19 infection: the INTERCOVID multinational cohort study. *JAMA Pediatr.* 2021;175(8):817-826.

Zhou M, Wong CK, Un KC, et al. Cardiovascular sequalae in uncomplicated COVID-19 survivors. *PLoS One.* 2021;16(2):e0246732.

The First Few Days at Home

■ GETTING HOME

Patients who survive an episode of critical illness are less commonly discharged directly home. Instead, many more are transferred to another facility for continued but less complex care or for rehabilitation. Discharge from one of those facilities is the immediate step prior to getting home. Of course, travel from such a facility to the patient's home—or the home of another family member or friend—requires transportation.

■ TRANSPORTATION

Depending on individual patient needs, sometimes family's or friend's private vehicle transportation is fine. For others, especially those who require ongoing care needs at home that depend on devices, specialized transportation is more ideal. In general, ambulance-like transport services are utilized to help with not only travel, but also entry into the home space. Sometimes only a wheelchair is needed, while for others stretcher transport might be required.

■ EQUIPMENT

If a patient needs specialized equipment such as a hospital bed, a feeding pump, oxygen, or other related care devices, those are delivered the day before the patient is slated to arrive home. This ensures that all necessary care items, including wound care supplies, are in place prior to home transportation. Family members should determine where they would like the equipment to be placed within the home. It is important to assess whether there are electrical outlets for power-requiring devices that are accessible in the location where the devices are to be used. Personal assistive devices such as a cane or a walker are common when muscle mass is lost after prolonged critical illness, and after injury or surgery leading to limb amputation.

■ MAKING THE TRANSITION HOME SUCCESSFUL

Planning is key for this major transition. It is important to recognize that immediately upon arrival home patients who survive critical illness may not be able to do all of the things they previously did. This is true for those who have developed the post-intensive care syndrome (see chapter on PICS). Therefore, family and friends, but most importantly patients, should adjust their expectations to match their strength, endurance, and cognitive and psychosocial abilities on the day they arrive home. This is often quite frustrating for the patient as the transition home signals "recovery" and they expect that they can simply resume their normal life activities.

Since many require ongoing care, there are a variety of things that patients and caregivers can do to help with that process. These undertakings should start on the first day of arrival home. They include, but are not limited to, the following:

1. Make a folder of all hospital and secondary facility paperwork including discharge summaries; plan to bring them to all first-time healthcare appointments after hospital discharge.

2. Make a list of current medications, when they are to be taken and the pharmacy that fills those prescriptions.

3. Create a calendar listing of all healthcare-related appointments; an electronic calendar that can be shared among family members or other caregivers is ideal in case responsibility for transportation needs to be shifted. Most patients will not be able to safely drive themselves.

4. If transportation services are required to get to appointments, post essential phone numbers and email addresses in a visible location in case the time of appointment needs to be adjusted.

5. Make a list of all clinicians that the patient is supposed to see and what each of those clinicians is supposed to assess or do.

6. Limit visitors and out-of-home activities during the first few days as the transition may be quite exhausting.

7. Check with the patient's automobile insurance agency to determine when they will cover the patient driving, especially if their hospital care involved surgery in the abdomen, chest, spine, or brain.

8. Plan on lighter as opposed to heavier meals for the first few days at home as the home diet will be quite different from the hospital one. Gastrointestinal upset is not uncommon.

9. Create a single place where questions for any of the clinicians that the patient is going to see can be noted and then taken to an appointment to get answered. Questions that are urgent should be pursued when they arise by phone or email or patient portal (when one exists). Emergencies of course, should be addressed using 9-1-1.

◼ CONVALESCENCE

Remember that the first few days at home are the next phase of the patient's recovery journey. For many, that journey can span weeks while for others it may take years. The time frame for recovery depends on the patient as well as any required procedures or operations that are planned during the recovery phase. There is no single time frame that fits everyone, and patience is substantially required during convalescence.

The First Primary Care Visit

Having survived the ICU as well as any additional care facilities prior to coming home, you are now ready to prepare for your first Primary Care office visit! This is a visit for which it is important to prepare as it is the first time that your Primary Care Clinician (PCC) will see you—and your family—after hospital discharge. You will immensely help your PCC by doing the following:

1. Bringing your discharge paperwork with you.
2. Preparing a list of the medications you are currently taking, and ask whether any of the new ones are still necessary.
3. Bringing a family member with you to provide history and perspective that you cannot provide (you may not remember a lot of what happened during your ICU stay).
4. Considering whether you:
   a. Feel as if you are back to your usual strength.
   b. Believe that you are thinking clearly and as well as you did before you became ill or injured.
   c. Enjoy relationships or activities as much as you did before being hospitalized.
5. Your family member that accompanies you should think about those same questions to provide an "external" perspective as well.
6. Prepare a list of questions regarding your current condition, especially things that are not going as well as you would like after hospital discharge.

Some of these questions—especially numbers 4 and 5 above—relate to the post-intensive care syndrome (PICS). Your PCC can help with specific referrals to aid with recovery, including managing a major consequence of critical illness—depression. When you cannot return to your normal activities, and especially if you are dependent on family members, depression is common and not a personal failing. You are not alone as many other patients struggle in exactly the same way. An ICU survivor support group is a great way for you *and your family* to address these kinds of issues, including PICS.

No question is unreasonable. Your PCC may need to discuss your current condition with clinicians who cared for you in the hospital before rendering a treatment decision. Don't be surprised if they do not have an immediate answer for what to do since recovery after needing critical care is complex and can take months to even years to fully recover. As a general rule, the older you are, the slower is your recovery—especially if you need additional surgery to restore normal function. If you live remote from the facility that provided you complex care, ask your PCC about using Telehealth to help assess or coordinate unfamiliar aspects of your care. Remember that your PCC is trained to assess and manage a broad array of medical conditions, but will need to rely on specialists for unique aspects of care that support your recovery.

Resources for Patients and Families

Agency/Organization	Content	QR Code	Resource URL
Society of Critical Care Medicine	SCCM THRIVE: Online resource for post-ICU-discharge		https://www.sccm.org/MyICUCare/Resources/Discharge-From-the-ICU
"After PICU"	Website: Comprehensive resources for children and families following a critical illness		www.afterpicu.com
American Academy of Pediatrics	Website: Dozens of individual resources for parents and families with search functionality		www.aap.org
American Thoracic Society	Website with multilingual resource for critical illnesses and interventions		https://www.thoracic.org/patients/patient-resources/topic-specific/critical-illness.php
American Thoracic Society	Website with multilingual resources dedicated to symptoms, diagnosis, and treatment of COVID-19		https://www.thoracic.org/patients/patient-resources/covid-19.php
American Thoracic Society	Brochure to educate patients and families on post intensive care syndrome		https://www.thoracic.org/patients/patient-resources/resources/post-intensive-care-syndrome.pdf
American Thoracic Society	Managing the ICU Experience: A Proactive Guide for Patients and Families		https://www.thoracic.org/patients/patient-resources/managing-the-icu-experience/
Atlantic Health System	After the ICU: Resources and information to help you and your family thrive after a critical illness		https://www.atlantichealth.org/content/dam/atlantichealth-v2/trauma-and-critical-care/MMC-42445-21-Thrive%20After%20the%20ICU%20(1).pdf

Agency/Organization	Content	QR Code	Resource URL
Certification Board for Music Therapists	Ensures access to safe, effective music therapy services		https://www.cbmt.org
Critical Care Recovery	Online resource with links to multiple opportunities including survivor stories and psychosocial educational material		https://www.criticalcarerecovery.com/
Every Deep-Drawn Breath	A critical care doctor's perspective on healing, recovery, and transforming medicine in the ICU. Proceeds benefit the CIBS Center Endowment for Survivorship		https://www.icudelirium.org/every-deep-drawn-breath
Health Talk	HealthTalk creates content by having professional researchers interview and share the stories of real people dealing with health concerns		www.healthtalk.org
ICUsteps	ICUsteps supports patients and relatives affected by critical illness. They promote recognition of physical and psychological consequences of critical illness and encourage research into treatment and prevention		www.icusteps.org
ICUDelirium	A resource for patients and families experiencing post-intensive care symptoms including the results of delirium		https://www.icudelirium.org/patients-and-families/overview
Johns Hopkins Medicine	Breathing Exercises after Critical Illness (including COVID-19)		https://www.hopkinsmedicine.org/health/conditions-and-diseases/coronavirus/coronavirus-recovery-breathing-exercises
Johns Hopkins Medicine	Bouncing Back from COVID-19; Your Guide to Restoring Movement		https://www.hopkinsmedicine.org/physical_medicine_rehabilitation/coronavirus-rehabilitation/_files/impact-of-covid-patient-recovery.pdf

Agency/Organization	Content	QR Code	Resource URL
Kaiser Permanente	A Family Guide to the ICU: a printable resource for families experiencing critical illness		https://mydoctor.kaiserpermanente.org/ncal/Images/Family%20Guide%20to%20ICU_tcm75-854750.pdf
Neurocritical Care Society	Family and Patient Resource Page for neurocritical care units		https://www.neurocriticalcare.org/resources/family-patient-resources
Neurocritical Care Society	Stories of Hope: Online Family Advocacy Resource including stories from real patients and care teams covering multiple topics, including recovery, advocacy, and more		https://currents.neurocriticalcare.org/stories-of-hope
Psychology Tools	Free Guide to Critical Illness, Intensive Care, and Post-Traumatic Stress Disorder; Available in 13 languages		https://www.psychologytools.com/articles/free-guide-to-critical-illness-intensive-care-and-post-traumatic-stress-disorder-ptsd/
Society of Critical Care Medicine	SCCM THRIVE—Post-intensive care syndrome (PICS) and the Family, an online resource		https://www.sccm.org/MyICUCare/Resources/Pediatric-Post-Intensive-Care-Syndrome-and-the-Fam
Society of Critical Care Medicine	SCCM: THRIVE—Redefining Recovery: Supplemental to THRIVE to educate survivors		https://www.sccm.org/MyICUCare/Resources/THRIVE-Redefining-Recovery
Substance Abuse and Mental Health Services Administration	Online resource providing guidance to mental health resources and the right questions to ask with respect to mental health		https://ncsacw.acf.hhs.gov/userfiles/files/SAMHSA_Trauma.pdf
University of Chicago Medicine Comer Children's Hospital	PICU Passport; an introduction to the ins and outs of being a patient and family in a pediatric intensive care unit. Includes a glossary of terms used in and outside of the ICU		https://www.sccm.org/getattachment/1723b336-1176-4f40-8766-0148c207114b/PICU-Passport

Resources for Primary Care Providers

Agency/Organization	Content	QR Code	Resource URL
Basic Resources and Clinician Toolkits			
ARDS Foundation	Resource webpage for the Acute Respiratory Distress Syndrome Foundation		https://ardsglobal.org/
Beth Israel Lahey Health	Post-ICU Care for Survivors of COVID-19: a resource for providers		http://bit.ly/3PTwWIY
Critical Care Explorations (Published Work)	Optimizing Critical Illness Recovery: Perspectives and solutions from the caregivers of ICU Survivors		https://journals.lww.com/ccejournal/Fulltext/2021/05000/Optimizing_Critical_Illness_Recovery__Perspectives.4.aspx
Johns Hopkins University School of Medicine	Tools and Review of ongoing research from the "Outcomes After Critical Illness and Surgery Group" (OACIS) at JHU		https://www.improvelto.com/
National Institute for Health and Care Excellence (NICE)	UK Resource for rehabilitation strategies for adults after critical illness		https://www.nice.org.uk/guidance/cg83
Society of Critical Care Medicine	Online Resource and webinar focused on practical lessons in recovery from critical illness		https://www.sccm.org/MyICUCare/THRIVE/I-Am-A-Healthcare-Provider
Society for Post-Acute and Long-Term Care Medicine	Directory of resources for a variety of situations in post-acute needs and long-term care needs of patients		https://paltc.org/

Agency/Organization	Content	QR Code	Resource URL
Society for Post-Acute and Long-Term Care Medicine	Resources on a variety of topics for long-term care needs		https://paltc.org/HealingTogether
Occupational Therapy Resources			
American Occupational Therapy Association	Main website for the US community of Occupational Therapists		https://www.aota.org/
Canadian Association of Occupational Therapy	Main website for the Canadian community of Occupational Therapists		https://caot.ca/site/adv/primarycare?nav=sidebar
Patient Communication and Education Tools			
Society of Critical Care Medicine	Online resources for families and primary care providers to facilitate communication and help with needs *during* and after critical illness		https://www.sccm.org/Clinical-Resources/ICULiberation-Home/ABCDEF-Bundles
Society of Critical Care Medicine	Patient Communicator App to facilitate ease of communication with patients who don't		https://www.sccm.org/MyICUCare/THRIVE/Patient-and-Family-Resources/Patient-and-Family
Physical Therapy Resources			
American Physical Therapy Association	Main Website for the US Community of Physical Therapists		www.apta.org
American Physical Therapy Association	Resource page on best recommendations for patients after COVID or other long-term illness		https://www.apta.org/patient-care/public-health-population-care/coronavirus/management-of-patients bit.ly/3jyTS4p
Post-Intensive Care Syndrome			
American Medical Association	AMA Webinar about COVID-19's long-post-infection challenges		https://www.ama-assn.org/delivering-care/public-health/what-doctors-wish-patients-knew-about-long-covid
British Medical Journal	Webinar on the management of Post-Acute COVID-19 in primary care, with parallels to critical illness recovery		https://www.bmj.com/content/370/bmj.m3026
Society of Critical Care Medicine THRIVE	Online resource and video describing critical illness recovery for families		https://www.youtube.com/watch?v=TO3palv4mYU

Agency/Organization	Content	QR Code	Resource URL
Speech and Language Pathology			
American Speech-Language Hearing Association	Main website for the US community of Speech and Language Pathologists/Therapists		https://www.asha.org/
Royal College of Speech and Language Therapists	Main website for the UK community of Speech and Language Pathologists/Therapists		https://www.rcslt.org/
Speech-Language and Audiology Canada (SAC)	Main website for the Canadian community of Speech and Language Pathologists/Therapists		https://www.caslpa.ca/
Support for Work Stress Burnout, Mental Health, Suicide Prevention			
American Thoracic Society	Fact sheet on burnout syndrome for health professionals		https://www.thoracic.org/patients/patient-resources/resources/burnout-syndrome.pdf
Centers for Disease Control and Prevention	Online resource for work stress and mental health needs for providers and clinicians		https://www.cdc.gov/niosh/topics/healthcare/workstress.html
Harvard Business Review	How to measure burnout accurately and ethically		https://hbr.org/2021/03/how-to-measure-burnout-accurately-and-ethically
Substance Abuse and Mental Health Services Administration	Resources for mental health crisis		https://www.samhsa.gov/find-help/988
Suicide and Crisis Lifeline	Online resource for crisis, suicide prevention, and other behavioral health needs		https://988lifeline.org/
Suicide and Crisis Lifeline Crisis Line	Help when someone needs it most		**Dial 988** or online http://bit.ly/3C3MmVj

About the Editors

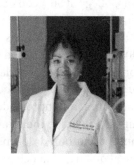

Meghan Lane-Fall, MD, MSHP, FCCM

Dr. Meghan Lane-Fall is an implementation scientist, anesthesiologist, and critical care physician. She obtained her bachelor's degree at UC Berkeley, her medical degree at Yale University, and a Master of Science in Health Policy Research at the University of Pennsylvania. Her clinical training in anesthesiology and critical care medicine was also completed at the University of Pennsylvania. Dr. Lane-Fall serves as the David E. Longnecker Associate Professor and Vice Chair of Inclusion, Diversity, and Equity in the Department of Anesthesiology and Critical Care at the Perelman School of Medicine at the University of Pennsylvania, with a secondary appointment in Epidemiology. Dr. Lane-Fall is the Executive Director of the Penn Implementation Science Center at the Leonard Davis Institute of Health Economics and Director of Penn's Implementation Science Certificate Program. Her social science lab focuses on improving perioperative and critical care patient safety and communication and is funded by the National Institutes of Health, the Agency for Healthcare Research and Quality, the Patient-Centered Outcomes Research Institute, and the American Heart Association. Dr. Lane-Fall also serves as the Vice President of the Anesthesia Patient Safety Foundation, is on the Board of Directors of the Foundation for Anesthesia Education and Research, and sits on the editorial boards of *Anesthesiology, Critical Care Medicine*, and *Global Implementation Research and Applications*. She lives in the Philadelphia suburbs with her husband and two children. She enjoys graphic design, technology, and logic puzzles in her free time. Her interest in critical care survivorship stems from her research on the experiences of trauma ICU survivors and her own experience as primary caregiver for her late father, who was admitted to an intensive care unit in the context of a protracted illness.

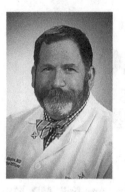 David S. Shapiro, MD, MHCM is the Chief Medical Officer and Vice President of Medical Affairs at Saint Francis Hospital in Hartford, Connecticut. Affiliated with the Frank Netter School of Medicine at Quinnipiac University and the University of Connecticut School of Medicine, he is an acute care surgeon and is board certified in General Surgery, Surgical Critical Care, and Hospice & Palliative Care Medicine. He has served as the president of the Connecticut Chapter of the American College of Surgeons, and is engaged with the American College of Surgeons nationally as a leading collaborator for STOP THE BLEED®. Dr. Shapiro has been a champion and contributor to violence prevention and interventions in New England, and has been an outspoken advocate for the LGBTQ+ population, both as patients and as professionals entering surgical careers. He is a founding member of the Association of Out Surgeons and Allies, a nonprofit dedicated to empowering LGBTQ+ surgeons and trainees to pursue their careers. He has received multiple awards for his work, and has authored dozens of published articles inclusive of his research on surgical quality, violence prevention, and innovations in the care of the injured patient. Following a degree at Boston College, he was awarded a degree in medicine and completed surgical residency at the University of Connecticut. He then served a fellowship at the Oregon Health Science University, and subsequently earned a degree in Health Care Management at the Harvard T.H. Chan School of Public Health. Dr. Shapiro is a published photographer, a traveler, a restauranteur, and dog lover. He lives in Hartford, Connecticut, and enjoys seeing parts of the world others avoid.

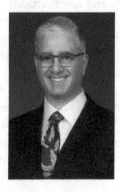 **Lewis J. Kaplan, MD, FACS, FCCM, FCCP**

Dr. Kaplan is a general, trauma, and critical care surgeon at the University of Pennsylvania in the Division of Trauma, Surgical Critical Care and Emergency Surgery and the Section Chief of Surgical Critical Care at the affiliated Corporal Michael J. Crescenz VA Medical Center. Education including a BA (Franklin and Marshall College; Biology; 1984) and an MD (Rutgers Medical School; 1988) was followed by Surgical residency (Medical College of PA, MCP;

1988-1995) and Surgical Critical Care Fellowship (University of Pittsburgh; 1996-1997). He has directed ICUs and critical care fellowships across three healthcare systems. At Yale (2002-2013) he established the first Emergency General Surgery service, as well as a Tactical Emergency Medical Service for a regional SWAT team with which he deployed. Dr. Kaplan serves in professional society leadership roles but most notably is a Past-President of the Society of Critical Care Medicine (2020-2021). He sits on multiple editorial boards (*Journal of Trauma and Acute Care Surgery, Critical Care Medicine, Surgical Infections, Injury*). His research interests include resuscitation, acid-base physiology, emergency general surgery, tactical emergency medicine services, mechanical ventilation, surgical infection, blood transfusion, and conflict management in critical care. He is married with three children. His middle child has autism, and he has undergone a variety of operations, including one which required care in an ICU. These life experiences have shaped and informed his desire to help craft a book that addresses the range of issues that accompany ICU survivorship.

Index

Note: Page numbers followed by *f* refer to figures; page numbers followed by *t* refer to tables.